MEGACITIES
& Global Health

EDITORS

Omar A. Khan, MD, MHS, FAAFP

Gregory Pappas, MD, PhD

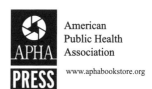

American
Public Health
Association

www.aphabookstore.org

American Public Health Association
800 I Street, NW
Washington, DC 20001-3710
www.apha.org

Georges C. Benjamin, M.D., F.A.C.P., F.A.C.E.P. (Emeritus), Executive Director
Judith C. Hays, R.N., Ph.D., Publications Board Liaison

Printed and bound in the United States of America
Typesetting: The Manila Typesetting Company
Cover and interior design: Jennifer Strass
Cover illustration: Monkey's Mount (Morro do Macaco) in Sao Bernardo do Campo, Sao Paulo, Brazil, October 12, 2005. Photo courtesy of Tatiana Cardeal, photographer.
Printing and Binding: Sheridan Press

Library of Congress Cataloging-in-Publication Data
Megacities and global health / editors, Omar Khan and Gregory Pappas ; foreword by Ida Susser.
  p. ; cm.
  Includes bibliographical references and index.
  ISBN-13: 978-0-87553-003-1 (alk. paper)
  ISBN-10: 0-87553-003-6 (alk. paper)
  1. Urban health. 2. World health. I. Khan, Omar A., 1973- II. Pappas, Gregory, 1952- III. American Public Health Association.
  [DNLM: 1. Urban Health. 2. Cities. 3. World Health. WA 380]
  RA566.7.M44 2011
  362.1'042–dc22
                                                                                    2010028991

05/2011

Contents

Foreword

Ida Susser, PhD

IN EXPLORING THE HEALTH challenges of megacities, this book superbly demonstrates the importance of combining urban theory with public health theory and practice.

Societies with less income inequality have populations in better health than do those with wider income gaps between rich and poor (Susser and Stein 2009). Gregory Pappas himself has shown that in the United States in the 1990s, increasing wealth inequalities were associated with increasing inequalities in health (Pappas et al. 1993). In addition, research indicates that a strong welfare state contributes to a healthier population (Judt 2010). Epidemiologists have clearly demonstrated that both class and the uneven development of capitalism are reflected in unequal morbidity and mortality (Wilkinson 1986; Wilkinson and Pickett 2010). Thus, there is little doubt that contemporary neoliberal policies, which increase the gap between rich and poor and also cut back the welfare state, negatively impact the health of populations. However, we still need to understand the processes that lead to inequalities in health. This volume addresses the dynamic interaction between the precipitous growth in megacities over the past three decades and the shocking disparities in health found in such new urban formations.

We can talk about a "right to the city" and a "right to health." Each of these shorthand concepts attempts to point to demands for social justice. However, while we may advocate such rights and trace our demands to the values of the enlightenment, or alternatively to cultural norms and values of egalitarian societies or indigenous peoples, understanding the complex interrelationship between such self-evident "rights" takes extensive research and analysis. As societies change, cities are transformed and the health needs of urban populations take on different dimensions.

The current neoliberal environment has, in fact, led to the "planet of the slums" described by Mike Davis in 2007, at the moment when more than half the world's population came to be living in cities (Davis 2007). Cities are growing through rural displacement caused by the influence of agribusiness and the loss of tariff protection for peasant farmers, as well as multiple factors such as debt, lack of legal title, gender subordination, and outright corruption, which have all led to the loss of rights to land. Corporate development of agriculture, depriving rural proletariat and peasantry of work and land, has combined with the relocation of manufacturing to the global south to force massive domestic and international migration into cities. Under neoliberal policies, meanwhile, services in most cities are shrinking and welfare states are fraying or decaying. The health challenges of megacities are a manifestation of such contradictions.

Cities in the global south have been in crisis since "structural adjustment" policies, implemented by Reagan and labeled the "Washington Consensus" at the International Monetary Fund (IMF) and the World Bank, were first implemented in the early 1980s (Stiglitz 2002). I remember clearly when Hector Abad Gomez, chair of the Department of Preventive Medicine and Public Health at the School of Medicine, University of Antioquia, Medellin, Colombia, gave a presentation in a series on Latin American cities in crisis at the City University of New York (Gomez 1989). He described the challenges to providing public health in Medellin, which although it had a population of just over 2 million at that time, had many of the challenges that have become so familiar in megacities. As Gomez noted, the borders of the municipality (which defined who was counted in municipal statistics) entirely excluded the informal settlements densely packed with new migrant populations and the emergence of large settlements without electricity or paved roads.

Gomez emphasized a particular aspect of health—violence—as a public health issue. At that historical moment, the drug economy and the violence associated with it became intertwined with the population of Medellin and the governance of that city. By 1983, in Medellin, homicide had become the second leading cause of death (after ischemic heart disease). Gomez documented the rise in mortality resulting from violence and argued for a public health approach which took the changing social context into account. Tragically, in 1987, soon after he gave the seminar in New York City, Gomez was assassinated, when, as president of the Human Rights Committee, he ran for mayor of Medellin. His paper was published posthumously (Gomez 1989).

At the same time as the social context of violence was changing in Colombia, it was also shifting in Naples, Italy (Belmonte 2005), New York City (Sharf 1997; Susser 1999; Mullings 2003), and Kingston, Jamaica (Robotham 2003). As Castells recognized in 1996, the new drug economy had become the underside of globalization (Castells 1996; Schneider and Schneider 2003). In 2000, Jane Schneider and I convened a conference on "Wounded Cities" (Schneider and Susser 2003) in which a paper on Medellin contextualized the drug economy and associated violence there within the global context (Roldan 2003). It became clear that the identification of violence as a public health issue in the early 1980s was a direct reflection of the changing context of Medellin within the global economy. This is a telling example of the importance of interdisciplinary understandings for both public health and urban studies. We can see here that Gomez was theorizing at the forefront of practical challenges and that his insights were key to understandings of the emerging new global order.

Following the events of the past decade in Mexico City allows us to see the full-blown effects of the drug trade, inequality, and domestic and international migration which were just beginning to make themselves felt in Medellin in the 1980s. As the North American Free Trade Agreement (NAFTA) policies have removed the last scrap of agricultural protection—even from the cultivation of rice and beans—agricultural peasants and laborers in Mexico have lost their rights to provide food for their own nation. Imported coffee, beans, rice, and vegetables, produced more cheaply than Mexican farmers can sell them, have left rural workers with little recourse but to migrate to Mexico City or illegally to the United States in search of work. Even the backbreaking local production of bricks, once an economic resource for the villages around Puebla, Mexico has lost its profitability as cheaper products are imported from elsewhere (Geraci 2011). In 2008, as the International AIDS Society (IAS) conference was planned in Mexico City, a rainbow coalition of 1 million rural laborers, some on tractors or donkeys, with transgender youth, sex workers, and grandmothers wearing t-shirts advocating condoms, marched into the city to protest the final steps of NAFTA. Of course, no matter what panels the IAS planned or policies they managed to implement, the lack of rural subsistence could only increase the numbers of people who had to seek employment in sex work or drug trafficking—thus increasing the global risk for the pandemic, crime, and violence (Susser 2009).

Gendered violence is also emerging as a public health issue in this historical context. Until the past few decades, domestic abuse was defined as a matter to be resolved within the confines of the patriarchal family, invisible or of no interest to the state. In New York City in the late 1980s, at the same time as social theorists began to document the feminization of poverty (Sidel 1986), we also saw a new manifestation of gendered conflict (Susser 1996). As services were cut and public assistance became even harder to receive, women had little access to day care and were supporting children alone, often without secure housing (Susser 1999). As Helen Rodriguez-Trias noted,

> assaults by husbands, ex-husbands, and lovers cause more injuries to women than motor vehicle accidents, rape, and muggings combined. Health officials estimate that each year more than 4 million women are battered and more than 4 thousand are killed by such "intimate assaults." Yet public health initiatives for preventing violence against women and helping women and children entrapped by violence are sadly lacking. (Rodriguez-Trias 1992, p. 663)

Rodriguez-Trias analyzed such violence as a public health issue. As the AIDS epidemic has pervaded South Africa, Rachel Jewkes and others have documented gendered violence as a central public health issue, as well as an important factor in the spread of AIDS among women (Jewkes 2002; Jewkes, Levin, and Penn-Kekana 2002; Jewkes et al. 2004). My own research on gender and AIDS in South Africa shows the way in which economic policies exacerbate not only income divisions, but gendered conflict, and, in fact, contribute to the spread of the AIDS epidemic. With the imposition of "structural adjustment" policies in the global South, the combined effects of unemployment, the need to migrate for work, and the lack of social services and adequate housing forced women to greater dependence on the few men who could find work (Susser 2009). This led to increased gender conflict, violence against women, and undermined the general health of the population.

Even more disturbing, as, following Castells (2001), Pappas notes the growth of the enormous conglomeration of populations in the Pearl River Delta of China, we have to take into account the second-class citizenship of rural migrants to cities in both China and Vietnam (Chae 2003). Under such regimes, there has been a lack of investment in agriculture, leading to a drop in the prices farmers can command. As farming becomes unsustainable rural workers have to leave in search of work. In fact, while the U.S. media has recently highlighted suicides among migrant workers in urban manufacturing, the highest rates of suicide anywhere may be among the rural women in China who have to stay behind with their children and in-laws while the men seek jobs elsewhere.

Meanwhile, with the increased investment of China in urban areas, cities have grown, sometimes leading to the seizing of agricultural land without compensation. Rural workers are pushed off their land often through violent processes and the unrestricted predation of local elites (Le Mons Walker 2006), what David Harvey might label accumulation by dispossession (2005). As they flock to the cities to work in new factories, migrants from rural areas of China are often forced to accept wages lower than they would receive in Africa or Latin America. Such policies allow Chinese goods to outsell the rest of the world (Kwong 2006). Rural migrants in both China and Vietnam have few rights to organize, with little protection or access to health care or any other benefits (e.g., education for their children) in the growing megacities where they work. Classified as rural, whatever services they are entitled to are restricted to the villages from which they have fled. Trapped by such regulations, young rural migrant workers, far from their rural communities, in shared marginal spaces with little food, sending remittances home to their families, have increasingly resorted to suicide. However, in 2010 workers all over China began speaking out against such conditions and receiving some recognition and response to their demands (Barboza 2010).

As this book demonstrates, in discussing megacities we are not simply talking about size. The uneven structuring of places, the municipalities, the organization of infrastructure, the zoning, the transportation, the pollution, and the massive impact of disasters (such as the earthquake in Port au Prince, Haiti) are politically determined characteristics which vary with the governance of the city (Susser and Schneider 2003). Struggles over the commons, the collective interests of urban populations in ecological decisions, water use, and water level frame the lives of inhabitants in the new megacities (Susser 2006). Will dams be strengthened or will the disaster of Katrina in New Orleans be repeated as already the lives of millions of people in Pakistan have been disrupted by water levels rising to flood cities? Will governments provide the infrastructure to fight fires or will, as threatened for Moscow, cities burn in the worsening drought conditions, with the added danger of burning nuclear waste thrown in? Such decisions with respect to collective interests will determine the health and survival of the millions who now inhabit the growing megacities of our era. This book outlines the destructiveness of neoliberal governance in the creation of megacities of displaced persons and scarce resources. It points as well to the ever-more crucial importance of supporting the commons, through adequate public health and education and environmental and occupational constraints, in the effort to sustain and possibly even improve the health of megacities populations in the next decades.

References

Barboza D. 2010. Another Death at Electronics Supplier. *Wall Street Journal*. Business Section. May 22:1.

Belmonte T. 2005. *The Broken Fountain*. 3rd ed. New York, NY: Columbia University.

Castells M. 1996. *The Information Age: Economy, Society and Culture*. Oxford, England: Blackwell.

Castells M. 2001. The space of flows. In: Susser I, editor. *The Castells Reader on Cities and Social Theory*. Oxford, England: Blackwell.

Chae S. 2003. Contemporary Ho Chi Minh City in numerous contradictions: reform policy, foreign capital and the working class. In: Schneider J, Susser I, editors. *Wounded Cities: Destruction and Reconstruction in a Globalized World*. New York, NY: Berg:227–251.

Davis M. 2007. *Planet of Slums*. New York, NY: Verso.

Geraci D. 2011. When Women Migrate: Children and Caring Labor in Puebla, Mexico [PhD dissertation]. New York, NY: City University of New York.

Gomez HA. 1989. Public health problems in Medellin. In: Edel M, Hellman R, editors. *Cities in Crisis*. New York, NY: City University of New York:103–115.

Harvey D. 2005. *A Brief History of Neoliberalism*. New York, NY: Oxford University.

Jewkes R. 2002. Intimate partner violence: causes and prevention. *Lancet*. 359:1423–1429.

Jewkes R, Dunkle K, Brown H, et al. 2004. Gender-based violence, relationship power, and risk of HIV infection in women attending antenatal clinics in South Africa. *Lancet*. 363:1415–1421.

Jewkes R, Levin J, Penn-Kekana L. 2002. Risk factors for domestic violence: findings from a South African cross-sectional study. *Soc Sci Med*. 55:1603–1617.

Judt T. 2010. *Ill Fares the Land*. New York, NY: Penguin.

Kwong P. 2006. China's Neoliberal Dynasty. *The Nation*. October 2.

Le Mons Walker K. 2006. "Gangster capitalism" and peasant protest in China: the last twenty years. *J Peasant Stud*. 33:1–33.

Mullings L. 2003. After drugs and the "war on drugs": reclaiming the power to make history in Harlem, New York. In: Schneider J, Susser I, editors. *Wounded Cities: Destruction and Reconstruction in a Globalized World*. New York, NY: Berg:173–203.

Pappas G, Queen S, Hadden W, Fisher G. 1993. The increasing disparity in mortality between socioeconomic groups in the United States, 1960 and 1986. *N Engl J Med*. 329: 103–109.

Robotham D. 2003. How Kingston was wounded. In: Schneider J, Susser I, editors. *Wounded Cities: Destruction and Reconstruction in a Globalized World*. New York, NY: Berg:111–129.

Rodriguez-Trias H. 1992. Women's health, women's lives, women's rights [editorial]. *Am J Public Health*. 82:663–664.

Roldan M. 2003. Wounded Medellin: narcotics traffic against a background of industrial decline. In: Schneider J, Susser I, editors. *Wounded Cities: Destruction and Reconstruction in a Globalized World*. New York, NY: Berg:129–149.

Schneider J, Schneider P. 2003. Wounded Palermo. In: Schneider J, Susser I, editors. *Wounded Cities: Destruction and Reconstruction in a Globalized World*. New York, NY: Berg:291–311.

Schneider J, Susser I, editors. 2003. *Wounded Cities: Destruction and Reconstruction in a Globalized World*. New York, NY: Berg.

Sharf JW. 1997. *King Kong on 4th Street: Families and the Violence of Poverty on the Lower East Side*. New York, NY: Westview.

Sidel R. 1986. *Women and Children Last*. New York, NY: Viking.

Stiglitz J. 2002. *Globalization and Its Discontents*. New York, NY: Norton.

Susser I. 1996. The construction of poverty and homelessness in U.S. cities. *Annu Rev Anthropol*. 25:411–435.

Susser I. 1999. Inequality, violence, and gender relations in a global city: New York, 1986–1996. S. *Identities Global Stud Cult Power*. 5:219–248.

Susser I. 2006. Castells: the city and the grassroots: an anthropological perspective. *Int J Urban Reg Plann*. 30(1):212–218.

Susser I. 2009. *AIDS, Sex, and Culture: Global Politics and Survival in Southern Africa.*, Oxford, England: Wiley-Blackwell.

Susser I, Schneider J. 2003. Introduction. In: Schneider J, Susser I, editors. *Wounded Cities: Destruction and Reconstruction in a Globalized World*. New York, NY: Berg:1–25.

Susser M, Stein Z. 2009. *Eras in Epidemiology: The Evolution of Ideas*. Oxford, England: Oxford University.

Wilkinson R. 1986. *Class and Health*. London, England: Tavistock.

Wilkinson R, Pickett K. 2010. *The Spirit Level*. New York, NY: Bloomsbury.

Acknowledgments

WE ARE BOTH EXTREMELY grateful to the time and attention given to this project by our liaisons at the American Public Health Association (APHA) Press. Special thanks to David Stockhoff, book production coordinator, for his attention to detail in all aspects of the book. The hard work of Brian Selzer (manager of production), Nina Tristani (director of publications), and David Hartogs (senior marketing manager), as well as the Publications Board of APHA, was also invaluable to this project. We especially thank Dr. Judith Hays for her tireless efforts at improving the manuscript; any errors remaining are those of the authors.

Omar Khan: The most important supporters of this work, and all my endeavors, have been my wife Salwa and son Zareef, as well as our extended family and friends. The intellectual foundations of this work were laid at APHA, where Greg and I convened discussions to review the major thematic areas of the book. The support of the Association has thus been invaluable in a number of ways. Many of the authors of this book are long-time colleagues. This project has thus been a globally dispersed and shared one, and despite our busy lives has allowed us to work more closely together. I would like to dedicate this book to those who live and work in megacities, whether slum dwellers or the public health professionals who strive to improve their lives. I hope that work such as this is a step towards bettering our collective human condition.

Greg Pappas: I would like to acknowledge Ida Susser and Mohammed Akhter for the encouragement I needed to undertake this project. I thank Omrana Pasha for her insights into Karachi, which helped me first realize how different that city was from what I first understood. I thank the Department of Community Health Sciences at Aga Khan University for mentoring me in megacities while I was living in Karachi. My mother and father have been the guiding lights of my life. Finally, I want to thank Imran Khan for listening to me struggle through the various stages of this book.

Introduction

Gregory Pappas, MD, PhD, and Omar Khan, MD, MHS, FAAFP

WHY A BOOK ON megacities and public health? Urban health has been well established for a long time and has provided a useful lens through which to view all aspects of public health. The roots of public health are found in Victorian London's efforts to address health problems created by the urban environment. What is new is the emergence of the megacity as a unique pattern of urban settlement and as the subject of research.

Megacities are urban centers with populations greater than 10 million. New York City was the first to reach megacity status in 1950; currently, there are about 25 megacities around the world. Size alone does not define megacities, however; megacities are the leading edge of the globalization that has spatially and socially transformed urban populations. Megacities are important to public health and should be a focus of inquiry for two reasons. First, megacities present unique challenges to the field challenges associated with size, but also with dynamic processes shared by all. When cities reach a certain size, a set of problems are created, many of which have associated health risks. Second, the megacities are strategically important in the global order; health challenges in megacities take on global significance, and public health has a role in sustaining global stability.

An extensive body of social science literature on megacities has developed over the past two decades and provides direction for thought and action in public health. Sociology, anthropology, geography, political science, and urban planning have made important contributions to our understanding of these emerging urban landscapes. Public health scholarship has called for greater use of social science but only recently begun to delve into the rich literature on these complex, fascinating, and troubling population centers (Susser, Watson, and Hopper 1985). During the past 30 years, global trends have transformed the early megacities and added new ones to the list (Castells 2000). The majority of megacities now are located in less-developed countries, having achieved this status only within the past 10 years.

Manuel Castells, one of the leading sociologists writing on megacities, has made the point that the study of these unique places is not merely a special topic in social science, but, more generally, is the starting point for understanding the transformation of the contemporary world. Castells suggests that the Pearl River Delta, an area of 40 to 50 million people including Hong Kong, Macao, and the Chinese industrial centers of Guangzhou, Huizhou, and Zhaoqing, is "likely to become the most representative urban face of the 21st century" (Susser 2002, p342). These population aggregates are centers of economic, social, political, and cultural activity in their own countries, of their regions, and in the world as a whole.

The Megacity Challenge to Public Health

Megacities are a new spatial form with importance to public health because of the important set of health risks associated with size and dynamic processes shared by this set of cities. One of the objectives of this reader is to stimulate the field of public health to consider the consequences of the rise of megacities, and the technological revolution which brought them into being, for the health of populations.

Megacities are major drivers of transformation in the world today, creating new challenges and opportunities for human existence. Megacity development has been part of a global revolution led by information technology, and, like other technological revolutions before it, has affected not just the economy but all dimensions of human endeavor. Telecommunications, information systems, advanced transportation technology, and new media systems have enabled integration of complex economic and social processes over vast landscapes, making possible what have come to be called megacities. Despite the great cultural and social diversity within megacities, they have developed into unified areas of production, labor markets, social and cultural life, and politics, with public health consequences including the spread of certain infectious diseases and air pollution (Castells 1998).

Although the 25 megacities have globally connected and share important risk and patterns, there is no standard epidemiological profile that describes them.

Patterns of health in Tokyo are different from those of Lagos, as would be expected from the dramatic difference in levels of development between these cities.

What megacities share are dynamics and processes—population size, density, geographic size, and many social patterns that create health risk. The tendency of systems towards collapse is another characteristic of megacities, one with obvious health implications. The health risks created by megacity dynamics are shared potentials. Through institutional development, many of the megacities have developed solutions to the "size problem," and, as part of an existing global network, the potential for learning between megacities is also great.

Strategic Importance of Megacities

The second part of the answer to the question, "Why a book on megacities and public health?" relates to the strategic importance of these places. Megacities are important to public health because they are critical to the global economy and political order. Protectioning the health of populations in megacities has far broader implications than protection of the health of individuals in those cities. Major health problems in megacities threaten to disrupt global economic and political stability. Put simply, megacities are important places to which public health must attend.

The health of people in these large population centers has significance for the entire planet; a health problem in one part of the world can spread rapidly to other parts of the world. The H1N1 events in Mexico City led to the declaration of a global influenza pandemic. The SARS epidemic spread globally after it reached the megacity of Hong Kong (Brookes and Khan 2005). Megacities, as media hubs, also attract terrorist attacks; Mumbai, Paris, and New York City were all targets of recent threats and attacks that received global attention. The spread of HIV globally through megacities has been well studied (Wallace and Wallace 1999). Disasters in megacities caused by earthquakes, tsunamis, severe storms, and political upheaval have catastrophic public health implications and cause economic and political consequences that extend far beyond local populations. Problems affecting megacities are magnified by the networked global media in these hubs.

Megacities are medical hubs for both countries and regions; the medical resources of megacities serve local populations as well as the needs of entire regions. Because of the activities of resident academic and research institutions, megacities are places where new health phenomena are often first noted. The identification of HIV/AIDS and recognition of the reemergence of tuberculosis occurred in megacities. Most megacities have some aspects of modern statistical systems with the capacity to monitor the health status of large populations. These systems enable science to identify trends that can have global significance; even mistakes made in the identification of trends have global significance.

Megacities and the Antiurban Bias in Development

Public health should also address megacities as part of a large effort to counter the historical antiurban bias of global health development. Of the 25 megacities, 20 are in the less-developed world (Brinkhoff 2010). This book directs readers to the extensive work on the well-documented health problems and inequalities in megacities in less-developed countries. Despite the fact that by 2007, more than half the population on the planet lived in cities, and despite extensive documentation of the needs of populations in cities, development assistance continues to show a historic bias against cities. To meet global health objectives, the needs of megacities in less-developed countries must be addressed.

One of the strong rationales for investment in health development around the world is the need to protect ourselves from diseases arising in other countries; that is, there is a need to protect the global population from diseases arising in individual countries (Institute of Medicine 2009). Toward this end, we need to build worldwide institutions that have the expertise to contain outbreaks of infectious diseases as well as to prevent and treat illness. Finally, there is growing recognition that poor health and inadequate health care in populations can lead to social and political destabilization, which leads to a more dangerous world, with potential setbacks in national security and other priorities. Megacities provide a staging platform from which the global fight against the outbreak of disease can be waged. The strategic importance of megacities in maintaining global order is clear, as is the role of public health in maintaining the stability of megacities. Research, funding, and development have not followed these clear imperatives, however.

Although most of the population growth in less-developed countries has been in urban areas, development assistance has continued to focus on rural areas. Between 1970 and 2000, urban areas received only 4% of all development assistance, a total of about U.S.$1.5 trillion (Worldwatch Institute 2006). The poor in cities are also largely overlooked in the distribution of foreign aid. Services for the poor, including housing, water, and sanitation, received even less: 11% of lending at the World Bank, 8% of lending at the Asian Development Bank, and 5% of lending at Japan's Overseas Economic Cooperation Fund. Global development programs of rich countries have a strong influence on research agendas and spending priorities of governments, universities, and nongovernmental organizations, which also have tended to focus on health problems in rural areas.

In a world of increased global health risks, economic disparities between countries, and profound challenges to national security, global health programs have become an important part of international diplomacy (O'Neill and Pappas 2009). The Obama administration has proposed to increase U.S. investment in global health to $63 billion (White House, Office of the Press Secretary 2009). New global health initiatives may provide the opportunity for implementing health projects in megacities and to move development assistance policy beyond its antiurban bias.

Origins of This Reader

This project, undertaken with the American Public Health Association (APHA) Press, began as a series of discussions that took place during the last few APHA annual meetings. At the 2008 meeting in San Diego, California, the editors of this volume convened a series of presentations—including case studies from Karachi, Dhaka, London, and New York City—to explore the topic of megacities and health. The project drew on the expertise of APHA membership with urban health interests and benefited from the guidance of Ida Susser and David Vlahov, who were instrumental in formulating perspectives and providing moral support.

Overview of Chapters

The remainder of this chapter summarizes the contents of this book. Most chapters follow the format of a didactic component with the additional context of a case study from a megacity.

Chapter 1 provides a conceptual framework for the study of megacities and health, drawing on the strong social science literature on megacities. The chapter makes the case for the study of megacities as a critical set of places and emphasizes the importance of lessons learned in some of those places that can be applied to others. Understanding trends in globalization and neoliberal policies are essential to understand how megacities have taken their present forms and how the battle for improved health must be waged.

Chapter 2 provides an overview of the urban ecology of megacities from Vlahov, who holds positions at the International Society of Urban Health (ISUH) and the New York Academy of Medicine (NYAM). This topic is particularly relevant, given that urban health was the theme of World Health Day 2010—in part, a recognition that half of the world's population now lives in cities—with important discussions taking place at conferences such as those sponsored by the ISUH and the NYAM.

Chapter 3 reviews the issues of overcrowding and population effects in the megacity of Dhaka, Bangladesh. It explores the complex interplay between poverty, migration, and environmental hazards within the context of one of the world's fastest growing megacities. M. Omar Rahman and colleagues Khondkar Ayaz Rabbani and Rahat Bari Tooheen makes a compelling case that population, environment, and development cannot be de-linked.

In Chapter 4, Mary Wilson discusses the increasing importance of emerging infectious diseases in megacity settings. Traditionally, emerging infectious diseases have not been studied within the urban context. However, given the variety of factors which promote their spread, this chapter presents emerging infectious diseases using a case study approach of dengue fever in Rio de Janeiro, Brazil. Specific factors such as size, location, population density, poverty, interactions with animals, and connectedness are reviewed as contributing to the possible rise and spread of emerging infectious diseases in megacities.

Chapter 5 provides an overview of megacity metrics, drawing on the work done at UN-HABITAT and the European Urban Health Indicator System. Arpana Verma proposes a conceptual framework for collection of metrics for the advancement of health and well-being in megacities.

Chapter 6 addresses the environmental hazards of megacities, drawing on experiences from Karachi, Pakistan. The chapter focuses on the unique problems of pollution in megacities that have not yet established monitoring and regulatory systems to control environmental hazards. Zafar Fatmi and Gregory Pappas relate the failure of the flow of lessons learned from megacities with well-organized environmental protection systems to others to the history of neoliberalism.

Chapter 7 provides a case study of the dynamics of HIV/AIDS in New York City, the oldest megacity in the United States, which also was one of the first to document the disease. In this geographic analysis, HIV/AIDS first became rooted in neighborhoods in the core of the city and spread along more commonly used transportation routes to other parts of the city and neighboring municipalities. This hierarchical diffusion strongly followed racial, ethnic, and class lines that are related to the historical transformation of megacities noted in this volume. Rodrick Wallace provides the link between the historical evolution of HIV and epidemiology that examines spatial change in infection rates over time.

Chapters 8 and 9 focus on megacities and disasters from two different perspectives. As Irshad Shaikh and Gregory Pappas explain, most of the world's megacities are at high risk of disasters either by location, vulnerability to serious weather, or other factors that relate to high population density. Their vulnerability is matched by their importance during responses to national disasters because of their inherent capacity to serve regional needs. In Chapter 9, Linda Young Landesman and Isaac Weisfuse study a massive power outage in the northeastern United States, the impact it had on the prototypical U.S. megacity—New York City—and subsequent responses. Lessons learned for the longer term are discussed as well.

Chapter 10 discusses the health issues in another established Western megacity—London—from a planning perspective. It starts by reviewing the development and growth of London (along with its historic tropical diseases); the author goes on to discuss the challenges presented to current development schemes and how spatial planning for London affects the health of those who live or work there. Neil Blackshaw makes a powerful argument for integrating health into city planning, especially in megacities, as an essential feature.

In Chapter 11, Dennis Andrulis and Nadia Siddiqui present a case study of Los Angeles, a city that has undergone social and geographic transformations during the past decades, similar to other megacities. A clear set of health patterns has emerged in Los Angeles following these social and economic changes. The old city center with concentrated poverty has become gentrified, forcing out poor residents; the suburbs have increasingly become home to poor and marginalized communities.

Chapter 12 provides a big-picture discussion of the primary care issues that arise in megacities, as well as some possible models and innovations in such settings. Primary care has been shown to reduce costs and improve health, yet its implementation in megacities has met with varying success. Omar Khan and Thomas Peterson analyze the barriers present, and suggest revisiting the precepts of community-oriented primary care by aligning community resources and needs with public health objectives.

A discussion of the important health challenges faced by Mexico City round off this collection. In Chapter 13, Carlos Castillo-Salgado frames the discussion by describing the health system in the city and then analyzing urban health problems and solutions through the lens of community action and national policy. The call for better health is linked to a plea for improved data and health assessment—a theme resonating with several other chapters in this book.

In all, this collection provides a rich overview of the complexity of the varied issues faced by megacities in the context of health. The didactic approach combined with the case studies in the chapters makes it clear that no one set of issues defines all these cities. There are lessons to be learned and applied from the many examples that emerge from these chapters to the health issues of megacities worldwide.

References

Brinkhoff T. 2010. The principle agglomerations of the world. Available at: http://www.citypopulation.de/world/Agglomerations.html. Accessed June 20, 2010.

Brookes T, Khan OA. 2005. *Behind the Mask: How the World Survived SARS, the First Epidemic of the Twenty-First Century.* Washington, DC: American Public Health Association.

Castells M. 1998. Introduction: looking at megacities as if people mattered. In: *Why the Megacities Focus? Megacities in the New World Disorder.* The Megacities Project 1998. Publication MCP-018. Available at: http://www.megacitiesproject.org/pdf/publications_pdf_mcp018intro.pdf. Accessed August 1, 2010.

Castells M. 2000. *End of Millennium. The Information Age: Economy, Society and Culture.* Vol. III. Cambridge, MA: Blackwell.

Institute of Medicine. 2009. *The U.S. Commitment to Global Health: Recommendations for the New Administration.* Washington, DC: National Academies.

O'Neill J, Pappas G. 2009. Health diplomacy: lessons for global health from PEPFAR. *Internet J World Health Societal Polit.* 7(1). Available at: http://www.ispub.com/journal/

the_internet_journal_of_world_health_and_societal_politics/volume_7_number_1_33/ article/health-diplomacy-lessons-for-global-health-from-pepfar.html. Accessed September 22, 2010.

Sassen S. 2001. *The Global City: New York, London, Tokyo.* Princeton, NJ: Princeton University.

Susser I, editor. 2002. *The Castells Reader on Cities and Social Theory.* Oxford, England: Blackwell.

Susser MW, Watson W, Hopper K. 1985. *Sociology in Medicine.* 3rd ed. New York, NY: Oxford University.

Thompson DF. 2008. The role of medical diplomacy in stabilizing Afghanistan. *Defense Horizons.* (63):1–8. Available at: http://www.fas.org/man/eprint/meddip.pdf. Accessed September 22, 2010.

Wallace D, Wallace R. 1999. *A Plague on Your Houses: How New York Was Burned Down and National Public Health Crumbled.* New York, NY: Verso.

White House, Office of the Press Secretary. 2009. Statement by the President on the Global Health Initiative. May 5. Washington, DC: The White House, Office of the Press Secretary. Available at: http://www.whitehouse.gov/the_press_office/Statement-by-the-President-on-Global-Health-Initiative. Accessed June 15, 2010.

Worldwatch Institute. 2006. *State of the World 2007: Our Urban Future.* New York, NY: Norton.

1

Conceptual Framework: Megacities and Public Health

Gregory Pappas, MD, PhD

THE SOCIAL SCIENCES HAVE long provided a source of perspectives and conceptual frameworks in public health research and practice, offering an excellent place to begin the public health study of megacities. Social and cultural determinants of health, now concepts fundamental to the field, have been understood in terms drawn from the social sciences (Susser, Watson, and Hopper 1985; Frenk 1993). The limited or inappropriate use of the social sciences, however, has led to weak public health scholarship and inadequate interventions (Muntaner, Lynch, and Smith 2000; Pearce 1996). By failing to reach more deeply into the rich literature of the social sciences, public health frameworks continue to be conceptually weak and programmatically limited.

Public health students and practitioners are sometimes discouraged by their readings of social science, finding the certainties of biological sciences preferable to the rancor of debates in sociology, anthropology, and related disciplines. What some in public health have missed, however, is that the subject of social science, society itself, is inherently open to debate (Crompton 1993). The very terms of the study of society are part of a struggle playing out in public health. It is not lack of precision or lack of development that leads to protracted debates in the social sciences, but the contested nature of its subject and terrain.

Public health is not immune to this struggle, nor does it make the adoption of social science in public health less useful. What is required is the application of the social sciences with greater awareness of the controversial nature of its domain and a clear statement of assumptions as public health enters into the debate. This recognition of values inherent in a social science–oriented conceptualization of public health issues refines and clarifies our inquiry. I set out a set of assumptions related to values that promote increasing self-actualization of individuals and groups and the assumption that this development will lead to improved population health (Giddens 1990).

Integration of insights into megacities gained from two decades of social science literature has only recently begun. This chapter develops a conceptual framework for public health, providing a comprehensive understanding of megacities by drawing from a wide range of social sciences. After a presentation of the demography of megacities, a review and synthesis of the literature on megacities is provided. First, an understanding of neoliberalism and globalization is used to provide the historical and political context in which the megacities have developed. Second, megacities are identified as unique places in the global order to which public health must attend. The 25 megacities are at the cutting edge of the many dimensions of global developments. In a third section, these themes are drawn together into a framework to associate megacity processes and dynamics with health risks. The concept of dysfunction related to excessive size provides a frame through which to view the wide diversity of megacities (Angotti 2005). Finally, this chapter 1 discuss the limitations of the social engineering approach, which public health shares with urban planning, and the critical role of politics in megacities and the evolution of social movements in them.

Demography of Megacities

A megacity is defined by the United Nations as a metropolitan area with a total population of more than 10 million people. The terms "megapolis" or "megalopolis" are also used but lack standard definitions. Some definitions set a minimum population density of 2000 persons per square kilometer (Brockerhoff 2000). Half of today's 25 megacities reached megacity status in just the past 10 years.

Although the rise of megacities is a comparatively recent phenomenon, megacities themselves are part of a long demographic trend in the growth of urban populations. In 1800, only 3% of the world's population lived in urban centers. Beijing became the first city in the modern era to have a population of 1 million. By 2007, more than half the Earth's population was living in cities.

In 1950, New York City became the world's first megacity, followed by London, Paris, and Tokyo. By 2000, there were 18 megacities. Increasingly, these cities are located in less-developed countries. Currently, Tokyo, with a population of 33.8 million, is the largest city in the world—larger than many countries—followed by São Paulo (18.3 million), Mexico City (18.3 million), New York City (16.8 million), and Mumbai (16.5 million).

The growth of urban areas and megacities is fastest in less-developed countries (United Nations Population Fund 2007). Fertility rates in these countries remain higher than rates in more-developed countries. Rapid industrialization in many less-developed countries draws migrants into cities, as was the pattern during earlier eras in other parts of the world. The hope of higher incomes and improved services in urban areas—particularly improved education, health care, sanitation, and communication—draws people from rural areas, where these services are less available. In some countries, economic change and political unrest have forced rural populations from their land.

Population growth in urban areas has led to amalgamation; as they grow, neighboring cities and towns begin to touch and merge, and rural areas become semiurban. One of the most advanced agglomerations, known as the Pearl River Delta, has a population of 50 to 60 million people. The economic and commercial centers of the region include Hong Kong, Macao, and the Chinese industrial centers of Guangzhou, Huizhou, and Zhaoqing. Integration of this vast area, which extends across international borders, progressed rapidly after the British turned over Hong Kong to China.

Determining the population of a megacity is complicated by differences in how borders of the city are determined and problems in census taking. Depending on the borders used, Tokyo is estimated to have a population of between 12 and 36 million. The Tokyo metropolitan area, which includes about 12 million people, has become part of a larger unit, the Kanto District (including three prefectures and many cities), which has a population of more than 41 million. For consistency, this chapter uses Thomas Brinkhoff's definitions and estimates for megacities (Table 1.1). These population estimates are based on projections for the reference date of January 1, 2010, and can be considered comparable. These figures may vary from official or government statistics for reasons including varying definitions of borders, accuracy of sources, and projection methods.

Table 1.1   Population of the 30 Largest Cities, by Rank: 2010

Rank	Name	Country	Population
1	Tokyo	Japan	33,800,000
2	Seoul	South Korea	23,900,000
3	Mexico City	Mexico	22,900,000
4	Delhi	India	22,400,000
5	Mumbai	India	22,300,000
6	New York City	United States	21,900,000
7	São Paulo	Brazil	21,000,000
8	Manila	Philippines	19,200,000
9	Los Angeles	United States	18,000,000
10	Shanghai	China	17,900,000
11	Osaka	Japan	16,700,000
12	Kolkata	India	16,000,000
13	Karachi	Pakistan	15,700,000
14	Guangzhou	China	15,300,000
15	Jakarta	Indonesia	15,100,000
16	Cairo	Egypt	14,800,000
17	Buenos Aires	Argentina	13,800,000
18	Moskva	Russia	13,500,000
19	Beijing	China	13,200,000
20	Dhaka	Bangladesh	13,100,000
21	Istanbul	Turkey	12,500,000
22	Rio de Janeiro	Brazil	12,500,000
23	Tehran	Iran	12,500,000
24	London	United Kingdom	12,300,000
25	Lagos	Nigeria	11,400,000
26	Paris	France	10,000,000
27	Chicago	United States	9,850,000
28	Shenzhen	China	9,400,000
29	Wuhan	China	9,000,000
30	Lima	Peru	8,850,000

Source: Brinkhoff 2010.

The number of people living in megacities is a matter of controversy with political implications, particularly in less-developed countries (Forstall, Greene, and Pick 2004). Because censuses frequently determine both numbers of elected officials and flows of tax revenue, there are frequently political controversies around determination of population size in megacities. As an example, the 1998 census in Pakistan initially reported a total of 9.4 million people in the city of Karachi. Later, the census commissioner confessed that another 2 million people lived in Karachi who were counted but not included in the census report. The explanation for this decision was that these people were allegedly Afghans and Bengalis and not Pakistani citizens; therefore, they do not consume resources. Other parts of the country included illegal residents, however. The political implication of a much larger Karachi plainly was at issue. The population of Karachi in 1998 was probably 11.4 million, and on that basis it was estimated to be about 15 million in 2007. United Nations estimates, however, were based on the official figure of 9.4 million. Other megacities in less-developed countries have similar problems with accurate enumeration. Census undercounts also have important implications for epidemiology; census data are frequently used as denominators for calculation of disease prevalence and can introduce serious errors in prevalence estimation when denominators are based on inaccurate census data.

Current population projections indicate a rapid increase in the number of megacities around the world during the next decade. This will be followed by a leveling off in the growth of new megacities, although the transformation of urban landscapes is projected to continue its dramatic pace. Globally, urban areas will grow disproportionately compared with rural areas, and by 2030 it is projected that three of five people on the planet will live in cities (United Nations Population Fund 2007). In Asia, several population centers are predicted to continue to grow, with Jakarta, Indonesia, reaching 24.9 million people; Dhaka, Bangladesh, reaching 26 million; Karachi, Pakistan, reaching 26.5 million; Shanghai, China, reaching 27 million; and Mumbai, India, reaching 33 million. Lagos, Nigeria, has grown from 300,000 in 1950 to an estimated 15 million in 2010 and may grow to 25 million by 2015.

The Context of Megacities Development: Neoliberalism and Globalization

Demography uses a population cutoff of 10 million to define when urban areas become megacities; however, sheer size may not be the most useful identifying characteristic for public health purposes. The development of megacities, their growth in number, their transformation, and health consequences must be understood in the context of the particulars of the history of the last three decades. Neoliberalism and globalization are two closely related terms which help us understand this period of megacity development.

Global change has been dominated by policies promoting deregulation of many sectors of society and government disinvestment in basic human needs

(Navarro 2007). As a set of beliefs, neoliberalism sees the source of economic growth and progress in global markets and barriers created by governments. In practice, however, neoliberalism has been associated with government support of powerful business concerns over local industry or popular demand (Chomsky 2003). Widening social and health disparities and the emergence of a host of maladies associated with living in megacities have resulted from these global policies. Thus, the critique of neoliberalism provides an overarching framework with which to understand the spatial, economic, and social transformation of cities around the world, particularly in the context of public health.

Neoliberalism has characterized the current phase of globalization, but globalization cannot be understood purely in economic terms. According to Anthony Giddens, modern institutions have globalized, creating four dimensions or drivers of change: the world economy, the international division of labor, the nation-state system, and world military power (Giddens 1990). For Giddens, the world economy is a set of relations and flows of capital. Globalization of the economy has led to an international division of labor (i.e., different countries playing difference roles with some providing raw materials, others providing labor and production, and still others directing financial flow) is an independent realm fueled by technological development and politics. The nation-state system is the third dimension, made up of global institutions that direct societies and direct the flow of information around the world. Militaries, the fourth dimension, with global reach and networks of cooperation, constitute a force independent of (but affected by) the other three dimensions. Each of these globalizing forces has distinct health consequences (Pappas, Hyder, and Akhter 2003). Public health has suffered from an antiquated conceptual framework which reduces globalization to economic forces alone (Labonté and Schrecker 2007).

Megacities as Special Places on a Globalizing Planet

Megacities can be regarded as 25 discrete places on the globe—unique places with particular histories and global roles. However, they are more than a subset of cities, because they constitute the engine of globalization. These 25 cities, with their vast populations, are connecting points for the global economic forces, military plans, information flows, and divisions of labor mentioned previously. They are also magnets within countries and regions for the flow of people and resources. People are drawn to large urban areas because they want to participate in the global economic system present in megacities, which act as depositories of segments of populations—in particular, underserved and underemployed people fighting to survive.

Three ideal types—*global cities*, *information cities*, and *dual cities*—drawn from the literature describe the ways that megacities have evolved and function. These concepts are not intended to create categories in which to place specific megacities, but rather to identify roles they play in the global order and to analyze the social forces that determine conditions of life and health in megacities. That is, no megacity is totally a global city, an information city, or a dual city; instead, each megacity can be understood as being formed by the forces that have been conceptualized to describe megacity phenomena.

Global Cities

Global cities is the term Saskia Sassen uses to describe the large urban centers that serve as headquarters for major corporations that command huge financial, technological, and informational capacity. Her book, *The Global City*, is a study of New York City, London, and Tokyo (Sassen 1998) that identified those cities' roles in the evolution of globalization. First, they are command posts for policy implementation for the global economy. Second, they are financial and consulting hubs that direct production and consumption. Third, they are sites of innovation for new businesses and industries. Finally, global cities provide huge markets for the financial and consulting services upon which the global economy depends.

Financial and consulting services have eclipsed production jobs in global cities. In New York City, there are more than 350 foreign banks; one of every four bank employees works in a foreign bank. Financial institutions in cities such as Hong Kong, Singapore, and Los Angeles function around the globe. Emerging markets have added São Paulo, Moscow, Seoul, Jakarta, and Buenos Aires to the ranks of global cities.

Information Cities

Information cities are part of an emerging understanding of a broader change in society, the shift toward an information-based society (Castells 2000); they can be understood as a further development of the concept of the global city. An information-based society is based on the creation, distribution, diffusion, use, integration, and manipulation of information as an important economic, political, and cultural activity (Castells 2004). Wealth in an industrial society, the predecessor to an information-based society, was created out of industrial production. Wealth in an information-based society is created through the economic exploitation of knowledge. In the information-based society, the current phase of global development, industrial production has not disappeared but has been radically transformed, and is directed globally through the use of information technology out of global hubs, predominantly located in megacities.

Closely related concepts are *postmodern society*, *knowledge society*, and *network society*, the latest phase of economic development. A high level of control of the global economy, politics, culture, and military takes place in the information cities. The network of information cities direct global flows and allocate certain roles among various megacities and associated regions or hinterlands. Industrial production, agriculture, or extractive industries are increasingly directed and controlled by the information cities through flows of capital, information, and people. Megacities play important roles in an information-based society, providing major hubs for these flows.

The Dual City

The notion of the *dual city* draws into our understanding of megacities the widening inequalities that have accompanied their growth. Arundhati Roy, in her book *Power Politics*, presents a vivid image of the underside of globalization: emaciated Indian workers digging ditches by candlelight to lay fiber-optic cables (Roy 2002). Marginalization of large segments of urban populations by the information revolution is an integral part of megacity development and globalization. Megacities have developed a complex social mosaic with stark patterns of inequalities and social exclusion. One billion people—one sixth of the world's population—now live in shanty-town breeding grounds for social problems such as crime, drug addiction, alcoholism, poverty, and unemployment (Davis 2006). Older megacities have become increasingly unequal, and new megacities have grown up with complex ethnic and social integration and disintegration.

The concept of dual cities also helps us understand the place of megacities like Karachi and Lagos in the global order. These megacities are both repositories of large, marginalized populations and unique places in the international division of labor. Karachi is the major port for provision of military supplies to Afghanistan; Karachi also receives from Afghanistan more than half of the world's heroin (Steinberg, Hobbs, and Mathewson 2004). Much of the violent struggle in Pakistan has been over control of these transportation links.

The megacity of Lagos, with 15 million residents, is a financial hub of Nigeria, the world's fifth-largest oil producer; it is also a global node for Internet scams and other illegal operations. People have poured into Lagos looking for ways to benefit from the huge amounts of money that flow through the city. Lagos is a critical hub of control of Nigerian oil reserves and is increasingly marked by violence. Packer writes of Lagos: "It's hard to decide if the extravagant ugliness of the cityscape is a sign of vigor or of disease—a life force or an impending apocalypse" (Packer 2006). All megacities are dual cities in part, but some in particular form the underbelly of globalization.

Defining Megacities in Terms of Dysfunction

Health risks in megacities can be understood from the perspective of dysfunction related to large size and rapid growth (Angotti 2005). *Dys-economies of scale* or dysfunctions in urban places occur when the advantages of size of place are outweighed by the disadvantages. Although economists have long seen cities as the engine of the wealth of nations, by the late twentieth century it became clear that cities are not the panacea for the development of human society. The downside of large, concentrated populations has led to a literature on optimal or *efficient* size (Capello 2000).

The history, special status, and process and dynamics of megacities described in the above sections have created a set of dysfunctions that are associated with health risks. These dysfunctions can be easily understood within the more general context of the social determinants of health on which much of public health relies (Commission on Social Determinants of Health 2008). Dimensions or dynamics in megacities include population size, density, rates of growth, and the integration and disintegration of systems (Table 1.2).

The dimensions, determinants, and health risks shown in Table 1.2 should not be thought of as a typology, as these are not static categories. Instead, Table 1.2 should be seen as presenting causal pathways forming a web or a matrix in which dysfunctions have health consequences. These dynamic processes are embedded

Table 1.2   Web of Causation: Megacity Dynamics, Social Determinants, and Health Risks

Megacity Dynamics	Social Determinants	Health Risks
Population size and density	Hazards of built environment, water, food, electricity outages, large population dynamics, critical mass	Spread of infectious diseases (e.g., dengue, tuberculosis), food and water supply quality problems, pandemic risk
Rate of growth	Overwhelmed infrastructure, solid waste management, pollution	Environmental health risks
Geographic size	Movement problems, jurisdictional issues	Travel injury, delays in services and health care
Integration/dispersion	Increasing social inequalities and marginalization, social isolation, feminization of poverty, communal tensions, relaxation of social supervision, criminality	Health disparities, HIV/AIDS, substance abuse infant mortality, domestic abuse, homicide

in the restructuring of the economy under neoliberalism and the emergence of an information-based society.

Dysfunctions of megacities create risks for human health and indeed, health outcomes have been used to define the dysfunctions of megacities (Susser 2002). Excess morbidity and mortality can be associated with dys-economies of scale described in the following three sections of this chapter. Most of the older mega-cities have developed specific infrastructures to accommodate large population size and avert health risks. By contrast, many of the megacities that have been un-able to develop such infrastructures and institutions are more likely to experience dys-economies of scale, or dysfunction. Yet, megacities of all kinds share a set of risks that lead to health problems if they are not addressed.

Health Consequences of Megacity Population Size, Density, and Rates of Growth

Megacity population size, density, and rates of growth create health risks by over-whelming municipal capacity to meet the needs of populations for housing, wa-ter, electricity, solid waste management, and basic services (fire/rescue, police, and health care). The public health problems of the nineteenth century have re-turned to today's megacities, despite scientific knowledge and well-developed technologies for the control of these diseases (Bashir 2002). Old scourges like tuberculosis, cholera, and other causes of diarrhea have returned and are joined by new problems, including air pollution, chronic diseases, and new infectious diseases (including dengue). Many of the megacities were built quickly and poorly planned without accommodation for parks and other recreational spaces. Lack of urban space for recreation has been evaluated as a risk for obesity, hypertension, and diabetes (Lovasi et al. 2009).

Air pollution related to motor exhaust, industrial production, and household cooking fires has increased in megacities in many parts of the world. Air pollution levels in many megacities today rival those of the "Great Smog" in London in 1952, in which over 4000 people died and 10,000 became ill (Davis 2002). Megacities have unique pollution hazards, because they bring together multiple air pollutants that may have synergistic effects on health (Molina et al. 2004). Megacities are now some of the most polluted places on the planet and yet are home to millions.

Solid waste management in megacities has reached dimensions never before imagined. In resource-poor settings, much of the trash produced in megacities is collected by people working in an informal network; trash is collected, processed, and resold in squalid settings. Plastic recycling, however, requires a more sophisticated recycling process that has not yet been widely established in cities like Karachi, Cairo, and Manila, which struggle with simple removal of waste. Plastic bags are frequently not recycled and have become a major hazard in megacities; thin plastic bags end up clogging sewage and water drains, making already overwhelmed systems even more hazardous. Tons of bags pile up and become overwhelming; to clear these piles, they are frequently burned within city limits, releasing carcinogenic dioxins and smoke, causing and exacerbating diseases. The problem contributes to regional environmental destruction with implications for climate change (Harshal and Pandve 2008).

Dengue presents a case of an infectious disease that illustrates megacity health dynamics (Horton 1996). Dengue hemorrhagic fever is caused by a mosquito-borne virus that was a rare tropical disease until the advent of megacities. The mosquitoes that spread the virus (*Aedes aegypti*) have found new environments to occupy in tropical megacities, areas in which plentiful rainfall creates countless breeding niches. Poorly-maintained areas of a city in which water is allowed to stand—in trash, discarded automobile tires, stagnant drains, and water tanks—create places for the mosquito to breed. Even megacities in deserts (e.g., Karachi) have annual outbreaks of dengue hemorrhagic fever, because water is stored inside or near homes. These man-made mosquito breeding sites interact with the large numbers of susceptible humans living in crowded neighborhoods, allowing this once-rare disease to take hold.

Health Consequences of Megacities' Geographic and Social Distances

The geographic size of megacities creates a unique set of problems. Physical movement becomes a major problem when roads and transport systems do not keep pace with population needs. Supersized cities create long and unpleasant transit times for businesses, workers, students, and teachers. Problems reaching work, school, and clinics are all common features of megacities with poorly developed transportation infrastructures. Travel time also delays basic city services by impeding police, fire, and emergency medical personnel. Routine weather conditions or news heard on the radio can cause major traffic problems that make travel impossible for hours. These long delays in transport (e.g., sitting in vehicular traffic) intensify pollution-related health problems. Public transportation lines have attracted terrorist attacks (e.g., the metro attacks in Moscow, Paris, and Tokyo), since megacities provide high-impact targets with large populations and proximity to global media.

Social distances and the dynamics of networks within megacities are themselves unique and have consequences for health. This concept finds its clearest example in the spread of infectious diseases. Critical numbers of people who are vulnerable and are in close proximity to others increase the opportunity for the spread of disease. HIV/AIDS is the best-understood example. Networks of people who share sex or needles are discrete and must be of a certain minimum size to sustain infection in populations. Megacities sustain many types of networks, many of which may overlap. The opportunity for the spread of infections is unparalleled in this collection of networks.

Megacities provide the "critical mass" numbers that make many trends possible. Mark Penn, a prominent pollster, suggests in his 2007 book, *Micro Trends,* that networks of as few as 100,000 people can create social groups that pressure companies, markets, and policymakers to address their unmet needs. The pioneering work by Christakis and by Collins have opened new avenues of research for exploring the ways in which networks contribute to emerging health patterns in populations (Christakis 2007; Collins 2004).

Information technology networks intensify these social forces in megacities. Although many have noted that electronic networking connects people and activities at great distances, perhaps the more profound connectivity occurs within urban settings. Megacities are highly networked internally and bridge many social distances, allowing trends to emerge, but the full significance of these forces has yet to be fully explored within the field of public health.

Integration, Disintegration, and Health Inequalities

Integration and disintegration of populations in space are critical features of megacities and provide a way to describe them physically and socially. These megacity patterns offer a context for understanding the prominent inequalities that mark the urban landscape. Megacities have grown in numbers, size, and wealth, but these changes did not happen through the simple expansion of smaller cities. Megacities have grown by enriching some areas and bypassing or abandoning others; the consequence of the restructuring of megacities is a complex mosaic of distinct and unequal neighborhoods and groups, with enormous inequalities in conditions for the people living there. Parts of cities are tightly knit together in an information web, while other parts are skipped over, even physically walled off and economically marginalized. Increases in social and economic inequalities, the feminization of poverty, and the rise of criminality have all been clearly associated with policies which discourage regulation and support of basic human needs (Castells 2004).

This patchy social development pattern in megacities has resulted in clear population health patterns. Disparities in health between classes and racial/ethnic groups have grown during the past decades in most countries (Farmer 1999). Patterns of integration and disintegration in megacities result in patterns of inequalities in health and have consequences for social networks (Ravallion, Chen, and Sangraula 2007). Lower income and poor living conditions are associated with poor health status and increased mortality (Mercado et al. 2007). Three examples show how health inequalities are associated with the megacity dynamics related to integration and disintegration: the spread of and inequalities associated with HIV/AIDS, the feminization of poverty and related health problems, and the social distribution of death caused by heat stroke and hepatitis C.

HIV/AIDS was first discovered in two megacities, New York City and Paris. Although the origins of the virus are uncertain, it is clearly the unique environment of megacities that allowed it to take hold and spread through human populations globally. Megacities provided a perfect set of conditions—large, dense social networks—in which HIV could make its appearance. Once HIV took root in the core of megacities blighted by changing economic and social conditions created by neoliberal reform, it then spread out across the landscape to suburbs and smaller cities via transportation lines (Wallace and Wallace 1999).

Poverty itself, however, is not the strongest predictor of HIV infection in megacities; the poorest parts of New York City do not have the highest levels of HIV/AIDS. Instead, the highest levels of HIV infection are found in the neighborhoods that have been the most disrupted. Disruptions in poor parts of New York City were caused by fires that grew out of control partly as a result of slow response times by the fire department, which had recently closed several stations in those areas due to budget cuts (Susser 1982). The withdrawal of these services and the subsequent fires were caused by neoliberal policies (i.e., disinvestment by government in basic human needs). The disruption of these communities led to high rates of syndemic problems: HIV/AIDS, drug addiction, crime, and infant mortality (Singer et al. 2006). Wallace and Wallace (2009) described the process with the terms *spatial* and *hierarchical diffusion*. This restructuring of the economic and social landscape of New York City by neoliberal policies represents the underside of the rise of the information society described by Castells (1978). Poor neighborhoods were marginalized as New York City was transformed from a light industrial capital to a financial hub.

The feminization of poverty is another consequence of the restructuring of the global economy that has left many women and their children vulnerable to physical and emotional harm (Susser 1996). The rise of domestic abuse is one of the symptoms of this trend. Megacities around the world have documented a rise in domestic abuse: cities as different as New York City and Karachi have similar levels of domestic abuse, as almost half of women in both cities experience a lifetime prevalence of domestic abuse (Fikree, Razzak, and Durocher 2005; El-Bassell et al. 2007). The forces leading to the global rise of domestic abuse—increases in substance abuse, HIV, and economic stability—are similar across megacities. The global rise of abuse tracks with the global rise in substance abuse, HIV/AIDS, and economic inequality.

Social networks in megacities have been associated with complex health risks associated with patterns of integration and disintegration. The deaths caused by the 1995 heat wave in Chicago did not follow expected socioeconomic lines (Klinenberg 2002): it was not the poor who died in the Chicago heat wave but people who did not have strong social networks. The spread of hepatitis C provides another example of the complex relationships between social networks and diseases. Once associated primarily with intravenous drug use, hepatitis C has recently become a major problem in megacities as systems of infection controls in health care facilities break down (Tanaka et al. 2004; Shepard, Finelli, and Alter 2005). Untrained and unlicensed practitioners in filthy clinics have led to the spread of this fatal disease through networks of families and in particular neighborhoods. Again, the poorest are not always the worst affected, because injections and procedures can be afforded by people who have the resources to obtain them but lack adequate information to protect themselves. Neoliberalism is responsible for a general weakening of government authority through decreases in regulation and welfare expenditure, which has in turn led to poor governance and the creation of disastrous health systems (Pappas et al. 2009).

The Megacity and the Limits of Social Engineering

The discussion of the health issues in megacities presented up to this point may lead the reader to the conclusion that these are somehow natural or inevitable consequences of human development and urban population dynamics. Social science–grounded studies of megacities dramatically point in the opposite direction. The evolution of megacities and their associated problems are the results of decisions made by people, whose decisions can be changed. This realization returns our focus to further discussion of neoliberalism and the political responses emerging from megacities, responses that frequently take on the dimension of social movements.

The hard lessons regarding political realities and the extensive knowledge that can be found in political science only rarely comes into public health education or public health science, but in his classic text *Megacities Lectures*, David Harvey, one of the preeminent American social scientists studying cities, exposes a number of myths about urban places that also help us understand the centrality of politics to policies that have determined the development of health patterns of populations in megacities (Harvey 2000). Harvey opened the way for an approach to city reforms that are essentially political. In his view, economic problems are not the genesis of megacity maladies. Instead, political decisions have led to the growth of megacities and to economic failures. Another myth lies in the faith in technology: Harvey emphasized that technological solutions rarely address problems faced by the masses and, regardless, cannot be implemented without a political process of support. Community solidarity is not the outcome of a policy any more than are religious or military dictatorships, another prominent myth described by Harvey as directing thought about megacities. Forms of solidarity in megacities, be they communitarian or authoritarian, are the results of political struggles. In short, we cannot understand megacity patterns or their problems without recognizing the ways politics affect policies and programs (Pappas 2010).

Harvey's myths have implications and are warning signs for public health and its partner, urban planning, both forms of social engineering. Earlier phases of urban planning have primarily been technical and professional, largely assuming that rational planning can solve the woes of rapid and erratic city development (Castells 1978). Almost all megacities have extensive plans that have continuously been developed and revised during the past decades, but few of those plans have been implemented or followed. The limitation of urban planning is related to the constraints of our collective understanding of how urban places work. Planning without consideration of politics—local, national, and global—has not worked.

A new generation of urban planners has rejoined social science in search of a broader paradigm. Recent approaches have offered the opportunity to explore innovative policy approaches, including work with marginalized communities, while building on the traditional urban analysis and methods. Not surprisingly, new forms of urban planning rely heavily on information technology and incorporate a variety of community into the process. Building coalitions among low-income tenants, community-based organizations, and development professionals, as well as the potential links to organizing among labor, women, and social service providers, provide the context in which effective planning is being proposed.

Policies are at the heart of much of what went wrong in megacities during the past 30 years, and these policies are rooted in politics. During this period, state intervention into the provision of basic needs for populations and for development of urban habitation has been replaced by what economists have called *laissez-faire* development, which has supposedly allowed markets to determine the direction of economic development. What has happened instead is that powerful business concerns, working through the political process, frequently undermine market forces (Chomsky 2003). The promise that wealth will "trickle down" to the population, allowing people to meet their basic needs by purchasing goods and services, has not been realized. A gradual dismantling of the welfare state around the world has been promoted as part of the global adoption of these market-oriented policies, but the horrendous conditions of everyday living in most of the megacities are the result.

Although past megacity development has been heavily influenced by these political forces, political responses to conditions in megacities has also begun to emerge. Social movements with global implications frequently originate or take off in megacities (Susser 2002). These movements are the responses to the negative consequences of globalization and megacity development and frequently have public health dimensions.

The term *antiglobalization movement* is perhaps a misnomer for much of this social protest of the past decades, since activists struggling against the consequences of neoliberalism are themselves frequently working on a global scale, using the globally linked technologies to speak to power. "Globalization for whom, to benefit whom?" might instead be the best umbrella under which to collect the many and diverse critics of globalization (Pappas, Hyder, and Akhter 2003). Whether these many voices and movements can find a common voice is a major question for the future, but it is likely that the answer to these questions will emerge from the megacities.

Contemporary urban social movements have developed around health threats, environmental degradation, destruction of local cultural traditions, and sexual identity (Badshah and Perlman 2002). These struggles are frequently waged against the state, or against powerful institutions that communities see as responsible for their problems. The political responses to global restructuring have taken diverse forms and include communal violence, religious militancy, revolutionary social movement, environmental action, and many acts of urban resistance (e.g., the anti-IMF food riots of the 1980s).

Identity politics have played an important role in many cities and strongly fueled social movements. Gay communities have organized in megacities to challenge oppressive conditions around housing, safety issues, health issues, and basic freedoms. More recently, this political struggle has globalized. Groups of people who adopt gay identity have been formed in megacities worldwide. The stunning decriminalization of homosexuality in India came as a result of political work that began in the megacities of Delhi, Calcutta, and Mumbai, where communities of men who have sex with men (MSM) organized around HIV prevention efforts (Voice of America 2009). These social organizations, working to prevent disease and save lives among an extremely marginalized population, have been attacked by conservative state forces (including the police) for the simple act of promoting safe sex using government-approved materials and methods. After a decade of coalition building and fighting in the courts, the colonial-era penal code that prohibited homosexuality on the grounds that it was "unnatural" was struck down. The courts were persuaded that homosexuality was not a sickness or unnatural by well-developed scientific arguments (essentially, homosexuality is found in nature and therefore not unnatural). These arguments, while specifically tailored to the situation, were drawn from global networks that have addressed similar debates in other countries.

Megacities have for decades supplied a critical mass of men independent of traditional families who have come together to form communities of their own. Information technology in megacities has allowed creation of online communities of gay men who have been able to discover each other despite oppressive settings, since their online identities protect them from public exposure and danger. As much as gay liberation in the United States and Europe was catalyzed by HIV/AIDS, community protection against this infectious disease also brought together sexual minority communities in India (Pappas et al. 2002). The debate within Indian megacities between "gay" and MSM groups attests to the vibrancy of these communities as well as their connection to the wider network of gay communities with hubs in megacities.

Summary

More than a decade of social science study has provided the basis for a public health understanding and approach to a megacities as a rapidly growing and changing phenomenon. Megacities are more than just the largest cities. They have a unique place in the global order, their own dynamics, and associated health consequences. One of the key determining factors in their growth, and in the global social and economic transformation that has accompanied their growth, is neoliberalism. The period of neoliberalism's dominance has been marked by the deregulation of many sectors of society and disinvestment by governments in basic human needs. The concepts of global cities, information cities, and dual cities have been used to understand how megacities function and how they are related.

Megacities have been characterized by dysfunction related to their size and associated processes. Issues of size, density, rates of growth, geographic size, and issues related to integration and dispersion of megacity functions come together to create dys-economies of scale: beyond a point, the levels of organization achieved by most megacities exceed the many benefits that urban settlements create. Health problems are both a consequence of this dysfunction and a means of assessing the extent of the adverse effects of large city size. Unique environmental health risks, traffic-related hazards, the rise of certain infectious diseases, and health issues related to widening inequalities are all issues for megacities that can be understood through the lens of social determinants of health.

Finally, megacities must be understood in relation to the limits that a social engineering approach brings to their study. Although planning, as a signature of social engineering, is critically needed, planning failures do not arise from technical inadequacies. Rather, political realities have stalled the implementation of technological solutions. For example, sewerage treatment solutions for large populations have been well understood for over a century now, but most megacities struggle to provide even basic levels of sanitation and clean water. Political issues related to governance and the broader abandonment of government solutions to social ills have reached an impasse in many places. Social mobilization to generate political responses to urban health problems may hold the potential for improving health in megacities.

References

Angotti T. 2005. New anti-urban theories of the metropolitan region: "planet of slums" and apocalyptic regionalism. Presented at: Conference of the Association of Collegiate School of Planners; October 27 (revised December 12); Kansas City, MO.

Badshah A, Perlman J. 2002. Megacities and the urban future: a model for replication best practices. In: Bridge G, Watson S, editors. *The Blackwell City Reader*. Malden, MA: Wiley-Blackwell:549–558.

Bashir SA. 2002. Home is where the harm is: inadequate housing as a public health crisis. *Am J Public Health*. 92:733–738.

Brinkhoff T. 2010. The principle agglomerations of the world. Available at: http://www.citypopulation.de/world/Agglomerations.html. Accessed June 20, 2010.

Brockerhoff MP. 2000. An urbanizing world. *Popul Bull*. 55:3–44. Available at: https://prb.org/Source/ACFAC3F.pdf . Accessed August 4, 2010.

Capello R. 2000. Beyond optimal city size: an evaluation of alternative urban growth patterns. *Urban Stud*. 37:1479–1496.

Castells M. 1978. *City, Class, and Power*. New York, NY: Macmillan.

Castells M. 2000. *End of Millennium. The Information Age: Economy, Society and Culture*. Vol. III. Cambridge, MA: Blackwell.

Castells M. 2004. *The Network Society: A Cross-Cultural Perspective*. Northampton, MA: Edward Elgar.

Chomsky N. 2003. *Hegemony or Survival*. New York, NY: Holt.

Christakis N, Fowler JH. 2007. The spread of obesity in a large social network over 32 years. *New Engl J Med*. 357:370–379.

Collins R. 2004. *Interaction Ritual Chains*. Princeton, NJ: Princeton University.

Commission on Social Determinants of Health. 2008. *Closing the Gap in a Generation: Health Equity Through Action on the Social Determinants of Health*. Final Report. Geneva, Switzerland: World Health Organization.

Crompton R. 1993. *Class and Stratification: An Introduction to Current Debates*. Cambridge, UK: Polity.

Davis DL. 2002 A look back at the London smog of 1952 and the half century since. *Environ Health Perspect*. 110:A734–A735.

Davis M. 2006. *Planet of Slums*. New York, NY: Verso.

El-Bassel N, Gilbert L, Wu E, et al. 2007. Intimate partner violence prevalence and HIV risks among women receiving care in emergency departments: implications for IPV and HIV screening. *Emerg Med J*. 24:255–259.

Farmer P. 1999. *Infections and Inequalities: The Modern Plagues*. Berkley, CA: University of California.

Fikree FF, Razzak JA, Durocher J. 2005. Attitudes of Pakistani men to domestic violence: a study from Karachi, Pakistan. *J Mens Health Gend*. 2:49–58.

Forstall RL, Greene RP, Pick JB. 2004. Which are the largest? Why published populations for major world urban areas vary so greatly. Presented at: City Futures Conference; July 8–10; University of Illinois at Chicago. Available at http://www.uic.edu/cuppa/cityfutures/papers/webpapers/cityfuturespapers/session3_4/3_4whicharethe.pdf. Accessed August 1, 2010.

Frenk J. 1993. The new public health. *Ann Rev Public Health* 14:469–490.

Giddens A. 1990. *The Consequences of Modernity*. Stanford, CA: Stanford University.

Giddens A. 2009. *Sociology*. 6th ed. Cambridge, UK: Polity.

Harshal T, Pandve HT. 2008. The Asian brown cloud. *Indian J Occup Environ Med*. 12:3–94.

Harvey D. 2000. *Megacities Lecture 4: Possible Urban Worlds*. Amersfoort, Netherlands: Twynstra Gudde Management Consultants.

Held D, McGrew A, Goldblatt D, Perraton J. 1999. *Global Transformations: Politics, Economics and Culture*. Stanford, CA: Stanford University.

Horton R. 1996. The infected metropolis. *Lancet*. 347:134–135.

Klinenberg E. 2002. *Heat Wave: A Social Autopsy of Disaster in Chicago*. Chicago, IL: University of Chicago.

Labonté R, Schrecker T. 2007. Globalization and social determinants of health: introduction and methodological background (part 1 of 3). *Global Health*. 3:5. Available at http://www.globalizationandhealth.com/content/3/1/5. Accessed August 1, 2010.

Lovasi GS, Hutson MA, Guerra M, Neckerman KM. 2009. Built environments and obesity in disadvantaged populations. *Epidemiol Rev*. 317–320.

Mercado S, Havemann K, Sami M, Ueda H. 2007. Urban poverty: an urgent public health issue. *J Urban Health*. 84(Suppl 1):7–15.

Molina LT, Molina MJ, Slott R, et al. 2004. Critical review supplement: air quality in selected megacities. *J Air Waste Manage Assoc*. 55. Available at: http://secure.awma.org/journal/pdfs/2004/12/onlineversion2004.pdf. Accessed June 28, 2010.

Muntaner C, Lynch J, Smith GD. 2000. Social capital and the third way in public health. *Crit Public Health.* 10:107–124.

Navarro V. 1999. The political economy of the welfare state in developed capitalist countries. *Int J Health Serv.* 29:1–50.

Navarro V, editor. 2007. *Neoliberalism, Globalization, and Inequalities: Consequences for Health and Quality of Life.* Amityville, NY: Baywood.

Packer G. 2006. This is Lagos: in Nigeria's megacity. Available at: http://www.worldhum.com/travel-blog/item/this_is_lagos_george_packer_in_nigerias_megacity_39061110. Accessed August 1, 2010.

Pappas G. 2010. Pakistan's hygiene hijinks. *Anthropol Now.* 2:40–47.

Pappas G, Ghaffar A, Masud T, et al. 2009. Governance and health sector development: a case study of Pakistan. *Internet J World Health Societal Polit.* 7(1). Available at: http://www.ispub.com/journal/the_internet_journal_of_world_health_and_societal_politics/volume_7_number_1_33/article/governance-and-health-sector-development-a-case-study-of-pakistan.html. Accessed August 2, 2010.

Pappas G, Hyder AA, Akhter N. 2003. Globalization and health: toward a new framework for public health. *Soc Theory Health.* 1:91–107.

Pappas G, Khan O, Wright J, et al. 2002. Men who have sex with men (MSM) and HIV/-AIDS in India: the hidden epidemic. *AIDS Public Health Policy.* 16:4–17.

Pearce N. 1996. Traditional epidemiology, modern epidemiology, and public health. *Am J Public Health.* 86:678–683.

Penn MJ, Zalesne EK. 2007. *Micro Trends.* London, England: Penguin.

Ravallion M, Chen S, Sangraula P. 2007. New evidence on the urbanization of global poverty. *Popul Dev Rev.* 33:667–701.

Roy A. 2002. *Power Politics.* Cambridge, MA: South End.

Sassen S. 1998. *The Global City: New York, London, Tokyo.* Princeton, NJ: Princeton University.

Shepard CW, Finelli L, Alter MJ. 2005. Global epidemiology of hepatitis C virus infection. *Lancet Infect Dis.* 5:558–567.

Singer MC, Erickson PI, Badiane L, et al. 2006. Syndemics, sex and the city. *Soc Sci Med.* 63:2010–2021.

Steinberg MK, Hobbs JJ, Mathewson K. 2004. *Dangerous Harvest: Drug Plants and the Transformation of Indigenous Landscape.* New York, NY: Oxford University.

Susser I. 1982. *Norman Street: Poverty and Politics in an Urban Neighborhood.* New York, NY: Oxford University.

Susser I. 1996. The construction of poverty and homelessness in U.S. cities. *Ann Rev Anthropol.* 25:411–435.

Susser I. 2002. *The Castells Reader on Cities and Social Theory.* Oxford, UK: Blackwell.

Susser MW, Watson W, Hopper K. 1985. *Sociology in Medicine.* 3rd ed. New York, NY: Oxford University.

Tanaka Y, Agha S, Saudy N, et al. 2004. Exponential spread of hepatitis C virus genotype 4a. *Egypt J Mol Evol.* 58:191–195.

United Nations Population Fund (UNFPA). 2007. *State of the World Population: Unleashing the Potential for Urban Growth.* Washington, DC: UNFPA.

Voice of America. 2009. UN: Decriminalization of Homosexuality in India Will Boost AIDS Prevention. Available at: http://www1.voanews.com/english/news/a-13-2009-07-02-voa54-68701677.html. Accessed August 4, 2010.

Wallace D, Wallace R. 1999. *A Plague on Your Houses: How New York Was Burned Down and National Public Health Crumbled.* New York, NY: Verso.

World Health Organization (WHO). 2009. *Megacities and Urban Health.* Geneva, Switzerland: WHO. Available at: http://www1.voanews.com/english/news/a-13-2009-07-02-voa54-68701677.html. Accessed August 1, 2010.

2

Urban Health in the Context of Twenty-First-Century Megatrends

David Vlahov, RN, PhD

THE NINETEENTH CENTURY WAS the era of empires and the twentieth was the age of nation-states, but now the twenty-first is the century of the city. The megatrends of the twenty-first century primarily will be played out in cities and include demographic shifts, globalization, climate change, and health inequities. For better or worse, the predominant mode of living is urban, globalization is most concentrated in cities, and climate change arises from and affects cities. Health inequalities are expanding in cities, with poverty becoming urbanized, creating ever-increasing vulnerable populations. How cities are to be understood and managed is an immediate priority for protecting and promoting the population's health.

Demographic Shifts

Demographic shifts involve three elements: migration, fertility, and mortality. Migration involves "push–pull" factors that can be economic, cultural, political, or environmentally based. Examples of "push" factors include few opportunities, discrimination, political fears, natural disasters, and desertification. Examples of "pull" factors include job opportunities and better living conditions. These movements occur between and within countries, with the predominant pattern being short distances. Migration can even be observed in the form of daily commuting, which also has implications for the environment and health.

Throughout history, rural-to-urban migration has been a predominant pattern and is especially salient with the recognition, beginning in 2008, that for the first time in human history, the majority of the world's population now live in cities. Virtually all population growth during the next 30 years will occur in urban areas. By 2030, about 60% of humans will be urban dwellers, rising to about 75% by 2050 (Montgomery 2008).

Megacities are a highly visible example of this trend. In 1975, only five cities worldwide had 10 million or more inhabitants, of which three were in developing countries. The number will increase to 23 by 2015, all but four of them in developing countries. The growth rate of megacities in the developing world will be much higher than in the developed world (e.g., anticipated growth from 2000 to 2015 for Calcutta is 1.9%, vs New York City's 0.7%).

Urban growth is expected to occur slowly in megacities and faster in midsized cities (Satterthwaite 2000). By 2015, an estimated 564 cities around the world will contain 1 million or more residents. Of these, 425 will be in developing countries. Although large cities of developing countries will account for 20% of the increase in the world's population between 2000 and 2015, small cities (less than 5 million inhabitants) will account for 45% of this increase (United Nations Population Division 2000). Although megacities are the most visible examples of urban concern, they represent only about 6% of the world's urban population. These projections highlight the importance of viewing urban health as an international and global issue.

Creating healthy and sustainable cities represents a complex challenge. As a result of the need to accommodate population growth, most of the new city growth occurs through horizontal expansion of small and midsized cities. At face value, this trend might seem to mitigate risks associated with overcrowding, but in fact it brings health challenges as well. For example, horizontal growth requires longer commutes, which present sedentary-lifestyle and traffic-related health risks. Horizontal growth threatens land needed for food and water supply and therefore has implications for sustainability.

Other demographic shifts include fertility and mortality, which have shown a global decline. Urban settings provide female literacy and employment that changes the basis for valuation of women from bearing and raising children to being productive contributors to the family. Contraception and family planning, generally more available in cities, also contribute to this transition. Declines in mortality have been observed with modernization and availability of preventive and curative care. One net effect of this is the aging of the population. By 2025, the global population of people older than 60 years will be 1.2 billion, double the number in 2000; this number is expected to more than double again by 2050. More prominent now in developed countries, this trend will be increasingly observed in developing countries. It will be most pronounced in cities, where most older people will live. How cities are organized and governed will shape how these challenges are managed.

Globalization

Globalization refers to processes that increase interdependence across borders, and although the phenomenon is not new, the pace and extent of it is. It is driven by advances in and the spread of technology; unprecedented flows of information; increased ability to travel; the migration of people, goods, and services; and creation or destruction of jobs and economic opportunity. All of these are first apparent in cities and can result in conditions that are positive or negative for health. Cities are also fundamental drivers of national economies, and certain cities host the markets and the national and multinational companies that dominate the global economy. If global economic and trade regimes address issues of fairness and equity, and national and urban governance are strong, the effects of globalization can be positive for the social, physical, and economic development of cities, taking advantage of the concentrations of population to provide efficient and accessible educational as well as health and social services. Globalization can also create unique conditions in cities for individuals and families to take advantage of economic development opportunities to increase their income, meet other entrepreneurs, or gain competitive advantage.

However, the early warning signals of the negative effects of globalization can too often be seen in cities with large populations of immigrants who are without employment and appropriate housing, education, and health services. Migrants might join the city's formal economy if the rules were designed to include and benefit them, but where this is not the case, they build an informal economy that creates their own form of advantage. Poor urban immigrants often develop or enter an informal economy of microenterprise that can account for up to 40% of a country's GDP, including remittances to relatives in depressed rural regions.

Globalization may have a considerable cultural impact, most profoundly in urban settings. As noted in the 2007 United Nations Population Fund Report,

> Since the 1950s, rapid globalization has also been a catalyst of cultural change most strongly felt in cities. Advanced telecommunications and the influx of media from other regions of the world are at the core of the urban transition and have enormous impact on ideas, values and beliefs. Such transformations have not been as uniform or seamless as social scientists predicted. Urbanites may lose contact with traditional norms and values. They may develop new aspirations, but not always the means to realize them. This, in turn, may lead to a sense of deracination and marginalization, accompanied by crises of identity, feelings of frustration and aggressive behavior. Many people in developing countries also associate the processes of modernization and globalization with the imposition of Western values on their own cultures and resent them accordingly (United Nations Population Fund 2007, p. 25).

How cities are organized and governed will shape how these challenges are managed.

In this context, globalization can arise from and contribute to crime and terrorism in cities in a way that migrates to other cities. Criminal gangs are a special form of terrorism and they can have a global network. Although early forms of street gangs are viewed as only promoting criminal aims, in their later and more mature stage of development, such as the criminal and para-states that are now in direct conflict with the dominant international order, they develop political agendas. Criminal group formation and growth occur frequently in cities. One example is Mara Salvatrucha-13, or MS-13, formed by immigrants who fled the civil war in El Salvador in the 1980s (Bunker and Bunker 2010). The number "13" relates to the 13th letter of the alphabet, or "M," a reference to "La Eme," or the Mexican Mafia, a California-based prison gang that exercises control over MS-13 members and other street gangs whose members pay taxes in exchange for protection. This group of immigrants found discrimination, virtually no access to benefits, and little opportunity for advancement in the United States, a situation which was resolved by engaging in criminal activity. Prisons provided networking for the development of MS-13, which has operated for the past 15 years in and around Los Angeles. The gang is estimated to have several thousand members in multiple U.S. cities, as well as throughout Central America and Mexico, and is known for its brutality.

In a more classic example, cities have been the centers for the globalization of infectious diseases throughout history. Cities concentrate people and serve as transportation hubs, both of which facilitate transmission of infectious diseases. SARS, an acute viral respiratory infection caused by a coronavirus designated "SARS-CoV," is an example in recent times of a newly emerging infection that was transmitted rapidly through global transportation between major cities. The disease was first reported in Asia in February 2003, initially as an atypical pneumonia that was sometimes fatal, in the southern Chinese province of Guangdong. The presumed initial source was transmission of the virus through trade in the civet, a catlike mammal sold in "wet markets" (markets at which live animals are sold); however, human–human transmission by respiratory droplets was subsequently considered the major mechanism of transmission. Global dissemination began in February 2003 when a physician from Guangdong, China, visited Hong Kong and stayed in the Metropole Hotel. The physician subsequently came down with a respiratory illness that proved to be fatal and was later named SARS; the hotel occupants on the same floor subsequently became index cases for epidemics in Singapore, Toronto, Hong Kong, and Hanoi. The SARS epidemic ended in mid-2003 with a total of 8436 diagnosed cases (Zhou and Yan 2003).

SARS was almost exclusively an urban disease that was transmitted primarily within hospitals and households, and in the early phases of the epidemic there was great confusion about its cause, treatment, and prevention. Attempts to control the infection included airport screening, quarantines, hand hygiene, and masks. Health care workers were particularly vulnerable and accounted for approximately 10% of cases. Although airport screening was aggressive, the retrospective analysis suggested little benefit despite the enormous negative impact on tourism and global travel to the metropolitan areas that were heavily affected. Reducing person-to-person spread (e.g., hand washing, use of masks) best achieved ultimate control of the epidemic.

Climate Change

A third twenty-first-century megatrend is climate change (McMichael, Woodruff, and Hales 2006). Emissions of carbon dioxide and other greenhouse gases are projected to increase temperatures globally in the coming century. Cities generate 80% of all carbon dioxide and significant amounts of other greenhouse gases. They contribute to climate change mainly through energy generation, vehicle use, industry, and burning of biomass as fuel. The densely built environment of cities creates an "urban heat island" effect, in which, due to absorption of heat by buildings and concrete surfaces, urban temperatures can be 3° to 4°C higher at any time than in adjacent rural areas. Increased temperatures lead to less outdoor activity and, indirectly, greater emission of greenhouse gases with air conditioning. Climate change can include temperature-related, extreme weather–related, and air pollution–related health effects. These effects include water-, food-, vector-, and rodent-borne diseases, food and water shortages, and population displacement. For example, as noted by Kjellstrom and Monge (2010), increased mortality during heat waves has been reported from many cities worldwide in the United States (Luber and McGeehin 2008), Europe (the most extreme being in France in August 2003; Poumadere et al. 2005), and developing countries (Hajat et al. 2005). In France, 15,000 people died during the 2-week heat wave in 2003, and a similar number died in other countries of central and southern Europe. Extreme-heat mortality is primarily an effect of overload on the cardiovascular system as a result of physiologic reactions to heat exposure (Parsons 2003). In addition, acute hospital admissions and emergency ambulance transport for heart disease, asthma, and acute kidney diseases increase during a period of extreme heat (Knowlton et al. 2009; Hansen et al. 2008; Kjellstrom et al. 2010).

One of the effects of increasing temperatures in cities is an increasing level of ground-level ozone, a result of motor vehicle emission interactions with solar ultraviolet radiation (Bell et al. 2007); and ozone formation is both faster in diffusion and greater in area when air temperatures increase. Ozone increases incidence and mortality of heart and lung diseases and causes respiratory distress symptoms (WHO 2006). Climate change is likely to create more extreme-weather incidents (Intergovernmental Panel on Climate Change 2007), which will cause droughts that can lead to more limited water and food supplies. Extreme-weather events can also manifest as floods and windy typhoons or hurricanes.

Cities are frequently situated on coasts and rivers, where they are vulnerable to climate-related changes in the form of rising sea levels, storm surges, and flooding. Floods can lead to landslides blocking roads and damaging houses, and both electricity and water supply. Floods have damaging health impacts that include drowning, injuries, and disruptions of health services (McMichael et al. 2003). The most vulnerable to these disruptions will be poor people and people with preexisting chronic diseases or disabilities. The effects of flooding after Hurricane Katrina in New Orleans, Louisiana, on poor people, who lacked transport for evacuation, showed what might occur in affected urban areas (Sharkey 2007). Changes in temperature and humidity can also affect dispersion of infectious diseases. Mental health stress associated with increasing temperatures can be heightened.

Health Inequalities and Inequities in Cities

Although it is generally understood that city dwellers, on average, enjoy better health than do their rural counterparts, this may reflect the practice of aggregating data that provide an average of all urban residents—rich and poor—rather than disaggregating population groups by income or other measures of socioeconomic status. For example, in developing countries, slums without legal status are often overlooked in official reports used for projecting service coverage within cities; therefore, the slum populations are frequently uncounted, distorting the urban average. As a result, the different worlds of city dwellers and the substantial health challenges of the urban poor go overlooked. These differences in health outcomes within urban areas disaggregated by absolute or relative poverty are seen worldwide and for a wide variety of health outcomes. Likewise, differences in health outcomes are seen by geographic area–specific levels of infrastructure and services within cities. A child who lives in a slum in Kenya is far more likely to die before the age of 5 years than is his or her compatriot living in another part of the city that is not a slum (African Population and Health Research Center 2002). In 1990, life expectancy of Black men in Harlem, an urban area of concentrated disadvantage in New York City, was lower than among men in Bangladesh (McCord and Freeman 1990). An oft-quoted study from Glasgow, Scotland, shows dramatic differences in life expectancy by neighborhood, with lower-income neighborhoods approaching life expectancies in the cities of developing countries (Macintyre, McKay, and Ellaway 2005).

Inequalities in cities are projected to become worse. As noted already, half of the world's population is urban and the proportion is projected to increase, with two thirds becoming urban by 2030, and three quarters by 2050. Most of this projected growth is expected to be in urban slums. Poverty is becoming urbanized, and poor health is associated with individual and area poverty. *Health inequalities* refer to differences or disparities between groups. A related term is *health inequities,* which refers to inequalities that can be corrected but are allowed to stand as a result of distorted power and decision-making arrangements. The typical approach to public health is to seek to improve the health of all residents, but additional efforts are needed to address the inequities that preserve inequalities in environment and health status.

As the four megatrends—globalization, demographic shifts, climate, and growing inequities—originate in, proceed through, and generate effects on cities, they create environments that are complex both to understand and to govern. A prominent feature of urban settings is that the disparities themselves are intensely local, with the rich in penthouses and the poor living on the street below. The megatrends, however, operate differentially on the poor.

The Urban Environment—The Urban Lens

It is important to have a framework for approaching urban health action. Urban health is not defined as addressing diseases unique to urban settings, but rather as the living conditions and influences on those living conditions that shape behavior and health itself. Those living conditions are not necessarily unique to cities, but the characteristics of size, density (with proximity and association), diversity, and complexity shape risk and approaches to addressing health in cities. Together, they provide an "urban lens" through which to view a variety of influences. Size provides scalability—presumably, the larger the population size, the more scalable a public health program or intervention, although program quality is a separate dimension to consider. Density is frequently thought of as synonymous with overcrowding and its related health risks; in fact, density, with adequate space per person, provides levels of proximity and association that create efficiencies of scale for opportunities and services. The trend toward urban areas with lower density may translate into less overcrowding, but comes with other risks, including greater expenditure on utilities, longer commutes, and social isolation.

Diversity refers to a mix of populations found in cities that bring social and cultural richness, but can also lead to cultural clashes (Massey 1996). Diversity necessitates tailoring interventions to meet the needs of different subpopulations; it also refers to the rich variety of services within urban settings that can provide both specialization and a greater variety of service options.

Finally, cities can be characterized by their complexity. Multiple systems interact; pluralistic political structures create competing stakeholders; cities are inextricably linked to other levels of sociopolitical organization, such as neighborhoods, metropolitan regions, and nation-states, each of which make demands and offer resources to the other levels; and local political and social forces create wide variations in the contexts in which public health programs are delivered.

The implications of size, density, diversity, and complexity, which vary between different urban areas, are that simple interventions are rarely sufficient to solve problems, programs may have unintended as well as intended outcomes, and generalization from one setting to another can be problematic. This contextual complexity requires a similar level of intervention complexity—an intersectoral governance approach that integrates different sectors within government and with business and community participation. Urban complexity also requires special attention to disaggregating data to the level of neighborhoods in order to identify and then address health inequities within urban populations.

Living Conditions as Determinants of Health

Urban living conditions describe the characteristics that shape the day-to-day lives of urban residents. They include population characteristics such as individual behavior and demographics (e.g., socioeconomic status), the urban physical environment, the social environment, and the service system. These urban characteristics can be viewed both as the "preexisting conditions"—which public health interventions seek to change—and as intermediate outcomes—the pathways by which interventions lead to improvements in health. The WHO Commission on the Social Determinants of Health acknowledged the centrality of "living conditions" in addressing health inequalities and inequities (Commission on Social Determinants 2008).

The urban physical environment includes geologic and climatic conditions of the site where the city is located, the air city dwellers breathe, the water they drink and in which they bathe, the indoor and outdoor noise they hear, the parkland inside and surrounding the city, and the built environment. The built environment includes housing, public facilities, highways, and streets. Planning and urban design may also influence water quality through runoff, eliminate or add green space, influence motor vehicle use and accident rates, and contribute to the urban heat island. The urban infrastructure is also part of the physical environment and determines how a city provides water and energy to its citizens and how it disposes of garbage (Melosi 2000).

Urban social environment describes the structure and characteristics of relationships among people within a community. Components of the social environment include social networks, social capital, segregation, and the social support that interpersonal interactions provide. Comprehensive definitions of many of these factors are given elsewhere (Berkman and Kawachi 2000). A city's social environment can both support and damage health through a variety of pathways (Leviton, Snell, and McGinnis 2000; Freudenberg 2000; Geronimus 2000; Yen and Syme 1999). For example, social norms in densely populated urban areas can support individual or group behaviors that affect health (e.g., smoking, diet, exercise, sexual behavior; King et al. 2003). Social supports can buffer the impact of daily stressors and provide access to goods and services that influence health (e.g., housing, food, informal health care; Berkman et al. 2000).

Health and Social Services

Another important aspect to urban health is the array of health and social services available (Casey, Thiede Call, and Klingner 2001; Felt-Lisk, McHugh, and Howell 2002). Even the poorest urban neighborhood often has dozens of social agencies, each with a distinct mission and service package. Services available vary by type, mix, quantity, and quality.

A conceptual framework that provides broad categories, such as physical, social, and health care and social service environments permits us to isolate and measure seemingly discrete factors that affect urban populations. In reality, the effects of the physical, social, and service environments are more difficult to separate. For example, decent shelter that comes with land security and tenure provides people with a home, security for their belongings, safety for their families, a place to strengthen their social relations and networks, a place for local trading and service provision, and a means of accessing basic services.

Municipal government, markets, and civil society influence living conditions. Municipal government influences the health of urban populations by providing services, regulating activities that affect health, and setting the parameters for urban development; it has the capacity to modify the urban physical and social environments and to deliver or oversee the delivery of public health, health care, and social services. Government activities in many sectors affect health, including those in public education, public transportation, recreation, public safety, criminal justice, welfare, housing, and employment. Local, national, and global markets play a central role in shaping the conditions that determine the health of urban populations. Markets allocate housing, food, employment opportunities, medical care, and transportation and, because of privatization, increasingly play a role in education, public safety, and other sectors previously confined to the public realm. Civil society defines the space not controlled by government or the market where residents interact to achieve common goals. These in turn are shaped by national and international trends such as migration, globalization, and decentralization. For example, in many developing countries there is very little decentralization, and most decisions are made at the national level. Although living conditions affect behavior and health, it is these other influences that shape living conditions.

The depiction of these upstream factors as structures is helpful up to a point. Addressing unhealthy and unequal living environments at the local level requires multiple partners. The term *urban governance*, formerly equated with urban management, has come to be understood as both government responsibility and civic engagement. Generally, it refers to the processes by which local urban governments—in partnership with other public agencies and different segments of civil society—respond effectively to local needs in a participatory, transparent, and accountable manner (United Nations Population Fund 2007). Complex urban problems cannot be addressed with single programs or policies, but rather by applying models of healthy urban governance that provide an approach to managing an array of programs and policies. Healthy urban governance brings together multiple sectors of government, along with civil society and business, to jointly identify priorities and solidify commitments to action.

Governance

To meet the challenges that come with the megatrends and to optimize health in cities, quality of governance is a critical factor. The form of government of individual cities, especially megacities and national capitals, is often defined by national policy and practice. The more recent practice of decentralization of government within countries—that is, from the center to peripheral governmental bodies in regions and districts—does not always bring resources for urban management, thereby failing to consider the special needs of cities. The relationship between national or regional government and city government can be critical to the ability of cities to innovate and create systems to manage health. Such innovation is needed, because although governments have the ultimate responsibility for assuring the conditions in which their people can be as healthy as they can be, government needs partners to accomplish this.

Achieving the goal of healthy populations requires new forms of governance—the alignment of multiple interests to achieve a "shared goal" or "joined up" governance (Harpham 2009)—models that allow governmental health leaders to work effectively with their colleagues across the governmental sectors that influence health, and with nongovernmental sectors in civil society, including nongovernmental organizations, advocacy groups, business, academia, and the media. Good urban governance responds to local needs in a participatory, transparent, and accountable manner in treating current issues and planning horizons that extend beyond current needs. A number of cities have taken steps to create specific mechanisms for participatory governance to enable communities and local governments to partner in building healthier and safer cities (Montgomery 2009; Caiaffa et al. 2010). The WHO has facilitated this process through the Healthy Cities program, which includes developing political commitment to a process of achieving Health in All Policies, addressing health beyond health care (for example, by encouraging active transportation). The WHO has outlined tools to achieve Health in All Policies that include city health profiles and health impact assessments (Vlahov et al. 2010).

Summary

Cities are traditionally the economic engines for a country and increasingly are shaping the world. Urbanization encompasses the megatrends affecting global health: globalization, demographic shifts, climate change, and health inequities. Cities offer advantages and opportunities as well as threats to health for its residents. Although individual behavior shapes health and illness, the urban environment shaped by upstream influences can impact both behavior and health.

Inequities in the decision-making process of governments that exclude elements of society can preserve and maintain inequalities that impact all urban dwellers. Megacities present complexities in governance, owing to the occurrence of size, density, and diversity where inequalities and inequities are pronounced. Good urban governance that brings together the health and other sectors with authentic community participation is essential to meet these challenges and improve the health of urban populations.

References

African Population and Health Research Center. 2002. *Population and Health Dynamics in Nairobi's Informal Settlements: Report of the Nairobi Cross-Sectional Slums Survey 2000*. Nairobi, Kenya: African Population and Health Research Center.

Bell M, Goldberg R, Hogrefe C, et al. 2007. Climate change, ambient ozone, and health in 50 U.S. cities. *Clim Change.* 82:61–76.

Berkman L, Glass T, Brissette I, Seeman TE. 2000. From social integration to health: Durkheim in the new millennium. *Soc Sci Med.* 51:843–857.

Berkman L, Kawachi I, editors. 2000. *Social Epidemiology*. New York, NY: Oxford University.

Bunker R, Bunker PJ. 2010. Urban terrorism. In: Vlahov D, Boufford JI, Pearson C, Norris L, editors. *Urban Health: Global Perspectives*. San Francisco, CA: Jossey-Bass/Wiley:192–206.

Caiaffa WT, Nabuco AL, de Lima Friche AA, Proietti FA. 2010. Urban health and governance model in Belo Horizonte, Brazil: a case study. In: Vlahov D, Boufford JI, Pearson C, Norris L, editors. *Urban Health: Global Perspectives*. San Francisco, CA: Jossey Bass/Wiley:438–452.

Casey M, Thiede Call K, Klingner JM. 2001. Are rural residents less likely to obtain recommended preventive healthcare services? *Am J Prev Med.* 21:182–188.

Commission on Social Determinants of Health. 2008. *Closing the Gap in a Generation: Health Equity Through Action on the Social Determinants of Health*. Final Report. Geneva, Switzerland: World Health Organization.

Felt-Lisk S, McHugh M, Howell E. 2002. Monitoring local safety-net providers: do they have adequate capacity? *Health Aff (Millwood).* 21:277–283.

Freudenberg N. 2000. Health promotion in the city: a structured review of the literature on interventions to prevent heart disease, substance abuse, violence and HIV infection in U.S. metropolitan areas, 1980–1995. *J Urban Health*. 77:443–457.

Geronimus AT. 2000. To mitigate, resist, or undo: addressing structural influences on the health of urban populations. *Am J Public Health*. 90:867–872.

Hajat S, Armstrong BG, Gouveia N, Wilkinson P. 2005. Mortality displacement of heat-related deaths: a comparison of Delhi, São Paulo, and London. *Epidemiology*. 16:313.

Hansen AL, Bi P, Ryan P, et al. 2008. The effect of heat waves on hospital admissions for renal disease in a temperature city of Australia. *Int J Epidemiol*. 37:1359–1365.

Harpham T. 2009. Urban health in developing countries: what do we know and where do we go? *Health Place*. 15:107–116.

Intergovernmental Panel on Climate Change. 2007. *Fourth Assessment Report*. Cambridge, MA: Cambridge University. Available at: http://www.ipcc.ch/publications_and_data/publications_and_data_reports.htm. Accessed August 16, 2010.

King G, Flisher, AJ, Mallett R, et al. 2003. Smoking in Cape Town: community influences on adolescent tobacco use. *Prev Med*. 36:114–123.

Kjellstrom T, Butler AJ, Lucas R, Bonita R. 2010. Public health impact of global heating due to climate change–potential effects on chronic non-communicable diseases. *Int J Public Health*. 55:97–103.

Kjellstrom T, Monge P. 2010. Global climate change and cities. In: Vlahov D, Boufford JI, Pearson C, Norris L, editors. *Urban Health: Global Perspectives*. San Francisco, CA: Jossey-Bass/Wiley:60–80.

Knowlton K, Rotkin-Ellman M, King G, et al. 2009. The 2006 California heat wave: impacts of hospitalizations and emergency department visits. *Environ Health Perspect*. 117:61–67.

Leviton LC, Snell E, McGinnis M. 2000. Urban issues in health promotion strategies. *Am J Public Health*. 90:863–866.

Luber G, McGeehin M. 2008. Climate change and extreme heat events. *Am J Prev Med*. 35:429–435.

Macintyre S, McKay L, Ellaway A. 2005. Are rich people or poor people more likely to be ill? Lay perceptions, by social class and neighbourhood, of inequalities in health. *Soc Sci Med*. 60:313–317.

Massey DS. 1996. The age of extremes: Concentrated affluence and poverty in the twenty-first century. *Demography*. 33:395–412.

McCord C, Freeman HP. 1990. Excess mortality in Harlem. *N Engl J Med*. 322:173–177.

McMichael AJ, Campbell-Lendrum D, Ebi K, et al. 2003. *Climate Change and Human Health: Risks and Responses*. Geneva, Switzerland: World Health Organization.

McMichael AJ, Woodruff RE, Hales S. 2006. Climate change and human health. *Lancet*. 367:859–869.

Melosi M. 2000. *The Sanitary City: Urban Infrastructure in America From Colonial Times to the Present*. Baltimore, MD: Johns Hopkins.

Montgomery MR. 2008. The urban transformation of the developing world. *Science*. 319:761–764.

Montgomery MR. 2009. Urban poverty and health in developing countries. *Popul Bull*. 64:1–16.

Montgomery MR, Stren R, Cohen B, et al., editors. 2003. *Cities Transformed: Demographic Change and its Implications in the Developing World*. Washington, DC: National Academies.

Parsons K. 2003. *Human Thermal Environments: The Effects of Hot, Moderate and Cold Environments on Human Health, Comfort and Performance*. 2nd ed. New York, NY: CRC.

Poumadere M, Mays C, Le Mer S, Blong R. 2005. The 2003 heat wave in France: Dangerous climate change here and now. *Risk Anal*. 25:1483–1494.

Satterthwaite D. 2000. Will most people live in cities? *BMJ*. 321:1143–1145.

Sharkey P. 2007. Survival and death in New Orleans: an empirical look at the human impact of Katrina. *J Black Stud*. 37:482–501.

United Nations Population Division. 2000. *World Urbanization Prospects: The 1999 Revision*. New York, NY: United Nations.

United Nations Population Fund (UNFPA). 2007. *State of the World Population: Unleashing the Potential for Urban Growth.* Washington, DC: UNFPA.

Vlahov D, Boufford JI, Pearson C, Norris L, editors. 2010. *Urban Health: Global Perspectives.* San Francisco, CA: John Wiley.

World Health Organization (WHO). 2006. *WHO Air Quality Guidelines for Particulate Matter, Ozone, Nitrogen Dioxide and Sulfur Dioxide. Global Update 2005. Summary of Risk Assessment.* Geneva, Switzerland: WHO.

Yen IH, Syme SL. 1999. The social environment and health: a discussion of the epidemiologic literature. *Ann Rev Public Health.* 20:287–308.

Zhou G, Yan G. 2003. Severe acute respiratory syndrome epidemic in Asia. *Emerg Infect Dis* [serial online]. 9:1608–1610.

3

Slums, Pollution, and Ill Health: The Case of Dhaka, Bangladesh

M. Omar Rahman, MD, DSc, MPH, Khondkar Ayaz Rabbani, MSc, and Rahat Bari Tooheen, MPH, MDM

THE WORLD'S POPULATION IS becoming increasingly urbanized. According to projections by the United Nations Population Division, by the year 2030 most of the developing world will contain more urban than rural dwellers (Montgomery 2008). Megacities (loosely defined as urban areas with over 10 million residents) are a prominent feature of urbanization in the developing world, and two thirds of the world's megacities are located in developing countries (Cohen 2006; United Nations 2008; Saier 2007; Hossain 2008; Rasheed 2008; Kraas 2007). However, the relationship between the characteristics of megacities and the health of their residents is not always clear. Rapidly increasing populations in megacities have been linked to increased environmental pollution (deteriorating air, water, and soil quality), poor housing, high population density and crowding, and poor services such as water and sanitation. Within megacities, slum dwellers have been cited as a particularly vulnerable group. Although increased environmental pollution can plausibly be linked to adverse human health impacts, especially among slum dwellers, this relationship is confounded by the underlying poverty and lack of education of this group, which could independently lead to poor health and nutritional status.

Approximately 280 million people currently reside in megacities, and this number is likely to rise to 350 million in the coming years (Munich Re Group 2004). According to Kraas, megacities are "the new phenomena of the worldwide urbanization processes" and have been associated with globalization (Kraas 2007, p. 80; Kasarda and Crenshaw 1991). Between 2007 and 2050, the population living in urban areas is projected to pass from 3.3 billion in 2007 to 6.4 billion in 2050 (United Nations 2008). In the developing world, by 2050, as much as two thirds of the population will likely be urban (Montgomery 2009). According to the Asian Development Bank (2002), about half of the urban poor will be residing in slums.

Urbanization is one of the major transformations occurring in Bangladesh (World Bank and Bangladesh Centre for Advanced Studies [BCAS] 1998). By 2020, the population of Bangladesh is expected to reach 185 million, with the urban population accounting for 80 million people (43%); the capital alone, Dhaka, is expected to reach approximately 20 million inhabitants (United Nations Population Division 2009; World Bank and BCAS 1998). According to the World Bank (2007), if the rate of rural–urban migration into Dhaka continues, Dhaka will be the third-largest city by 2020. According to the United Nations, Dhaka ranked ninth among all cities in 2007 but by 2025 will be the fourth-largest megacity (Table 3.1). Urbanization in Bangladesh is projected to increase, with 40 to 60% of urban populations living in the slums by 2020 (Podymow et al. 2007).

Table 3.1 Ranking of the World's Ten Largest Megacities: 2007 and 2025

	2007		2025	
	Rank	Population	Rank	Projected Population
Tokyo, Japan	1	35.7 million	1	36.4 million
New York, United States	2	19.0 million	8	20.6 million
Mexico City, Mexico	3	19.0 million	6	21.0 million
Mumbai, India	4	19.0 million	2	26.4 million
São Paulo, Brazil	5	18.8 million	5	21.4 million
Delhi, India	6	15.9 million	3	22.5 million
Shanghai, China	7	15.0 million	9	19.4 million
Kolkata, India	8	14.8 million	7	20.6 million
Dhaka, Bangladesh	9	13.5 million	4	22.0 million
Buenos Aires, Argentina	10	12.8 million	10	13.8 million

Source: United Nations 2008.

Most migrants come from rural areas searching for opportunities for new livelihoods, translating to improvements in living standards (Afsar 2000; World Bank 2007). Significant numbers of the migrants live in slums and squatter settlements and experience extremely low living standards and high unemployment (Hossain 2008). The urban sector in Bangladesh is experiencing the most severe impact of population growth, and Bangladesh, as one of the world's poorest countries, faces tremendous challenges in coping with the infrastructure and service requirements for its rapidly growing urban population (Rasheed 2008). From the frequent breakdowns in municipal services like water, gas, and electricity, it is clear that Dhaka has become almost unmanageable (Siddiqui et al. 2000), with the lack of a coherent urban policy being a major contributor (World Bank 2007).

The increasing gaps in essential services and the attendant rise in environmental pollution that are associated with rapid urbanization have been linked by various authors to decreasing health status among urban residents of megacities, particularly those living in slums. According to Takano (2007), rapid urbanization is associated with health problems linked to environmental factors; Redman and Jones (2005) point out that densely packed cities, combined with poor sanitation and inadequate solid waste removal, create the necessary components for the spread of infectious disease. Specific aspects such as concentration of housing in below-standard construction, and complex and aging infrastructure, have been identified by Wenzel, Bendimerad, and Sinha (2007) as contributing to the vulnerability of megacities.

Like many megacities, Dhaka is struggling to find solutions to its massive domestic waste problem, water supply needs, and the adverse impact of air pollution stemming mainly from motor vehicle emissions that have exponentially increased in recent years (Akter, Azad, and Sultana 2002; Nasiruddin 2006; Begum et al. 2010). Dhaka is reported to be the fastest growing megacity in the world, receiving up to 400,000 poor migrants from rural areas annually (World Bank 2007). These poor rural migrants, constituting approximately one third of Dhaka's population, reside in slums and squatter settlements characterized by very poor environmental conditions. We used Dhaka as a case study to look at the complex relationship between megacities, associated environmental pollution, and consequent impacts on the health status of urban dwellers—particularly slum dwellers, keeping in mind the confounding effects of the underlying poverty and lack of education of this subgroup.

Dhaka City: Growth and Population Density

The partitions of Bengal (1905–1911), of the subcontinent into India and Pakistan, and the post liberation period were important events that increased the political importance of Dhaka (Siddiqui et al. 2000). Because of the rivers lying to the south and west of Dhaka, expansion of the city can only occur in the north and, to a certain extent, to the east (Siddiqui et al. 2000). After Dhaka became the capital of East Pakistan in 1947, the next 25 years of Pakistani rule (1947–1971) saw a heavy influx of population to Dhaka from rural areas, and areas to the north and east were developed (Siddiqui et al. 2000). The legal and administrative boundaries of the city were greatly extended (Islam 2003). Figure 3.1 shows a recent map of Dhaka.

The growth in population, area, and density of Dhaka from the beginning of the Pakistan period to the present (1951 onwards) are presented in Table 3.2. Data on the physical growth of Dhaka are difficult to obtain because of the varied and scattered nature of the literature on the subject. Table 3.2 should be interpreted with caution, because new areas around the city are continuously being developed. But in any case, it is clear that Dhaka continued to grow in size and population from the mid-twentieth century onward, with the largest and most dramatic increase in population occurring after 1980. This increase may have resulted from expansion in the area of Dhaka—much of the recent development of Dhaka as a national capital began after 1980, and the city developed quickly. Figure 3.2 illustrates the population growth of Dhaka from 1951 to the present.

The population density (persons/km^2) of Dhaka has continued to grow, except for the period from 1980 to 1990 (Figure 3.3), during which the inclusion of new development areas in and around Dhaka actually increased the total area of Dhaka at a faster rate than its population grew. However, the overall trend after 1990 is clear: both the population and density of Dhaka are increasing at a very high rate.

Rural–urban migration has been the major contributing factor to the growth of slums in Dhaka, and has impacted the population density in the city as well (Rasheed 2008; Siddiqui et al. 2000; Siddiqui 2004). Although Bangladesh has the highest population density in the world, at more than 1000 persons per square kilometer, the population density in the slums is roughly 200 times greater at more than 20,500 persons per square kilometer, making the slums of Dhaka one of the most densely populated slums in Bangladesh (Centre for Urban Studies et al. 2006). Among megacities in Asia, Dhaka has the highest population density but the lowest GNP per capita (in 2009 U.S. dollars; Table 3.3).

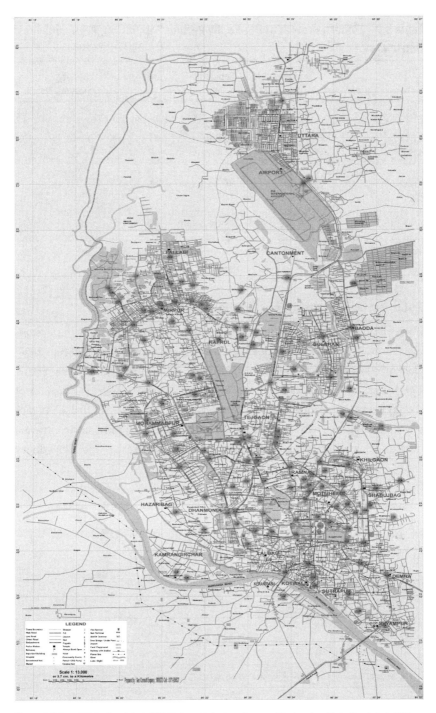

Figure 3.1 Map of Dhaka, Bangladesh. With kind permission from Geoconsult Engineering, Dhaka, Bangladesh: 2010.

Table 3.2 Modern Growth of Dhaka, by Period: Population, Area, and Density

	Year	Population	Area, km²	Density, persons/km²
Pakistan period	1951	411,279	85	4838.5
	1961	718,766	125	5750.1
	1974	2,068,353	336	6155.8
	1981	3,440,147	510	6745.3
	1991	6,887,459	1353	5090.5
Postliberation to present	2001	10,712,206	1530	7001.4
	2006	11,813,728	1629	7251.1
	2007	12,295,728	1629	7548.0
	2008	12,797,394	1629	7856.0

Sources: Islam 2003; Hossain 2008; Bangladesh Bureau of Statistics 2009; Rahman and Tariquzzaman 2001.

Pollution and Environment in Dhaka

It is well documented that rapid urbanization of cities, particularly in developing countries, leads to a host of environmental problems (Chen and Kan 2008; Cohen 2006; Galea, Freudenberg, and Vlahov 2005; Grimm et al. 2008; Pernia 1993). As a city undergoes rapid increases in size and population, the capacity of the city to provide adequate services for its citizens is diminished. Dhaka, as a rapidly expanding megacity, is no exception and is faced with many environmental hazards, such as air, water, and soil pollution (Alam, Karim, and Chowdhury

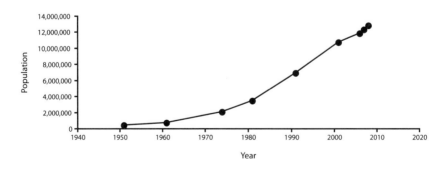

Sources: Statistical Pocketbook of Bangladesh 2008, 2009; Hossain 2008; Islam 2003; Rahman and Tariquzzaman 2001.

Figure 3.2 Change in the population of Dhaka: 1951–2008.

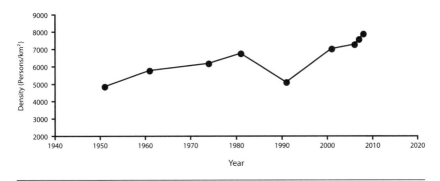

Sources: Hossain 2008; Islam 2003; Rahman and Tariquzzaman 2001; Bangladesh Bureau of Statistics 2009.

Figure 3.3 Change in population density of Dhaka, 1951–2008.

2002; Rasheed 2008; United Nations Environment Programme [UNEP] and BCAS 2005). Increases in population of Dhaka in the last few decades have strained the utility services of the city, including electricity, gas, water, and waste disposal systems. The city's environment is greatly affected by poor water and sanitation services, and most of it is in a continuous state of deterioration (UNEP and BCAS 2005). Table 3.4, adapted from Rasheed (2008), summarizes the major environmental issues faced by the inhabitants of Dhaka on a daily basis.

In terms of a healthy environment, one crucial factor for the residents of a city is the quality of the air. Exposure to air pollutants is an increasing

Table 3.3 Comparison of Dhaka, Mumbai, and Bangkok: Population, Area, Density, and Gross Domestic Product

	Dhaka	Mumbai	Bangkok
Population in 2010	10.1 million	21.3 million	8.3 million
Projected 2025 population	22.0 million	26.4 million	8.5 million
Area[a]	246 km^2	777 km^2	2,202 km^2
Density[b]	40,100 km^2	24,900 km^2	3,600 km^2
National GDP/capita (2009)[c]	$1,600	$3,100	$8,100

Sources: Acharya and Nangia 2004; Demographia 2010; Index Mundi 2010; Westin and Westin 2008; Ziv and Cox 2007.

[a]Land area estimate based on map or satellite photograph analysis.

[b]Density calculated using population midpoint between base and current year.

[c]2009 U.S. dollars.

Table 3.4 Environmental Problems of Dhaka

Domain	Status
Water	Inadequate water supply; polluted tap water with high bacteria contamination; risk of intestinal diseases from drinking tap water
	Poor sanitation facilities or lack of public sanitation facilities; open defecation in some neighborhoods; low ratio of toilets to residents in slums/squatter settlements
	Inadequate storm drains; existing drains are clogged and in poor condition; frequent street flooding and waterlogging
	Water bodies inside the city are shrinking or disappearing because of unplanned and unauthorized land filling; rivers around the city are shrinking or disappearing because of illegal encroachment
	Untreated effluent discharge by industry pollutes rivers around the city
Soil	Inadequate and inefficient waste management; disorganized collection of waste; inadequate recycling of waste; unavailability of disposal sites; high exposure to disease vectors from open dumping
	Unplanned and unregulated land development; high pressure on vacant public lands from squatter settlements
	Vulnerability of poorly constructed buildings to earthquakes; inadequate emergency services in city; poorly maintained fire fighting and rescue equipment
Air	Pollution from large number of transport vehicles; use of low-quality fuel causing air pollution; poorly maintained vehicles; poor traffic management
	Air pollution from industries in and around Dhaka; lack of supervision of pollution emitted from factories; lack of infrastructure and testing laboratories to measure air pollution
	Pollution from brick kilns, which provide bricks for the construction of buildings in Dhaka; lack of supervision and monitoring of air pollutants

Source: Adapted from Rasheed 2008.

problem as a result of the diversity of pollutants, the adverse effects observed given a broad range of air pollution levels, and the vast number of people at risk (World Health Organization 2002; Smith 2000; Chen and Kan 2008, Pope, Ezzati, and Dockery 2009; Ritz et al. 2002; Cropper et al. 1997). Because of economic development in cities, air pollution has been and continues to be a significant urban health hazard worldwide. An ever-increasing number of epidemiological studies have linked urban air pollution to increased risk for morbidity and mortality (Pope, Ezzati, and Dockery 2009; Peters et al. 2001; Agius et al. 2002). Urban air pollution has surfaced as a significant international environmental concern because of the large concentration of minority and low-income residents living in urban environments with unhealthy air quality. The World Health Organization (WHO) acknowledges that minority and low-income populations often have higher prevalence rates of diseases adversely affected by air pollution (Smith 2000). The WHO has also developed air quality guidelines that explicitly recognize the need to consider subpopulations that may be at considerably increased risk of suffering adverse health effects (World Health Organization 2000).

Several studies have examined the effect of air pollution on the health of city residents (Peters et al. 2001; Samet et al. 2000; Cropper et al. 1997). The classic study on the effect of air pollution on health is the Harvard Six Cities study conducted in the 1970s (Peters et al. 2001). This 16-year prospective cohort study of six cities in the United States showed that long-term exposure to small particulate matter (PM) was positively associated with both overall mortality and mortality from cardiopulmonary causes. A more recent study, conducted in 2000 in 20 of the largest U.S. cities, examined associations of the levels of the five major outdoor-air pollutants (ozone, particulate matter, nitrogen dioxide, sulfur dioxide, and carbon monoxide) with daily mortality rates (Samet et al. 2000). The results showed that the estimated increase in the relative rate of mortality from all causes was 0.51% (95% posterior interval = 0.07–0.93%) for each increase in larger particulate matter (PM). The estimated increase in the relative rate of death from cardiovascular and respiratory causes was 0.68% (95% posterior interval = 0.20–1.16%) for each increase in the PM level. There was weaker evidence that increases in ozone levels increased the relative rates of death during the summer, when ozone levels are highest, but not during the winter. Levels of the other pollutants were not significantly related to the mortality rate (Samet et al. 2000). Common sources of PM_{10} in urban environments include resuspended dust, soil, pollen, and spores, whereas common sources of $PM_{2.5}$ in urban environments include direct emission from combustion sources such as industrial processes, wood and coal burning, and motor vehicle exhaust (Pope and Dockery 2006).

Closer to home, in India, a time-series study on the impact of PM on daily mortality was conducted in Delhi. The study showed a positive, significant relationship between particulate pollution and daily nontraumatic deaths, as well as deaths from certain causes (respiratory and cardiovascular problems) and for certain age groups (Cropper et al. 1997). In general, these impacts are smaller than those estimated for other countries, where on average a 100-$\mu g/m^3$ increase in PM leads to a 6% increase in nontraumatic mortality. In Delhi, such an increase in PM is associated with a 2.3% increase in deaths (Cropper et al. 1997).

Until recently, monitoring of air pollution in Dhaka was conducted in an irregular fashion, mainly by a few academics for research purposes (Khaliquzzaman,

Tarafdar, and Biswas 1997; Azad and Kitada 1998; Karim et al. 1997; Akter, Azad, and Sultana 2002). A study was conducted during the winter of 1995–1996 that measured both sulfur dioxide and nitrogen oxide concentrations in 64 locations in Dhaka, using passive diffusion tube samplers (Azad and Kitada 1998). Passive diffusion tube samplers are ideal for identifying areas of high concentration and can give important spatial information about the source of pollutants. The study showed significant spatial variation in the concentration of pollutants in Dhaka. Sulfur dioxide, an emission from industry and brick kilns, was highest along the southeastern industrial zone, whereas nitrogen oxide, an emission from motor vehicles, was high in the city center and along the main roads (Azad and Kitada 1998). Another study by Karim et al. (1997) calculated the daily total emissions of some common air pollutants, like nitrogen oxides, hydrocarbons, carbon monoxide, particulate matter, and sulfur dioxides. The emissions were estimated using the daily fuel consumption and total traffic flows in Dhaka. According to the study, the estimated daily emission for nitrogen oxides was 42 tons per day and that of sulfur oxides was also 42 tons per day. The high influx of people into Dhaka from different parts of the country results in an increased demand for transportation, which increases the level of pollutants in Dhaka (Akter, Azad, and Sultana 2002). The number of vehicles registered in Dhaka has shown a steady yearly increase (Kundu et al. 2006; Figure 3.4).

The number of vehicles in Dhaka and their effect on air pollution was also studied for Dhaka from 1990 to 2000 (Akter, Azad, and Sultana 2002) Fuel

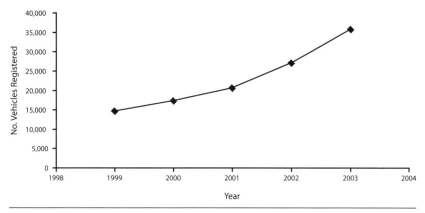

Source: Kundu et al. 2006.

Figure 3.4 Increase in number of vehicles registered in Dhaka: 1990–2000.

consumption was estimated from the number and type of vehicles in Dhaka; pollutant emissions were estimated from the fuel consumption data. The emission estimates from this study show a 13.87% increase in total nitrogen oxide emission every year from 1990 to 2000.

Any comprehensive study of the trends in air pollution for Dhaka require reliable daily ambient air quality data, which was unavailable until recently. In 2002, a continuous air quality monitoring station was established at the premises of the National Parliament Building, located at the center of Dhaka, as part of a World Bank-financed project called the Air Quality Management Project (Akhter, Quadir, and Khan 2003). Its monitors measure key air pollution indicators such as particulate matter, nitrogen oxides, carbon monoxide, sulfur dioxides, ozone, methane, and nonmethane hydrocarbons continuously for 24 hours, meeting the U.S. Environmental Protection Agency (U.S. EPA) Federal Reference Method specifications (Asian Development Bank 2006). The data are recorded as hourly averages from which 8-hour, 24-hour, and other averaging periods can be generated. Consistent monitoring of air pollution has been performed in Dhaka since then, and though enough time has not elapsed to provide sufficient data points to indicate scientifically rigorous long-term trends, the data does provide useful indications of the amount of air pollution that the residents may face (Nasiruddin 2006). There is also a clear seasonal variation of particulate matter concentrations, in which the highest concentrations of PM_{10} and $PM_{2.5}$ generally occur from November to February, during the mild winter, and the lowest concentrations generally occur from May to September, when rainfall totals are highest. There was a slight increase in particulate matter concentrations (both PM_{10} and $PM_{2.5}$) in the city from April 2002 to July 2006. The time interval is too small to draw any conclusions, but the increases in particulate matter concentrations were attributed to the increase in the number of motor vehicles in the city (Nasiruddin 2006).

To determine the source of particulate matter in air, the Bangladesh Atomic Energy Commission (BAEC) studied the trace element composition of particulate matter in Dhaka from 1993 to 1994, using the positive matrix factorization method (Biswas et al. 2000). The results showed that the sources of particulate matter include exhaust from motor vehicles, pollutants from gas and diesel burning, particles from metal smelting, and resuspended soil in the air. The study also showed that 29% of the $PM_{2.5}$ particles can be attributed to motor vehicles. In a follow-up study using the same methodology in 2001–2002, the results showed that motor vehicles account for a 38% of $PM_{2.5}$ particles (Begum et al. 2010).

Increases in motor vehicle density have been shown to be responsible for health problems including respiratory and heart disease, lung cancer, and acute bronchitis in children and adults (Ostro 2004; Brunekreef and Holgate 2002; Peters et al. 2001; Lagorio et al. 2006; Kampa and Castanas 2007). It is plausible to assume that the same holds true for Dhaka, and that increasing the number of motor vehicles will increase health problems for inhabitants. Unfortunately, from a public health perspective, very few studies have assessed the impacts of air pollution on the health of the inhabitants of Dhaka. Some estimates show that up to 10% of respiratory infections and disease in Bangladesh are attributable to urban air pollution (World Bank 2007) and that the economic loss associated with health problems due to air pollution may be as much as $270 million per annum, which accounts for as much as 7.5% of the city's annual gross product (Xie, Brandon, and Shah 1998). Lead levels in children at five primary schools in Dhaka were evaluated for sources of environmental exposure and potential risk factors for lead poisoning, with the source of lead thought to be primarily automobile exhaust (Kaiser et al. 2001). A total of 779 students, aged 4 to 12 years and representing a range of geographic and socioeconomic strata, participated in the study. The mean lead level was 15.0 µg/dL (range = 4.2–63.1 µ/dL), and most students (87.4%) had lead levels above the WHO guideline of 10 µg/dL. Among other correlations, elevated lead levels correlated with children living close to major roads (odds ratio = 2.30; 95% confidence interval = 1.23–4.29). The lead levels found in this study were similar to those found in inhabitants in other countries that use leaded gasoline. This has led to the conclusion that the combustion of leaded gasoline is the main source of lead exposure in Dhaka, resulting in ubiquitous contamination of the environment (Kaiser et al. 2001).

A prospective cross-sectional study was performed to compare peak expiratory flow rate (PEFR) among 100 adolescents living in rural areas (outside Dhaka) and 200 adolescents from industrial and nonindustrial areas of Dhaka (Akhter et al. 2008). The participants in the study were of both sexes, with ages ranging from 15 to 18 years. The mean percentage of predicted value of PEFR in male urban industrial adolescents was significantly lower than that of male rural adolescents (P < .05). The differences between the mean percentage of predicted value of PEFR between males in urban industrial and urban nonindustrial areas and urban nonindustrial and rural areas were not statistically significant. The observed values of female urban industrial adolescents were lower than those for urban nonindustrial and rural areas, but the difference was not statistically significant. In this study, it was speculated that male adolescents were more affected by urban air pollution as a result of higher exposure to these pollutants (Akhter et al. 2008). Further studies are needed to clearly understand the impacts of air pollution on health in Dhaka, not only to guide policy development but also to devise mitigation strategies. Pollution affects all inhabitants of the area where it occurs, and this is certainly true for air pollution. However, it is reasonable to assume that the health effects of air pollution will be more pronounced in areas where there is a high density of residents. In Dhaka, this will be in the slums.

Slums in Dhaka City: General and Health Scenario

The same living standards are not enjoyed by all urban residents of Dhaka. A huge growth of slums and squatter settlements accommodate a large number of people of the low-income group (Afsar 2000; UNEP and BCAS 2005). According to UNESCO, a slum is a contiguous settlement with inadequate housing and inadequate basic services. According to Centre for Urban Studies et al. (2006), slums are characterized by high population density and crowding, poor environmental services, and low socioeconomic status.

Significant numbers of residents of the city live in slums and squatter settlements and experience extremely low living standards (Hossain 2008). The slum population is increasing at an alarming rate, and prevailing conditions favor the spread of communicable diseases, a challenge for health authorities (Khan and Kraemer 2008). These slums and squatter settlements are either on government or private land and, according to Ahmed (2007), 80% of residents pay rent to the local gang leaders or "mafia." These gang leaders do not have ownership of the land, but the slum dwellers pay them for access to use the land. The true owners sometimes only get a small portion of the rent from the gang leaders. There is neither a legal nor a contractual status between the residents and true owners of the land and this is the main reason for the lack of government- and donor-funded allocations for the communities living in these settlements (Ahmed 2007).

A number of studies have demonstrated that people living in the slums and squatter settlements have poor health conditions. Studies have tended to concentrate on health outcomes that affect women and adolescents (Khan and Kraemer 2008; Nahar and Amin 2009; Uzma et al. 1999), but a few studies have examined the health outcomes of the overall adult population living in the slums (Podymow et al. 2007; Pryer, Rogers, and Rahman 2006; Pryer and Rogers 2006). Afsar's study (2002), a comprehensive work on rural–urban migration in Bangladesh, looked at well-being using several health indicators. The study found that health expenditures formed a small portion of the slum households' overall expenditure and, in terms of water supply and sanitation, a majority of slum households were using common water supply and toilet facilities. The UNEP and BCAS (2005) study of the environmental situation of Dhaka also reported water supply and sanitation pressures in the slum areas, with 55% of households receiving tap water and 9% having proper sanitation facilities.

Dhaka's rapid growth, large size, shortage of livable land, environmental conditions, and lack of governance with regard to basic urban utility services worsen the already-complex land and housing issues for the poor living there (World Bank 2007). Pryer and Rogers (2006) examined the nutritional status of adults in the Dhaka slum households; their results demonstrated that women were more likely to be undernourished than were men across all age groups, and that undernourished adults were more likely to reside in areas with poor housing and environmental conditions. A study conducted by Hossain (2008) looked at the extent of urban poverty in Dhaka and the slum dwellers living below the poverty line. The poverty line was determined using the Direct Calorie Intake (DCI) method and Cost of Basic Needs (CBN) method for determining urban poverty. The study showed that most of the slum population lives below the poverty line in terms of both DCI and CBN (Hossain 2008). The city's poor live in rudimentary housing and only one in twenty live in permanent housing (World Bank 2007). Rents are high, living space is crowded, and, although it is difficult to measure the provision of utilities with any certainty, it is almost certainly low given the temporary nature of most housing (World Bank 2007).

The 2006 Bangladesh Urban Health Survey (NIPORT, MEASURE, ICDDR,B, and ACPR 2008), which collected information on health problems and health care–seeking behavior from urban slum and non-slum residents, indicates the health scenario across the slums of Dhaka. A relevant feature of this survey is that it makes comparisons between slum and non-slum areas of Dhaka in detail, an aspect few other studies have undertaken. In terms of adult respondents who claimed to be

Table 3.5   Currently Unhealthy Men and Women in Slum Versus Non-Slum Areas of Dhaka: 2006 Bangladesh Urban Health Survey

| | Currently Unhealthy, % (No.) | |
	Women	Men
Slum	18.6 (3252)	11.6 (3286)
Non-slum	12.4 (1693)	7.4 (1846)

Source: NIPORT, MEASURE, ICDDR,B, and ACPR 2008.

currently unhealthy, a significantly higher proportion of men and women in the slum areas of Dhaka report being relatively unhealthy compared with men and women from the non-slum areas of Dhaka (11.6% vs. 7.4% for men, and 18.6% vs. 12.4% for women; Table 3.5). It is worth noting that women report much worse health than do men in both slums and non-slums, and that the relative health disadvantage between slums and non-slums is greater for women. One may speculate that this gender disparity is a result of the fact that women who live in slums have very little mobility because they do not work and stay in the slum all day—their primary responsibility is to take care of family and household duties. As a result, they are continuously exposed to the environmental factors that make slum living unhealthy.

Provision of clean water and safe disposal of wastewater is a basic necessity for the daily survival for all the residents of a city (Lundqvist et al. 2005). Tables 3.6 and 3.7 show that in Dhaka the drinking water and sanitation access situation in slum areas is substantially worse compared with non-slum areas. In slum areas, the household's drinking water source usually is located outside the household and must be shared between a large number of other families.

A similar situation has been observed for toilet facilities within the slums (Table 3.7), with a majority of slum dwellers using unsanitary latrines and sharing

Table 3.6   Drinking Water Availability in Slum Versus Non-Slum Areas of Dhaka: 2006 Bangladesh Urban Health Survey

	Households With Drinking Water Available, % (No.)
Slum	46.9 (1993)
Non-slum	87.1 (1460)

Source: NIPORT, MEASURE, ICDDR,B, and ACPR 2008.

Table 3.7   Households With Sanitary Toilet Facilities in Slum Versus Non-Slum Areas of Dhaka: 2006 Bangladesh Urban Health Survey

	Households With Sanitary Toilet Facilities, % (No.)
Slum	39.8 (1993)
Non-slum	60.7 (1460)

Source: NIPORT, MEASURE, ICDDR,B, and ACPR 2008.

them with a large number of other families. These findings are important in demonstrating that water and sanitation facilities within slum areas are overburdened and inadequately distributed, which may have health implications for the slum dwellers, thus making the lack of sanitation facilities a public health concern for Dhaka.

According to the 2006 Bangladesh Urban Health Survey, slum dwellers (35% of men and 27% of women) are more likely to be undernourished than their non-slum peers (19% of men and 13% of women) In both slums and non-slums, men had a higher mean BMI (body mass index) compared to women (NIPORT, MEASURE, ICDDR,B, and ACPR 2008). Stunted growth, as an indicator of malnutrition in early childhood, highlights the difference in nutrition status between slum and non-slum dwellers. Among children younger than 5 years of age, slum children are stunted (i.e., low height for age) compared with non-slum children across the entire age range (Table 3.8).

The mortality rates of children younger than 5 years old per 1000 live births are presented in Table 3.9. The data, collected from slum and non-slum areas in 2006, is presented in three periods of 0 to 4, 5 to 9, and 10 to 14 years preceding the survey. It is clear from the table that slum dwellers in Dhaka have significantly

Table 3.8   Stunted Growth in Children Younger Than 5 Years in Slum Versus Non-Slum Areas of Dhaka: 2006 Bangladesh Urban Health Survey

Age in Months	Stunted Growth, %	
	Slum	Non-Slum
6–11	44	15
12–23	61	46
24-35	64	9
36–47	57	34
48–59	57	37

Source: NIPORT, MEASURE, ICDDR,B, and ACPR 2008.

Table 3.9   Under-Five Mortality in Slum Versus Non-Slum Areas of Dhaka: 2006 Bangladesh Urban Health Survey

	Rates per 1000 Persons	
Years Preceding Survey (2006)	Slum	Non-Slum
0–4	80.7	31.0
5–9	90.5	53.2
10–14	131.7	68.1

Source: NIPORT, MEASURE, ICDDR,B, and ACPR 2008.

worse mortality rates than do their non-slum peers. What is also interesting to note is that the difference between the mortality rate between slum dwellers and non-slum dwellers in the recent years (0–4 years preceding the survey) is larger than previously (10–14 years preceding the survey). This shows that over the last 14 years, the gap in under-five mortality rates between slum children and non-slum children has worsened.

Discussion

Dhaka, as one of the fastest growing megacities in the world, provides an ideal case study to examine the health and environmental impacts of rapid urbanization (World Bank 2007). Rapid increases in population and, particularly, population density over the last three decades in Dhaka have led to a significant decline in the urban quality of life, characterized currently by very poor access to basic services such as appropriate housing, potable water, sanitation, and electricity. Concomitantly, environmental pollution in the form of worsening air quality and exposure to contaminated water and soil has become much more marked. In addition to the poor overall quality of urban life in Dhaka, slum dwellers are worse off than their non-slum peers in terms of access to basic services and exposure to environmental pollution.

Slum dwellers in Dhaka have much worse health and nutritional status compared with their non-slum peers. While it would not be implausible to infer that this slum versus non-slum health disadvantage is causatively associated with the increased environmental pollution experienced by slum dwellers, this association is confounded by other independent reasons for this health and nutritional disadvantage, insofar as slum dwellers are also much poorer and less educated than are their non-slum peers. Unfortunately, studies that tease out these important confounding relationships and determine the precise contribution of differential environmental pollution to health and nutritional differences are lacking. Such studies are imperative if we are to get a definitive sense of the true impacts of environmental pollution on health and nutrition.

Assuming that the poor health and nutritional status of slum dwellers in Dhaka is in part due to environmental pollution, it is not unreasonable to assume that targeted improvements in access to safe drinking water, proper sewerage, industrial waste disposal arrangements, and access to sanitary toilet facilities in slum areas would have a significant impact in improving the health and nutritional status of slum residents. But whereas water, sanitation, and waste disposal improvements are by their very nature locally specific, outdoor air pollution remediation is different in that it involves nontargeted, generalized citywide reductions. Air pollution in Dhaka stems mainly from motor vehicle emissions. While reductions in motor vehicle emissions will lead to an improvement in the respiratory health of all residents of Dhaka, it can be plausibly argued that slum dwellers are likely to benefit proportionately more than will their non-slum peers, because their underlying health and nutritional status is much worse. The issue of air pollution is an illustrative case of generalized citywide policy approaches to improving urbanized environmental conditions and the social, legal, and bureaucratic challenges constraining targeted localized improvements in the environmental conditions of slum areas in a megacity such as Dhaka.

To reduce air pollution from motor vehicles, Dhaka needs a comprehensive, efficient, and environmentally acceptable transportation system (Bari 2008; Karim 1998). Suggestions that have been put forth to reduce air pollution include gradual removal of old, polluting motor vehicles, building flyovers and underpasses over major intersections to facilitate smooth flow of traffic, increasing the number of public buses to ease congestion, phasing out rickshaws and other slow-moving vehicles from the main busy roads, and implementing a mass rapid transit system (Rahman and Tariquzzaman 2008). However, all of these suggestions require massive investments in infrastructure, which will be difficult for the country to afford.

Alternative approaches to solving the problem can be learned from the policy measures adopted by other countries to reduce the amount of air pollution. In Singapore, residents are required to purchase a certificate of entitlement before they can register a vehicle for use on the road (Hong 2001). There is a fixed quota of vehicles that can ply the roads, and the price of the certificate is determined by a public tendering system. Singapore has also adopted an electronic road pricing system (Hong 2001). Motorists pay a fee whenever they pass through a busy road during peak hours. The system is completely automated and has greatly reduced traffic congestion in the city (Hong 2001).

A similar but larger system is in place in London, which has implemented a congestion charge scheme in central London to reduce the level of congestion. The system has been in place since 2003, and has helped promote environmentally friendly transport options such as the use of public transport and bicycling. Another scheme being tried in different cities is a license plate rationing system. This program restricts a set of vehicles from entering a specified area on certain days based on the last digit of the vehicle's license plate. License plate rationing has been implemented in cities like Tokyo, Singapore, Mexico City, and São Paulo (Cambridge Systematics Inc. 2007). These and other policy or legislative measures would, in principle, help to reduce the number of motor vehicles in Dhaka and thus reduce air pollution significantly in the city. The major constraints for the effective implementation of these policies include the disproportionate political power of various constituencies who would be adversely affected by these changes, the pervasive corruption of transport regulatory officials, and the lack of a transparent legal framework which can impose and enforce penalties for violations.

One of the long-standing frustrations of urban researchers and activists is that, despite slum dwellers' being a significant proportion of urban residents, there have been very few concerted efforts around the world to improve the specific environmental infrastructure of slums and assure slum dwellers access to basic services (housing, water, sanitation, electricity). As a number of authors have argued, the plight of slum dwellers stems from the fact that, as far as municipal authorities are concerned, slum dwellers are not legitimate claimants of city services. They are viewed as illegally squatting on private or public land, and municipal governments have been very hesitant to provide services, as this would be seen as entrenching and legitimizing their "illegal" residence. In Dhaka as in most other cities, particularly in the developing world, slum dwellers are at best ignored, or at worse subject to random harassment by sporadic eviction drives. This municipal myopia is very problematic, as the reality is that, given the rapid pace of rural-to-urban migration in the developing world and the lack of available housing opportunities in cities, slum dwellers are unlikely to go away any time soon, no matter how much urban authorities may wish it so. Indeed, if recent history is any guide (particularly in the case of Dhaka), they are likely to be an increasing proportion of city residents. A more reasonable approach is for cities to stop marginalizing slum dwellers and start providing some rudimentary access to water, sewerage, sanitation, and other facilities as well as appropriately-crafted tenancy rights and protections (Durand-Lasserve 2006; de Soto 1996). It must be recognized that from a public health perspective, because of the fluid geographic boundaries between slums and non-slums and the employment of slum dwellers in non-slum residences and institutions, increasing environmental pollution in slum areas raises the risk of the rapid spread of infectious disease from slum to non-slum areas.

Summary

We have used Dhaka as an illustrative example to look at the complex relationship among the growth of megacities, associated environmental pollution, and consequent impacts on the health and nutritional status of urban dwellers—particularly slum dwellers. The data provided here suggest that slum dwellers are significantly worse off in terms of health and nutritional status compared with their non-slum peers. We can reasonably infer that this disparity is in part a result of differential environmental pollution, although its precise contribution cannot as of yet be determined because of a lack of appropriate data. We have suggested that improvements in the urban environmental situation require both generalized approaches (e.g., reducing overall motor vehicle emissions) to air pollution and targeted, locally-specific solutions to improve water and sanitation access. All of these require the requisite political will, an accountable regulatory system, and a transparent legal framework. Finally, we have highlighted the fact that any substantive improvement in the quality of life of slum dwellers requires an acknowledgement of the legitimacy of their claims for municipal services.

References

Acharya AK, Nangia P. 2004. Population growth and changing land-use pattern in Mumbai metropolitan region of India. *Caminhos Geogr.* 11:168–185.

Afsar R. 2000. *Rural–Urban Migration in Bangladesh: Causes, Consequences and Challenges.* Dhaka, Bangladesh: Dhaka University.

Agius R, Cohen GR, Beverland I, et al. 2002. Epidemiological study of susceptibility to cardiorespiratory death from particulate air pollution. *Ann Occup Hyg*. 46(Suppl 1): 452–455.

Ahmed IK. 2007. Urban poor housing in Bangladesh and potential role of ACHR. Bangkok, Thailand: Asian Coalition for Housing Rights (ACHR).

Ahmed MF, Tanveer SA, Badruzzaman ABM, editors. 2002. *Bangladesh Environment 2002*. Vol. 1. Dhaka, Bangladesh: Bangladesh Poribesh Andolon.

Akhter N, Molla MH, Akther D, et al. 2008. Effect of air pollution on peak expiratory flow rate in urban industrial and non-industrial adolescents. *J Med Sci Res*. 10:22–26.

Akhter S, Quadir SMA, Khan A. 2003. Trends in ambient air quality in Dhaka City. Presented at: Better Air Quality Workshop; December 17–19; Manila, Philippines.

Akter J, Azad AK, Sultana J. 2002. Traffic contribution to air pollution: a case study on Dhaka. In: Ahmed MF, Tanveer SA, Badruzzaman ABM, editors. *Bangladesh Environment 2002*. Vol. 1. Dhaka, Bangladesh: Bangladesh Poribesh Andolon.

Alam MA, Karim KMR, Chowdhury PS. 2002. The role of civil society to control the environmental degradation of Bangladesh. In: Ahmed MF, Tanveer SA, Badruzzaman ABM, editors. *Bangladesh Environment 2002*. Vol. 1. Dhaka, Bangladesh: Bangladesh Poribesh Andolon.

Asian Development Bank. 2002. Strategy to meet challenges of Asia's megacities [news release, May 9]. Available at: http://www.adb.org/Documents/News/2002/nr2002075. asp. Accessed July 20, 2010.

Asian Development Bank. 2006. Country Synthesis Report on Urban Air Quality Management: Bangladesh. Discussion draft, December 2006. Available at: http://www. cleanairnet.org/caiasia/1412/csr/bangladesh.pdf. Accessed July 28, 2010.

Azad AK, Kitada T. 1998. Characteristics of the air pollution in the city of Dhaka, Bangladesh, in winter. *Atmos Environ*. 32:11.

Bangladesh Bureau of Statistics. 2009. Statistical Pocket Book of Bangladesh 2008. Dhaka, Bangladesh: People's Republic of Bangladesh.

Bari M. 2008. Dhaka Needs Proper Transport Planning. *Financial Express* (Dhaka). January 19.

Begum BA, Biswas SK, Markwitz A, Hopke PK. 2010. Identification of sources of fine and coarse particulate matter in Dhaka, Bangladesh. *Aerosol Air Quality Res.* 10:345–353.

Biswas SK, Islam A, Tarafdar SA, Khaliquzzaman M. 2000. Monitoring of atmospheric particulate matter (APM) in Bangladesh. Presented at: Joint UNDP/RCA/IAEA Project Conference on Sub Project: Air Pollution and its Trends; November 13–15; Manila, Philippines.

Brunekreef B, Holgate ST. 2002. Air pollution and health. *Lancet.* 360:1233–1242.

Cambridge Systematics Inc. 2007. *Technical Memorandum: Congestion Mitigation Commission Technical Analysis, License Plate Rationing Evaluation.* New York, NY: New York City Economic Development Corporation and New York City Department of Transportation.

Centre for Urban Studies (CUS), National Institute of Population Research and Training (NIPORT), and MEASURE Evaluation. 2006. *Slums of Urban Bangladesh: Mapping and Census 2005.* Dhaka, Bangladesh; Chapel Hill, NC: CUS, NIPORT, and MEASURE Evaluation.

Chen B, Kan H. 2008. Air pollution and population health: a global challenge. *Environ Health Prev Med.* 13:94–101.

Cohen B. 2006. Urbanization in developing countries: current trends, future projections, and key challenges for sustainability. *Technol Soc.* 28:63–80.

Cropper M, Simon NB, Alberini A, Sharma PK. 1997. *The Health Effects of Air Pollution in Delhi, India.* Washington, DC: World Bank Development Research Group.

de Soto H. 1996. The missing ingredient: what poor countries will need to make their markets work. In: Anderson T, Hill PJ, editors. *The Privatization Process: A Worldwide Perspective.* Lanham, MD: Rowman and Littlefield: 19–24.

Demographia. 2010. World Urban Areas and Population Projections. Edition 6.1. Available at: http://www.demographia.com/db-worldua.pdf. Accessed August 8, 2010.

Durand-Lasserve, A. 2006. Treating people and communities as assets: informal settlements and the Millennium Development Goals: global policy debates on property ownership and security of tenure. *Glob Urban Develop* 2:1–15.

Galea S, Freudenberg N, Vlahov D. 2005. Cities and population health. *Soc Sci Med.* 60:1017–1033.

Grimm NB, Foster D, Groffman P, et al. 2008. The changing landscape: ecosystem responses to urbanization and pollution across climatic and societal ingredients. *Front Ecol Environ.* 6:264–272.

Hong TQ. 2001. Singapore's experience in control of vehicular emissions. Presented at: Clean Air Regional Workshop on Fighting Urban Air Pollution: From Plan to Action; February 12–14; Bangkok, Thailand.

Hossain S. 2008. Rapid urban growth and poverty in Dhaka City. *Bangladesh e-J Sociol.* 5:1–24.

Islam S, editor. 2003. *BANGLAPEDIA National Encyclopedia of Bangladesh.* Vol. 3, CHO–ENT. Dhaka, Bangladesh: Asiatic Society of Bangladesh.

Kaiser R, Henderson AK, Daley WR, et al. 2001. Blood lead levels of primary school children in Dhaka, Bangladesh. *Environ Health Perspect.* 109:563–566.

Kampa M, Castanas E. 2007. Human health effects of air pollution. *Environ Pollut.* 151:362–367.

Karim MM. 1998. Light Rail Transit in Dhaka. *Daily Star.* August 23.

Karim MM, Matsui H, Ohno T, Hoque MS. 1997. Current state of traffic pollution in Bangladesh and Metropolitan Dhaka. In: *Proceedings of the 90th Annual Meeting and Exhibition of the Air and Waste Management Association.* Toronto, Ontario: Air and Waste Management Association.

Kasarda JD, Crenshaw EM. 1991. Third world urbanization: dimensions, theories, and determinants. *Annu Rev Sociol.* 17:467–501.

Khaliquzzaman M, Tarafdar SA, Biswas SK. 1997. *Trace Element Composition of Size Fractionated Airborne Particulate Matter in Urban and Rural Areas in Bangladesh.* Bangladesh: Bangladesh Atomic Energy Commission. AECD/AFD-CH:6–48.

Khan MMM, Kraemer A. 2008. Socio-economic factors explain differences in public health-related variables among women in Bangladesh: a cross-sectional study. *BMC Public Health.* 8:254.

Kraas F. 2007. Mega cities and global change: key priorities. *Geogr J.* 173:79–82.

Kundu PC, Tarafder B, Mollah MRU, Hayat SR. 2006. *Report on Roadside Vehicle Emmission Testing Program in Dhaka.* Air Quality Management Project. Dhaka,

Bangladesh: Department of Environment, Ministry of Environment and Forest, Government of Bangladesh.

Lagorio S, Forastiere F, Pistelli R, et al. 2006. Air pollution and lung function among susceptible adult subjects: a panel study. *Environ Health.* 5:11.

Lundqvist J, Tortajada C, Varis O, Biswas A. 2005. Water management in megacities. *AMBIO.* 34:267–268.

Montgomery MR. 2008. The Urban Transformation of the Developing World. *Science.* 319:761–764.

Montgomery MR. 2009. Urban poverty and health in developing countries. *Popul Bull.* 64:2–16.

Munich Re Group. 2004. Megacities-*Megarisks: Trends and Challenges for Insurance and Risk Management.* Knowledge Series, Geo Risks Research Department. Munich, Germany: Munchener Ruck Munich Re Group.

Nahar S, Amin F. 2009. Unmet need of contraceptives among eligible couples of urban slum dwellers in Dhaka. *Ibrahim Med Coll J.* 3:24–28.

Nasiruddin M. 2006. Setting Ambient Air Quality and Vehicular Emission Standards: Dhaka's Experience. Presented at: Pakistan Development Partners Meeting on Clean Air; September 4; Karachi, Pakistan.

National Institute of Population Research and Training (NIPORT), MEASURE Evaluation, International Centre for Diarrhoeal Disease Research, Bangladesh (ICDDR, B), and Associates for Community and Population Research (ACPR). 2008. *2006 Bangladesh Urban Health Survey.* Dhaka, Bangladesh; Chapel Hill, NC: NIPORT, MEASURE Evaluation, ICDDR, B, and ACPR.

Ostro B. 2004. *Outdoor Air Pollution: Assessing the Environmental Burden of Disease at National and Local Levels.* Environmental Burden of Disease Series, No. 5. Geneva, Switzerland: World Health Organization.

Pernia EM. 1993. *Urbanization, Population Distribution and Economic Development in Asia.* Report No. 58. Manila, Philippines: Asian Development Bank.

Peters A, Dockery DW, Muller JE, Mittleman MA. 2001. Increased particulate air pollution and the triggering of myocardial infarction. *Circulation.* 103:2810–2815.

Podymow T, Turnbull J, Islam MA, Ahmed M. 2007. *Health and Social Conditions in the Dhaka Slums*. New York: International Society for Urban Health. Available at: http://www.isuh.org/download/dhaka.pdf. Accessed July 20, 2010.

Pope CA, Dockery DW. 2006. Health effects of fine particulate air pollution: lines that connect. *J Air Waste Manage Assoc*. 56:709–742.

Pope CA, Ezzati M, Dockery DW. 2009. Fine-particulate air pollution and life expectancy in the United States. *New Engl J Med*. 360:4.

Pryer JA, Rogers S. 2006. Epidemiology of undernutrition in adults in Dhaka slum households, Bangladesh. *Eur J Clin Nutr*. 60:815–822.

Pryer JA, Rogers S, Rahman A. 2006. Adult illness in Dhaka slum households. *Hum Ecol*. 14:33–38.

Rahman G, Tariquzzaman SM. 2001. *Squatter Settlement on the Flood Protection Embankment in Dhaka City*. Available at: http://www.commonwealth-planners.org/papers/ssdc.pdf. Accessed July 20, 2010.

Rasheed KBS. 2008. *Bangladesh: Resource and Environmental Profile*. Dhaka, Bangladesh: AH Development Publishing House.

Redman CL, Jones NL. 2005. The environmental, social and health dimensions of urban expansion. *Popul Environ*. 26:505–520.

Ritz B, Yu F, Fruin S, et al. 2002. Ambient air pollution and risk of birth defects in Southern California. *Am J Epidemiol*. 155:17–25.

Saier MH. 2007. Are megacities sustainable? *Water Air Soil Pollut*. 178:1–3.

Samet JM, Dominici F, Curriero FC, et al. 2000. Fine particulate air pollution and mortality in 20 U.S. cities, 1987–1994. *New Engl J Med*. 343: 1742–1749.

Siddiqui K, Ahmed J, Awal A, Ahmed M. 2000. *Overcoming the Governance Crisis In Dhaka City*. Dhaka, Bangladesh: Dhaka University.

Siddiqui K, editor. 2004. *Megacity Governance in South Asia*. Dhaka, Bangladesh: Dhaka University.

Smith KR. 2000. Environmental health—for the rich or for all? 2000. *Bull WHO*. 78:1156–1157.

Takano T. 2007. Health and environment in the context of urbanization. *Environ Health Prev Med*. 12:51–55.

United Nations Environment Programme and Bangladesh Centre for Advanced Studies. 2005. Dhaka State of Environment Report 2005. Available at: http://www.rrcap.unep.org/pub/soe/dhakasoe05.cfm. Accessed July 20, 2010.

United Nations Population Division. 2008. *World Urbanization Prospects, 2007 Revision.* New York, NY: United Nations.

United Nations Population Division. 2009. World Population Prospects: The 2008 Revision Population Database. Available at: http://esa.un.org/unpp. Accessed March 26, 2010.

U.S. Environmental Protection Agency (EPA). 1996. *Air Quality Criteria for Particulate Matter.* Vols. I–III. Washington, DC: EPA.

Uzma A, Underwood P, Atkinson D, Thackrah R. 1999. Postpartum health in Dhaka slum. *Soc Sci Med.* 48:313–320.

Wenzel F, Bendimerad F, Sinha R. 2007. Megacities—megarisks. *Nat Hazards.* 42:481–491.

Westin C, Westin N. 2008. *Projections of Urban Development.* IMISCOE Working Paper No. 25, Centre for Research in International Migration and Ethnic Relations. Stockholm, Sweden: Stockholm University.

World Bank. 2007. Dhaka: *Improving Living Conditions for the Urban Poor.* Bangladesh Development Series Paper No. 17. Dhaka, Bangladesh: World Bank.

World Bank and Bangladesh Centre for Advanced Studies. 1998. *Bangladesh 2020: A Long-Run Perspective Study.* Dhaka, Bangladesh Development Series. Dhaka, Bangladesh: Dhaka University.

World Health Organization (WHO). 2000. *Quality Guidelines for Europe.* 2nd ed. European Series No. 91. Geneva, Switzerland: WHO Regional Publications, Regional Office for Europe.

World Health Organization (WHO). 2002. *The World Health Report 2002, Reducing Risks, Promoting Healthy Lives.* Geneva, Switzerland: WHO.

Xie J, Brandon CJ, Shah JJ. 1998. *Fighting Urban Transport Air Pollution for Local and Global Good: The Case of Two-Stroke Engine Three-Wheelers in Dhaka.* Washington, DC: World Bank.

Ziv J, Cox W. 2007. Megacities and affluence: transport and land use considerations. Presented at: World Conference on Transport Research; June 24–28; Berkeley, CA.

4

Megacities and Emerging Infections: Case Study of Rio de Janeiro, Brazil

Mary E. Wilson, MD

MEGACITIES CONTINUE TO EXPAND rapidly in number and size globally. Several characteristics of megacities make them vulnerable to new and resurgent microbial threats. Megacities can serve as a source of microbes, a site of amplification, and a place in which introduced microbes can spread and disperse to other places. The global connectedness of megacities through travel and trade means that distant as well as local populations can be affected. Threats include infections that are spread from person to person, such as influenza, SARS, multidrug-resistant tuberculosis, and HIV/AIDS; infections that are spread through contaminated food and water, such as cryptosporidiosis, cholera, and typhoid fever; and vector-borne infections spread by urban mosquitoes, such as dengue fever, chikungunya, and yellow fever. The dynamics of spread vary depending on the specific pathogen and other factors, including socioeconomic status and local ecoclimate. Spread can be explosive (e.g., influenza) or can unfold over a period of years (e.g., HIV/AIDS). This chapter will briefly discuss a number of the types of risk and will focus in detail on one vector-borne viral infection, dengue fever, primarily in one place, the megacity of Rio de Janeiro, Brazil. The case of dengue illustrates how megacities facilitate emerging infections and also shows the value of understanding the particular ecology, biology, and risk attached to specific infectious organisms.

Characteristics of Megacities

Several characteristics of today's megacities are relevant when assessing risks from microbial threats (Smolinski, Hamburg, and Lederberg 2003; Wilson 2010a). These include size, density, location, mobility and linkages, human–animal interfaces, and poverty and inequalities. Cities are often imagined as an agglomeration of buildings, roads, tunnels, sewers, pipes, steel, bricks, cement, and mortar—the built environment—but they are also comprised of a vast and diverse biotic component: they are teeming with humans, animals, insects, and other fauna and flora. Separation between urban and rural environments is not cleanly demarcated, and forested areas with wild animals and extensive biodiversity may exist within cities. Agricultural activities, such as growing food animals and crops, may interdigitate with dense settlements at the periphery of urban areas (Montgomery 2008).

Size

The large size of the human population in megacities provides abundant opportunities for replication events by microbes. In fact, with the dengue virus, the number of lineages of the virus has increased roughly in parallel with the size of the human population during the past 200 years (Zanotto et al. 1996). This means that more humans are being exposed to an increasingly diverse population of viruses. More replication events provide more opportunities for the emergence of a variant that is more transmissible or more virulent or both. Higher viremia is associated with more severe disease with dengue infection (Vaughn et al. 2000), and the probability of a mosquito becoming infected is related in large part to the level of viremia in the host, so the mosquitoes can help to select and propagate viruses that produce higher viremia (Cologna, Armstrong, and Rico-Hesse 2005). Overall size (i.e., numbers) of the human population living in close proximity to one other also matters for the maintenance of many viral pathogens. The critical size of a human community able to sustain the endemic transmission of dengue virus is somewhere between 150,000 and 1 million people—and urban areas in tropical and subtropical areas continue to reach this size (Kuno 1995).

Location

The location of newly developing megacities has shifted from temperate areas to lower-latitude sites. Today, ten of the 25 largest cities lie at latitudes at or within the tropics (23° 26′ N to 23° 26′ S), and all but four are within zones considered subtropical (often defined as the climatic region adjacent to the tropics and extending to 40° of latitude in both hemispheres) or tropical (Table 4.1; Figure 4.1). The geoclimatic characteristics are relevant, because warmer climates are associated with greater microbial diversity. In general, the number of animal and plant species is higher in tropical areas and decreases at higher latitudes. This latitudinal gradient in species diversity applies to species that cause infectious diseases, including parasitic species, as well as for other species (Guernier, Hochberg, and Guégan 2004). Geoclimatic conditions help to explain the geographic variation in some infectious diseases (Wilson 2010a).

Table 4.1 Latitude of the 25 Largest Cities, by Rank: 2010

Rank	Megacity	Country	Latitude
1	Tokyo	Japan	35° 41′ N
2	Guangzhou	China	23° 20′ N
3	Seoul	South Korea	37° 33′ N
4	Mexico City	Mexico	19° 41′ N
5	Delhi	India	28° 38′ N
6	Mumbai	India	18° 58′ N
7	New York City	United States	40° 43′ N
8	São Paulo	Brazil	23° 33′ S
9	Manila	Philippines	14° 36′ N
10	Los Angeles	United States	34° 03′ N
11	Shanghai	China	31° 10′ N
12	Osaka	Japan	34° 42′ N
13	Kolkata	India	22° 34′ N
14	Karachi	Pakistan	24° 51′ N
15	Jakarta	Indonesia	6° 11′ S
16	Cairo	Egypt	30° 03′ N
17	Buenos Aires	Argentina	34° 40′ S
18	Moscow	Russia	55° 45′ N
19	Beijing	China	39° 54′ N
20	Dhaka	Bangladesh	23° 42′ N
21	Istanbul	Turkey	41° 00′ N
21	Rio de Janeiro	Brazil	22° 54′ S
21	Tehran	Iran	35° 42′ N
24	London	United Kingdom	51° 30′ N
25	Lagos	Nigeria	6° 35′ N

Sources: Brinkhoff 2010; Wikipedia 2010.

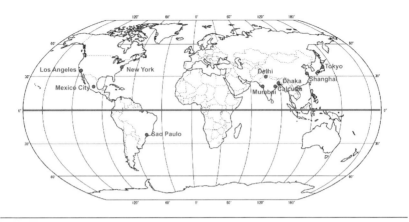

Source: UN Population Division. 2002. *World Urbanization Prospects.* New York, NY: United Nations.

Figure 4.1 Geographic locations of the ten largest cities: 2000.

Density and Poverty

Many of the recently appearing megacities in low-latitude areas are also characterized by high population density. High density can favor transmission of infections that are spread from person to person (Bell et al. 1963), and high density has
been associated with an increased risk for some urban vector-borne infections,
such as dengue fever. Of the 25 largest cities, all but six are located in countries
considered emerging and developing economies according to the International
Monetary Fund's *World Economic Outlook Report* (International Monetary Fund
2009). Poverty is also associated with a greater burden for many infectious diseases. In the poorest countries, infectious diseases continue to account for a substantial portion of morbidity and mortality. Among the 10.6 million deaths of
children aged 0 to 4 years globally in 2001, 99% occurred in children living in
low- and middle-income countries (Lopez et al. 2006). More than half of these
deaths were attributable to infectious diseases (acute respiratory infections, measles, diarrhea, malaria, HIV/AIDS). Approximately 24% of all deaths (all age
groups) globally are attributable to infectious diseases.

Interfaces With Animals, Other Populations

Many of the newly developing megacities have expanded rapidly and include
large populations living under conditions of dire poverty in slums or favelas,
often found at the periphery of the city or embedded within it. Large populations live under conditions of intense crowding and lack a reliable piped water

supply, waste management facilities, and clean drinking water. They also often have little or no access to medical or preventive health services. The food supply may be meager, irregular, of poor nutritional value, and contaminated with microbes and toxins. The air and soil are often highly polluted with smoke and environmental toxins. Animals for food (e.g., poultry, pigs, cattle), transport (e.g., horses, donkeys, mules), and pets often live inside or in close proximity to human housing. These can be a source of pathogens, such as influenza viruses, that infect humans. Pests—including large ones such as rats, mice, and other rodents, as well as small ones, including many potential vectors such as mosquitoes, fleas, and sandflies—are abundant; few or no barriers exist between them and humans (Wilson 1995a).

Populations of slums exist outside of many surveillance programs designed for early identification of diseases or outbreaks (Smolinski, Hamburg, and Lederberg 2003). Because many people who live in the favelas have migrated to urban areas for economic reasons, they often have family members living in rural areas. Many work in the city at tasks that bring them into frequent contact with large populations. Transportation networks—streets, subway systems, trains, buses, cars, and vans—are supplemented by bicycles, motorbikes, animal transport, and walking. Residents of favelas regularly move to and from the city center to the periphery, where they live, and to rural areas, where they visit families. These populations at high risk for many infectious diseases can serve as a bridge to link the city center and rural populations (Wilson 2003). All megacities are also served by major international airports, providing frequent and rapid links to populations throughout the world by air. Some are near seaports or rivers that allow travel by boat, and all have some system of highways that links them to cities and rural areas.

Mobility and Connectedness

The volume and speed of travel today are unprecedented in world history. United Nations (UN) World Transportation Organization figures show that the number of international tourist arrivals approaches 1 billion per year. In 2008, globally 47% of inbound tourists traveled by air, 42% by road, 7% by water, and 4% by rail (UN World Transportation Organization 2009). Air travel has eliminated spatial and temporal barriers, and humans can reach virtually any part of the Earth within the incubation period for most infectious diseases (Wilson 1995b, 2010b). This allows the juxtaposition of species that had never before had physical proximity.

A number of megacities are located on or near coastal areas at risk for flooding, cyclones, and adverse consequences of sea level rise. More than half of the megacities are located in areas with high or very high seismic hazard for earthquakes (Bilham 2006). Due to shoddy construction of many buildings, especially in the rapidly growing cities in low-income countries, earthquakes can be catastrophic in these regions. Severe floods, mud slides, and earthquakes disrupt basic services, displace populations, and may lead many individuals to migrate to new areas. All of these catastrophic events can place populations at increased risk for infectious diseases, including food and waterborne and vectorborne infections.

The burden and distribution of infectious diseases are shaped by socioeconomic, climatic, and environmental factors. An analysis of 335 emerging infectious disease events reported between 1940 and 2004 highlighted the role of zoonoses (Jones et al. 2008). Overall 60.3% of the emerging infections were considered to be zoonoses, the majority (71.8%) originating from wildlife. Important examples include HIV/AIDS, SARS, and Ebola virus infections (Lloyd-Smith et al. 2009). Potential hot spots for the emergence of new infections include low-latitude, developing-country areas with extensive human—animal contact. Avian influenza caused by H5N1 first appeared in areas of Asia with large, dense human populations that had frequent contact with poultry and other avian species. The virus has now become entrenched in some of the avian populations, though it has not yet acquired the capacity to transmit efficiently from human to human. Despite its high virulence for humans, it has not yet caused major outbreaks in human populations (Webster and Govorkava 2006).

SARS was caused by a virus that crossed the species barrier from animals and infected humans, probably via "wet markets," where live animals are sold for food, in southern China (Webby, Hoffman, and Webster 2004). Although the palm civet was initially identified as the proximate source of the first human infections, subsequent studies have uncovered the virus in bats, which are likely to be its natural reservoir hosts (Li et al. 2005). The virus was disseminated to multiple countries and caused major economic losses and disruption of global travel, with the most severe impact felt in Asian countries (Ali and Keil 2008). A few features of its appearance and dissemination are notable in relation to emerging infections and megacities. The virus originated from human–animal contact and spread globally in a remarkably short period of time, carried by international air travelers. Outside of China, the major impact was felt in a few large cities in developed countries that had received infected travelers, who then spread it largely in households and health care settings. Fortunately for humans, the biological characteristics of the virus—it typically caused symptoms in humans before they could transmit the virus—made it possible to contain the virus and halt transmission (Fraser et al. 2004) by instituting strict measures, including isolation and quarantine. Influenza viruses, by contrast, are much more difficult to contain because infected individuals may spread infection before they develop obvious symptoms.

Another notable feature of SARS was its capacity to spread within the built environment by unexpected means. At the Amoy Gardens, a multibuilding apartment complex in Hong Kong, a large community outbreak of SARS affected more than 300 residents in the spring of 2003. A careful analysis by epidemiologists assessing the temporal and spatial distribution of the first 187 human cases and by engineers studying the airflow dynamics in the buildings led to the conclusion that airborne transmission had occurred within the apartment complex (Yu et al. 2004). The spread was consistent with virus-laden aerosols (generated from an index case with high concentrations of SARS-associated coronavirus in feces and urine in drainage from toilets) being carried by a rising plume of warm air in the air shaft between buildings and then entering other apartments through open windows. It was thought that dried-up seals of floor drain traps allowed aerosols from drainage pipes to return to the bathroom and then reach the air shaft by the suction created by exhaust fans.

The experience with SARS suggests that features of the built environment may allow wide dissemination of well-known and novel pathogens in unexpected ways. Had a large SARS outbreak occurred in an area with limited resources, control of the epidemic might have been slow or impossible. Other diseases with airborne transmission, such as measles, Q fever, and tuberculosis (drug-susceptible and drug-resistant) could potentially be disseminated in unexpected ways in the built environment (Roy and Milton 2004). Transmission of measles, for example, occurred in a domed stadium (Ehresmann et al. 1995), and tuberculosis has been transmitted on naval vessels through shared air sources.

Case Study: Dengue

Dengue fever is caused by a mosquito-transmitted RNA virus in the family Flaviviridae. Four serologically distinct serotypes (DENV-1, DENV-2, DENV-3, DENV-4) cause dengue infections, which can range from asymptomatic or mild infection to dengue hemorrhagic fever (DHF) and dengue shock syndrome (DSS), each of which can be fatal. In one prospective study in Bangkok, 87% of dengue infections were subclinical (Burke et al. 1988). Patients with dengue fever typically have an acute, self-limiting illness lasting a week or less, though prolonged fatigue may follow acute infection. Common symptoms are severe headache and muscle aches ("breakbone fever"), and occasionally a rash. Symptoms typically begin 4 to 7 days after the bite of an infective mosquito, but a range of 3 to 14 days has been observed.

A small percentage of patients with dengue fever develop complications (DHF or DSS) that lead to hospitalization. Although there are no specific antivirus medications available to treat dengue infections, expert, supportive care with intravenous fluids can be lifesaving (Halstead 2007). Case fatality rates of 20% or higher have been reported, but in the best hospitals, where staff have experience in treating complicated dengue, mortality from complicated dengue is <1%. Dengue epidemics are costly, because of days of work or education lost and consumption of resources for medical care and control efforts.

Because four distinct serotypes cause dengue fever, an individual can experience up to four dengue infections. By contrast with infections caused by many pathogens, such as hepatitis A virus, in which infection results in immunity against reinfection or blunts the severity of a second infection, infection with one dengue serotype predisposes to severe disease if one is subsequently infected with a different serotype. After infection with one serotype, the immunity to that serotype is lifelong, but the protection against the three other serotypes is transient (a few months at most). Subsequent infection with a different serotype is associated with increased risk for complicated dengue. In two different studies, the risk for severe disease during infection with a second serotype ranged from 1.8% to 12.5% (Burke et al. 1988). In Singapore, where many residents have experienced one or more previous dengue infections, the percentage of dengue cases that manifested as DHF was 2.4% in 2006 and 2.1% in 2007 (Lee et al. 2010). Different dengue serotypes and genotypes may also vary in their capacity to cause severe disease, thus complicating predictions about risks for specific populations and regions (Guilarde et al. 2008; Fried et al. 2010). Host genetic factors also influence the clinical course (Blanton et al. 2008; Sierra, Koury, and Guzman 2007; Nguyen et al. 2008).

Dengue has expanded in number and severity of cases, both in Brazil and globally (Teixeira et al. 2009; Siqueira et al. 2005; Wilder-Smith and Gubler 2008; Gubler 2002; Martin et al. 2010). Dengue endemic or epidemic areas are now found in more than 100 countries, and all tropical and subtropical areas are at risk (Figure 4.2). An estimated 2.5 billion people live in dengue-endemic areas, and an estimated 50 to 100 million cases of dengue fever occur annually, making dengue the most common arbovirus infection globally. Many factors contribute to the increasing number of complicated dengue infections in tropical and subtropical areas; two critically important ones are urbanization in the tropics and subtropics and global traffic (Gubler 2004; Wilson 2010b). Although dengue viruses probably originated in nonhuman primates and continue to infect them in some areas, dengue viruses circulate almost exclusively in a human–mosquito–human cycle. This means that humans are the important host carrying the virus from one geographic area to another.

Mosquito Vectors

The predominant mosquito vector for dengue in most parts of the world is *Aedes aegypti*. It is remarkably well adapted to the urban environment, breeding in

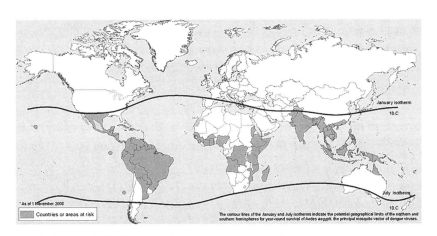

Source: World Health Organization, Public Health Information and Geographic Information and Geographic Information System, 2006.

Figure 4.2 Countries or areas at risk for dengue: potential geographic limits for the year-round survival of *Aedes aegypti* mosquitoes, the primary vector for dengue fever: 2008.

discarded plastic cups and cans, flower pots, drains, water tanks, discarded tires, trash, and in any other site that contains still water (Reiter 2007; Reiter et al. 1995). Construction sites, common in tropical cities, also offer abundant places for mosquito breeding. The eggs, larvae, and pupae are resistant to dessication, making it possible for them to survive dry periods (Lourenço-de-Oliveira 2008). High rates of vertical transmission (female mosquito to eggs) of the dengue virus also help to maintain the virus (Maciel-de-Freitas et al. 2006). The vector enters homes and prefers human blood to that of animals (Suwonkerd et al. 2006). It is a nervous feeder and, if interrupted while taking a blood meal, will leave to feed on other humans. Hence, one mosquito may transmit to multiple human hosts. *Ae. aegypti* females, which develop 120 to 140 eggs per blood meal, typically distribute their eggs among multiple oviposition sites (Reiter et al. 1995), complicating control efforts. If released at the edge of a forest, the mosquito will move to areas of human habitation (Maciel-de-Freitas et al. 2006).

Ae. aegypti mosquitoes are now present in tropical and subtropical areas throughout the world, likely introduced into the Americas from West Africa via the slave trade in the seventeenth century (Lounibos 2002). *Ae. aegypti* is one of the primary vectors for the yellow fever virus, which can cause fatal infection. In 1947, the Pan American Health Organization adopted a resolution calling for a hemisphere-wide *Ae. aegypti* eradication program to combat urban yellow fever. In 1958, Brazil was certified to have eradicated *Ae. aegypti*, but the mosquito reinfested the country in 1967. Despite initial success at re-eradication, Brazil was again reinfested in 1976. The first case of dengue fever in Brazil since 1923 epidemic in Rio de Janeiro occurred in early 1981 (Schneider and Droll 2001).

Another vector, *Aedes albopictus*, the so-called Asian tiger mosquito, is also present in Brazil; its distribution overlaps with *Ae. aegypti* in some areas. It is also able to transmit dengue, chikungunya, yellow fever, and other viruses that are human pathogens. *Ae. albopictus* has been broadly dispersed more recently than has *Ae. aegypti* (Lounibos 2002; Enserink 2008). It has gained new prominence in recent years because it has been the primary vector for chikungunya fever outbreaks in some areas (Charrel, de Lamballerie, and Raoult 2008; Reiter, Fontenille, and Paupy 2003). It has also been the primary vector for dengue fever outbreaks, for example, in Hawaii in 2001 (Effler et al. 2005) and Macao (Almeida et al. 2005). To date, *Ae. albopictus* has not been thought to be important in the transmission of dengue in Brazil.

Ae. albopictus was first documented in the United States in the early 1980s—most likely arriving in used tires shipped from Asia—and subsequently spread to at least 25 states in the continental United States (Reiter and Darsie 1984; Hawley et al. 1987). *Ae. albopictus* also invaded Brazil in the 1980s. By July 1985, *Ae. albopictus* infestations had been documented in three Brazilian states and 63 municipalities (Reiter 2010). Although mosquito vectors can be transported by air travel, modern container ships are known to have introduced *Ae. albopictus* and other alien mosquitoes into new areas. When 22,000 used tires arriving from Japan were carefully inspected, 25% were found to contain water, and five different species of mosquitoes were found among those tires, including *Ae. albopictus* (Craven et al. 1988).

About 90% of nonbulk cargo globally is moved in containers stacked on ships. An individual ship can carry more than 14,500 of these containers, which are often tightly packed and moved directly from container ship to truck, rail, or barge and then delivered unopened (Reiter 2010). Most are not inspected, so it is easy to see how exotic species of mosquitoes could accompany the cargo. Biological characteristics favor survival and introduction into new areas: the eggs are dessication resistant and can remain viable for a year or more (Knudsen 1995).

Tatem et al. examined a database on international ship and aircraft traffic and showed that the dispersal of *Ae. albopictus* and potentially other disease vectors can be predicted based on volume of traffic and climatic suitability (Tatem, Hay, and Rogers 2006). They found traffic volumes were more than twice as high on shipping routes to ports where *Ae. albopictus* was established in comparison with other ports where it has not yet invaded (Tatem, Hay, and Rogers 2006). Changing patterns of sea and air traffic could potentially change the likelihood of the introduction of vectors into other areas with climatic suitability, and increasing traffic to and from megacities in tropical areas could favor such dispersal.

In studies of *Ae. albopictus* and *Ae. aegypti* in Rio de Janeiro, both species were more abundant in close proximity to homes, with 98% of *Ae. aegypti* and 78.7% of *Ae. albopictus* found near homes (Lourenço-de-Oliveira et al. 2004). *Ae. albopictus* breeds in a wider range of containers than does *Ae. aegypti*—artificial containers, but also natural containers such as bromeliads, treeholes, and bamboo. By contrast with *Ae. aegypti*, which has a strong preference for human blood, *Ae. albopictus* feed on a wider range of hosts—many vertebrates, including birds and reptiles—although it prefers mammals (Honorio et al. 2003). If released in a forest, *Ae. albopictus* mosquitoes can fly as far as 1000 meters in a week to reach homes; when released near homes, they stay there and have a low tendency to disperse to forests (Maciel-de-Freitas et al. 2006). Nonetheless, *Ae. albopictus* mosquitoes can survive in more rural and forest environments, suggesting that they could potentially serve as a bridge vector to disseminate pathogens from forested regions (such as yellow fever virus) into urban areas. The forest could also serve as a refuge where they could survive if intensive spraying transiently made survival in the urban environment difficult.

Built Environment, Lighting, and Biting Behavior of Mosquitoes

Ae. aegypti are typically described as being most active in seeking blood meals in the periods after sunrise and before sunset. Another mosquito, *Anopheles gambiae*, an important vector of malaria in Africa, bites during the night, so the use of bednets, especially if treated with insecticide, can be extremely effective in reducing mosquito bites. Subspecies of *Ae. aegypti* that inhabit different geographic countries or regions may exhibit different behavior, so detailed study of the local mosquitoes is always valuable. Some studies suggest that the urban, built environment may change the biting behavior of *Ae. aegypti*. In a study carried out in Trinidad, West Indies, landing behavior (on humans) and light intensity were measured in rural and urban areas at both indoor and outdoor sites (Chadee 2004). Investigators observed a trimodal landing pattern for the *Ae. aegypti* in Trinidad, with peaks 1 hour after sunrise, 1 hour before noon, and 1 hour before sunset. Of note, in rural sites, outdoor biting stopped by 7:00 P.M. and only limited biting occurred indoors until 9:00 P.M. By contrast, in urban areas about 10% of the mosquito feeding occurred at night. Light intensity was also much greater in the urban environment, suggesting that patterns of mosquito biting may be altered in brightly lit urban environments and that this needs to be taken into account in developing vector control programs.

The built environment can also provide barriers to *Ae. aegypti* dispersal in urban areas. A genetic analysis of mosquitoes on either side of a highway found that the highway acted as a barrier to mosquito movement even though the mosquitoes were able to fly the distance to the other side (Hemme et al. 2010).

The urban environment may also provide protected habitats in which mosquitoes can survive harsh conditions such as low temperatures. For example, mosquitoes may be able to winter in the protected environment of a subway system in an area otherwise too cold for year-round survival. Since cities are "heat islands" and warmer than surrounding areas, cities may protect mosquito populations (Grimm et al. 2008). Warmer temperatures, up to a point, favor mosquito abundance and may influence biting activity (Focks et al. 1995). Higher temperatures shorten the mosquito gonotrophic cycle and accelerate viral dissemination within the mosquito vector, thus reducing the extrinsic incubation period (the time it takes after a mosquito ingests blood from a viremic host until the mosquito can transmit the virus to another person it bites). Shortening the extrinsic incubation period is associated with the potential for increased transmission. Warmer temperatures, whether because of global climate change or local factors, affect virus–mosquito interaction. Laboratory studies in Thailand found an inverse relationship between temperature and viral dissemination in mosquitoes. At 30°C the extrinsic incubation period for DENV-2 in *Ae. aegypti* was 12 days; this dropped to 7 days for mosquitoes incubated at 32° and 35°C (Watts et al. 1987). The extrinsic incubation period can also vary depending on the specific mosquito vector and strain of virus. Temperatures lower than 20°C can delay and disrupt larval hatching and development (Lourenço-de-Oliveira 2008).

Several of the megacities that exist today have developed in areas with insufficient water supplies and poor capacity to provide reliable piped water to residents. As a result, water is stored in or adjacent to homes in water tanks, which provide good breeding sites for mosquitoes (Figure 4.3).

Rio de Janeiro, Brazil's Second Megacity

Rio de Janeiro and São Paulo have similar geographic latitudes, but Rio de Janeiro, because it is warmer and more highly connected, is more likely to receive persons who are infected with the dengue virus in an environment that is especially favorable for transmission and from which the virus can spread. As such, populations in Rio de Janeiro could serve as receptor, amplifier, and disseminator.

The magnificent coastal city of Rio de Janeiro, with an estimated population of 12,500,000, lies in the tropics. It is marked by glorious beaches, magnificent peaks, forested areas, sleek high-rise buildings, and vast favelas. The Tijuca Forest, the world's largest urban forest (32 square kilometers or 12.4 square miles), is situated within Rio de Janeiro, flanked in part by favelas. The forest was declared a National Park in 1961, and receives many visitors from Rio de Janeiro and elsewhere. The climate of Rio de Janeiro is tropical with the hot, wet season spanning

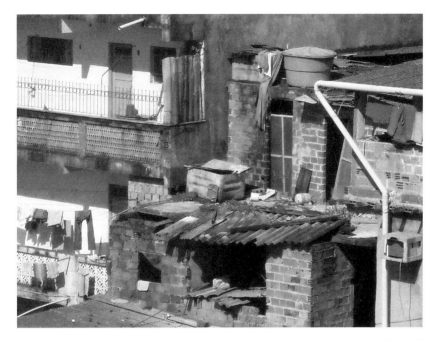

Figure 4.3 Water storage tanks in Salvador, Brazil, that provide breeding sites for *Aedes aegypti* mosquitoes. Courtesy of Felix Lam, photographer.

the months of December through May. The monthly average high temperature ranges from 27° to 33°C; the average monthly low temperature ranges from 17° to 23°C. The coolest months are May through September. The average annual rainfall is 109 centimeters.

Rio de Janeiro is highly connected with other parts of Brazil and the rest of the world. Most of Brazil lies within the tropics, and its total population is about 190 million; it has the largest area and population of all Ibero-American countries. In 2008, Rio de Janeiro received 2.8 million inbound international tourists. Brazil as a whole received more than 5 million international arrivals in 2008, with 73.1% arriving by air, 24.7% by road, and 2.2% by sea (UNWTO 2009).

The city is also highly connected to São Paulo, Brazil's other, even larger megacity (population 21 million), which received 1.7 million international arrivals in 2008. Although São Paulo lies at a similar geographic latitude (see Table 4.1), it is inland and situated at an altitude of 760 meters (2,469 feet) above sea level, giving it a slightly cooler climate than Rio de Janeiro (monthly mean high temperature ranges from 22° to 28°C and monthly mean low temperature ranges from 12° to 19°C), which is important in mosquito-borne infections, which are highly sensitive to temperature. Although temperatures are warm enough to permit dengue transmission within the city, to date São Paulo has not experienced the intensity of transmission observed in the city of Rio de Janeiro. Warming could make the city more vulnerable to more severe outbreaks of dengue and possibly other vector-borne infections.

Because Brazil will host the Fédération Internationale de Football Association World Cup games in June and July 2014, the Summer Olympic Games in August 2016, and the Paralympics in September 2016, travel to Brazil is expected to increase substantially over the next several years, and additional facilities to accommodate expanded tourism are being constructed. Arrivals increased from 4.7 million in 2001 to 7.2 million in 2008, and analysts forecast this number will increase to 9.2 million by 2014. The international airport in São Paulo already handles 12 million passengers per year, and with new construction, the capacity will increase to 29 million per year. The Summer Olympics are expected to draw athletes from 205 nations, including many that are endemic for dengue and other infections. Athletes and guests could potentially carry pathogens that can be transmitted by mosquitoes already present in Brazil. The 2014 World Cup will have venues in 12 cities throughout Brazil; eight of them are closer to the equator than is Rio de Janeiro, making them on average warmer and potentially more favorable for transmission of vector-borne infections, such as dengue fever.

Dengue in Rio de Janeiro

Rio de Janeiro experienced an epidemic of dengue fever in 1923 but was free of reported dengue for decades, presumably in large part because of *Ae. aegypti* eradication efforts. Dengue virus was reintroduced into Brazil in the early 1980s. The first cases were documented in northern Brazil in early 1981, caused by two different dengue serotypes, DENV-1 and DENV-4. It was only after DENV-1 reached Rio de Janeiro that widespread dissemination of dengue occurred in Brazil, where most of the population was susceptible to all dengue serotypes. The large size of the human population and high level of connectedness of this major urban area may favor dispersal. In Thailand, for example, Cummings et al. have described the appearance of the first of the new dengue serotypes in Bangkok, which were then followed by dispersal to smaller cities in the region (Cummings et al. 2004).

Between 1986 and 1993, dengue epidemics in Brazil occurred in localized areas (Siqueira et al. 2005). Since 1994, dengue has become endemic in many areas, and large epidemics, which have grown in size and severity, have been observed (Teixeira et al. 2009). More than 3 million cases of dengue were reported in Brazil from 2000 to 2005, representing 78% of all cases reported in the Americas (Teixeira et al. 2009). In Rio de Janeiro, epidemics now occur almost every year (Luz et al. 2008). When dengue infections exploded in the city of Rio de Janeiro in 2008, other cities in the state of Rio de Janeiro and other parts of Brazil were also affected. In the state of Rio de Janeiro in the first 4 months of 2008, more than 155,000 cases of dengue were reported (an incidence of 2543.7 per 100,000 inhabitants). More than 9000 persons were hospitalized and 110 people died; approximately half of the deaths were children. The large number of cases overwhelmed the medical facilities in many areas, and tents were set up to handle the high volume of ill patients. By the end of October 2008, more than 250,000 cases had been reported in the state of Rio de Janeiro; half of the cases (125,988) and 105 of the confirmed deaths were in the city of Rio de Janeiro. The largest number of cases (44%) occurred in adults aged 20 to 49 years. High rates of infection in working adults caused disruption of many activities. In recent years, the median age of those with severe dengue (DHF) has decreased in Brazil with more cases occurring in children (Teixeira et al. 2008).

In a study of survival of *Ae. aegypti* mosquitoes in two different parts of Rio de Janeiro, one a slum area with high human density, and the other an urban area with lower population density (each with population of just under 3000), investigators found that mosquitoes survived better in the slum area than in the less densely settled urban area (Maciel-de-Freitas et al. 2007). In this study, mosquitoes were marked, released, and recaptured. When released in a slum area during the wet season, one third of mosquitoes survived for periods that exceeded the extrinsic incubation period for the dengue virus; during the dry season, almost half survived for a similar period. These findings suggested that conditions were exceedingly favorable for dengue transmission. The investigators postulated that mosquitoes do better in an environment where a large number of humans makes it easy for the mosquito to find a blood meal. Another study in Rio de Janeiro found lower infestation rates and shorter adult female mosquito survival in high-income areas with low density of human population in comparison with suburban and slum areas with a higher density (David, Lourenço-de-Oliveira, and Freitas 2009).

Two features of tropical cities that are associated with vector breeding sites in many studies are water storage containers and trash that can hold water. When investigators inspected 747 containers in 300 dwellings in the state of Rio de Janeiro, they found that containers used to store water or classified as garbage (e.g., discarded plastic cups and bottles) accounted for the breeding sites of 90.2% of the larvae and 88.9% of the pupae of *Ae. aegypti* (Medronho et al. 2009). In another study in Rio de Janeiro, investigators inspected 1041 properties and found that domestic drains and discarded plastic pots were the most productive containers for mosquito development, collectively holding up to 80% of the pupae of *Ae. aegypti* (David, Lourenço-de-Oliveira, and Freitas 2009).

Similar findings have been observed in the city of Salvador, Brazil. This city, the epicenter of a 1995 dengue epidemic, is an area with high population density, low socioeconomic level, and poor sanitation conditions (Barreto et al. 2008). Sampaio et al. found that, in Rio de Janeiro, the neighborhood with the greatest increase in construction of buildings and condominiums had the highest dengue incidence (Sampaio, Kligerman, and Junior 2009). These were also the areas with the most trash, and other researchers have noted an association of vector breeding sites with trash. Investigators have also found a higher incidence of dengue in areas that lack running water, a circumstance that leads residents to store water in containers that are favorable breeding sites for mosquitoes (Teixeira and Medronho 2008).

Decorative bromeliads can harbor immature forms of *Ae. aegypti*, but limited studies have found low rates of infestation of these plants (Cunha et al. 2006; Mocellin et al. 2009). In an area of Rio de Janeiro where immature *Ae. aegypti* stages were found in artificial containers in nearly 5% of nearby homes, only two *Ae. aegypti* larvae and five *Ae. albopictus* larvae were among the 2816 mosquito larvae collected from 120 bromeliads (Mocellin et al. 2009).

Cities today are populated with apartments and high-rise buildings, yet this high-rise ecosystem has been little studied. Most of the studies of vector behavior (and most of intervention strategies) have addressed only the lowest levels of housing units. In a study in Trinidad, West Indies, investigators looked for eggs of *Ae. aegypti* at elevations from 0 to 60 meters (1 to 5 floors) in apartment buildings. They found more eggs at 13 to 24 meters of elevation than any other elevation, although about 7% of eggs were also found at the highest elevation studied (49 to 60 meters: Chadee 2004). Spraying of insecticide at ground level may reduce populations at lower levels, but apartment buildings provide all of the essentials for the mosquitoes: a source of blood meals (humans), shelter, congenial ambient temperature (if the buildings are not air conditioned), and breeding sites (e.g., flower pots, drains, and other sites with standing water). Investigators in Singapore found that when female *Ae. aegypti* and *Ae. albopictus* were released on the 12th floor of a 21-floor empty apartment building, they dispersed to all levels—including the highest and lowest floors (Liew and Curtis 2004). The presence of screens on the windows could impede movement. The presence of air conditioning would likely have strong inhibitory effect, because mosquito activity slows with lower temperatures. In many tropical cities, however, many high-rise buildings have neither screens nor air conditioning.

Because of the unique characteristics of the dengue virus, introduction of a new serotype (e.g., DENV-4) or genotype, or one that has not been present in Brazil for many years, could lead to devastating epidemics of dengue. In many Brazilian cities, more than half of the humans have already been infected by one or more dengue serotypes (>80% are seropositive in some cities; Teixeira et al. 2002), protecting them against those serotypes while making them more vulnerable to severe consequences if infection with a new serotype occurs. Currently DENV-1, DENV-2, and DENV-3 are circulating in Brazil, but other dengue serotypes are present in neighboring countries, and DENV-4 has never circulated widely in Brazil.

To try to estimate the probability that a traveler who is (or will become) viremic with dengue virus will enter Brazil and potentially spark an epidemic, it is useful to assess the numbers of travelers entering Brazil from dengue-endemic countries (Brazilians and non-Brazilians). Because a large percentage (87% in one study) of dengue infections are mild or asymptomatic, infected, viremic persons with unrecognized infection may travel to and from Brazil (Burke et al. 1988). In the most recent years, the number of travelers to Brazil from dengue-endemic countries in Asia has been small, but the number is likely to increase during the Olympics and World Cup events (Table 4.2). The likelihood of a viremic person being the source for local cases depends on several factors, including the level of immunity of humans to a given dengue virus, the abundance of local, competent mosquitoes, access of the mosquitoes to infected and susceptible persons, and environmental conditions, with temperature being the most important factor influencing virus replication and dissemination in the mosquito.

Fortunately, both the World Cup and Summer Olympic events have been timed to occur during the cooler months of the year in the southern hemisphere, a season less favorable to dengue transmission.

Besides dengue virus, other potential threats for introduction include chikungunya virus, which can be transmitted by *Ae. aegypti* and *Ae. albopictus*. The virus is endemic in parts of Africa, but since 2004 it has spread broadly, causing massive and explosive epidemics in the Indian Ocean region and India and other parts of Asia (Simon, Savini, and Parola 2008; Enserink 2008). In the summer of 2007, it caused an epidemic in Italy sparked by a person who had recently arrived from India and had an acute infection (Rezza et al. 2007). A mutation in the envelope protein gene of the chikungunya virus appears to allow the virus to replicate more efficiently in *Ae. albopictus*, which has been the vector implicated in several recent outbreaks, including the one in Italy (Tsetsarkin et al.

Table 4.2   Arrivals to Brazil, by Region of Origin: Nonresidents of Brazil, 2008

	No. (%)
Total	5,050,099 (100)
Regions	
Africa	75,824 (1.5)
Americas	2,883,839 (57.1)
East Asia and the Pacific	256,271 (5.1)
Europe	1,814,146 (35.9)
Middle East	25,967 [2007 data]
South Asia	19,456 (0.4)
Not specified	563 (0.0)
Regions containing dengue-endemic areas	
Africa	75,824 (1.5)
Caribbean	6268 (0.1)
Central America	41,800 (0.8)
North America: Mexico	77,193 (1.5)
South America: excluding Chile and Uruguay	1,631,901 (32.3)
Northeast Asia: China	78,514 (0.8)
Australasia: Australia	37,034 (0.7)
East Asia and the Pacific	46,773 (0.9)
South Asia: India	19,456 (0.4)

Source: UN World Transportation Organization 2009.

Note. In many countries, dengue transmission occurs only sporadically, seasonally, or in limited parts of the country; therefore, numbers overestimate those potentially exposed to dengue in those areas; for example, Argentina (only in the northern part of the country); Bolivia (almost half of the country), Paraguay (only small parts of the country), and Peru (about half of the country).

2007; Schuffenecker et al. 2006; Charrel, de Lamballerie, and Raoult 2007). It is notable that the geographic latitude of Castiglione di Cervia, one of the towns in the Ravenna region of Italy involved in the outbreak of chikungunya infections, is 44° N 27', well outside the tropics. The outbreak occurred during the hottest months of the year, and *Ae. albopictus* mosquitoes are abundant in that area. In order for a vector-borne infection to be introduced and spread, however, it is necessary to have seasonal synchrony of vector activity (Charrel, de Lamballerie, and Raoult). Although ecoclimatic conditions allowed this outbreak to occur in summer months, cooler fall and winter temperatures stopped the spread, and there has been no evidence that the virus has persisted in this region.

Brazil has the ecoclimatic conditions and vector presence that make it vulnerable to the introduction of a new dengue serotype or chikungunya virus. The relatively low volume of travel between Brazil and areas with ongoing activity of chikungunya may help to explain why sustained spread of chikungunya virus has not been observed to date in Brazil. A notable contrast is Singapore, where repeated introductions of chikungunya and dengue viruses have occurred despite extensive vector control programs (Leo et al. 2009). Singapore is a major travel hub, with more than 37 million air passengers passing through in 2008, including many arriving from areas with outbreaks.

To better understand the likelihood of spread of viruses into areas with competent vectors and susceptible human populations, modelers have assessed the basic reproductive rate and the number of infections expected as the result of one infection in a susceptible population, and have concluded that it is lower for yellow fever virus than it is for dengue virus (Massad et al. 2001, 2003) and lower for chikungunya than for dengue (Massad et al. 2008). Still, Rio de Janeiro (and other tropical urban areas) are at risk for urban yellow fever outbreaks, which could be disastrous (Monath 1999). Currently, yellow fever vaccine is not recommended routinely for residents of Rio de Janeiro and São Paulo, though it is included in childhood vaccination programs for many parts of Brazil where yellow fever is endemic.

It is fascinating to read an editorial published in 1913 in the journal *Lancet* at a time when Rio de Janeiro had a population of less than 1 million (Editors 1913). Yellow fever outbreaks were a regular occurrence in the city, and between 1877 and 1902 almost 35,000 deaths were attributed to yellow fever. After it was shown that mosquitoes transmit the yellow fever virus, authorities in Brazil adopted the "modern scientific methods" used successfully in Cuba and elsewhere. In Rio de Janeiro, yellow fever was almost eliminated by sanitary improvements that included a comprehensive drainage scheme, embanking the waterfront, and deployment of "mosquito brigades." This was decades before the yellow fever vaccine and pesticides such as DDT were available. When control measures were relaxed, mosquitoes began appearing in large numbers. Today, Rio de Janeiro and many other megacities in tropical and subtropical regions are heavily infested with *Ae. aegypti* (Lourenço-de-Oliveira 2008), and some also harbor *Ae. albopictus*, placing residents at high risk for outbreaks of dengue, chikungunya, and in some instances yellow fever. The vaccine that protects against yellow fever continues to be highly efficacious (rarely associated with severe adverse events); however, global supplies may prove insufficient if massive urban populations are threatened by outbreaks. Mosquitoes have become resistant to many insecticides, which hampers control efforts.

Climate change and its potential effect on the location and intensity of transmission of dengue virus and other vector-borne pathogens has received much attention of late. (Jetten and Focks 1997; Gubler et al. 2001; Lafferty 2009; Pascual and Bouma 2009). Vectors are clearly responsive to ecoclimatic factors (Bale and Hayward 2010), but many other factors, as discussed above (such as housing and living conditions), also influence transmission. At present, it is unclear how much climate change is contributing to increased transmission of dengue and how important a role this will play in the future.

Summary

Megacities are vulnerable to microbial threats because of a confluence of factors that include size, density, poverty, and their extensive connectedness with adjacent rural populations and urban populations throughout the world. Among the threats are those of vector-borne infections, such as dengue fever. Because most of the global population growth today is taking place in urban areas in low-latitude areas, an increasing number of people live in tropical and subtropical areas at risk for dengue fever. As shown by the example of Brazil, many megacities provide the ecological setting that can permit rapid spread of some vector-borne infections. Absence of reliable piped water supplies leads residents to store water in their homes. These containers and other features of the urban landscape provide ideal breeding sites for urban mosquitoes, *Ae. aegypti*, which can transmit viruses, such as the dengue, yellow fever, and chikungunya viruses, that cause serious infection in humans. The mosquito is now widely distributed in tropical and subtropical areas, is well adapted to contemporary urban life, and is complicated and costly to control. The large volume of human travel and global trade contribute to the movement of viruses and vectors in our increasingly connected world. Although perhaps not as facile as microbes, mosquitoes also have a short generation time (relative to humans) and can adapt to changes in the environment and human activity. The rise of megacities is likely to exacerbate the global challenge of emerging infections.

References

Ali SH, Keil R, editors. 2008. *Networked Disease: Emerging Infections in the Global City*. Oxford, England: Wiley-Blackwell.

Almeida AP, Baptista SS, Sousa CA, et al. 2005. Bioecology and vectoral capacity of *Aedes albopictus* (Diptera: Culicidae) in Macao, China, in relation to dengue virus transmission. *J Med Entomol*. 42:419–428.

Bale JS, Hayward SAL. 2010. Insect overwintering in a changing climate. *J Exp Biol*. 213:980–994.

Barreto FR, Teixeira MG, Costa MCN, et al. 2008. Spread pattern of the first dengue epidemic in the city of Salvador, Brazil. *BMC Public Health*. 8:51.

Bell DM, Weisfuse IB, Hernandez-Avila M, et al. 2009. Pandemic influenza as 21st century urban public health crisis. *Emerg Infect Dis*. 15:1963–1969.

Bilham R. Dangerous tectonics, fragile buildings, and tough decisions. 2006. *Science*. 311:1873–1875.

Blanton RE, Silva LK, Morato VG, et al. 2008. Genetic ancestry and income are associated with dengue hemorrhagic fever in a highly admixed population. *Eur J Hum Genet*. 16:762–765.

Brinkhoff T. 2010. The Principal Agglomerations of the World. Available at: http://www.citypopulation.de/world/Agglomerations.html. Accessed June 20, 2010.

Burke DS, Misalak A, Johnson DE, Scott TM. 1988. A prospective study of dengue infections in Bangkok. *Am J Trop Med Hyg*. 38:172–180.

Chadee DD. 2004. Observations on the seasonal prevalence and vertical distribution patterns of oviposition by *Aedes aegypti* (L.) (Diptera: Culicidae) in urban high-rise apartments in Trinidad, West Indies. *J Vector Ecol*. 29:323–330.

Chadee DD, Martinez R. 2000. Landing periodicity of *Aedes aegypti* with implications for dengue transmission in Trinidad, West Indies. *J Vector Ecol*. 25:158–163.

Charrel RN, de Lamballerie X, Raoult D. 2007. Chikungunya outbreaks–the globalization of vectorborne diseases. *N Engl J Med*. 356:769–771.

Charrel RN, de Lamballerie X, Raoult D. 2008. Seasonality of mosquitoes and chikungunya in Italy. *Lancet Infect Dis*. 8:5–6.

Cologna R, Armstrong PM, Rico-Hesse R. 2005. Selection for virulent viruses occurs in humans and mosquitoes. *J Virol*. 2005;79:853–859.

Confalonieri UEC, Wilson ME, Najar AL. 2006. Social and environmental vulnerability to emerging infectious diseases. In: *Interactions Between Global Change and Human Health*, vol. 106. Vatican City: Pontifical Academy of Sciences: 195–212.

Craven RB, Eliason DA, Francy DB, et al. 1988. Importation of *Aedes albopictus* and other exotic mosquito species into the United States in used tires from Asia. *J Am Mosq Control Assoc*. 4:138–142.

Cummings DAT, Irizarry RA, Huang NE, et al. 2004. Travelling waves in the occurrence of dengue haemorrhagic fever in Thailand. *Nature*. 427:344–347.

Cunha SP, Alves JRC, Lima MM, et al. 2002. Presence of *Aedes aegypti* in Bromeliaceae and plant breeding places in Brazil. *Rev Saude Publica*. 36:244–245.

David MR, Lourenço-de-Oliveira R, Freitas RM. 2009. Container productivity, daily survival rates and dispersal of *Aedes aegypti* mosquitoes in a high income dengue epidemic neighbourhood of Rio de Janeiro: presumed influence of differential urban structure on mosquito biology. *Mem Inst Oswaldo Cruz* (Rio de Janeiro). 104:927–932.

Editors. 1913. The threatened recrudescence of yellow fever in Rio de Janeiro [editorial]. *Lancet*. 182:819–820.

Effler PVL, Pang L, Kitsutani P, et al. 2005. Dengue fever, Hawaii, 2001–2002. *Emerg Infect Dis*. 11:742–749.

Ehresmann KR, Kedberg CW, Grimm MB, et al. 1995. An outbreak of measles at in international sporting event with airborne transmission at a domed stadium. *J Infect Dis*. 171:679–683.

Enserink M. 2008. A mosquito goes global. *Science*. 320:864–866.

Focks DA, Daniels E, Haile DG, Keesling JE. 1995. A simulation model of the epidemiology of urban dengue fever: literature analysis, model development, preliminary validation, and samples of simulation results. *Am J Trop Med Hyg*. 53:489–506.

Fraser C, Riley S, Anderson RM, Ferguson NM. 2004. Factors that make an infectious disease outbreak controllable. *Proc Natl Acad Sci U S A*. 101:6146–6151.

Fried JR, Gibbons RV, Kalayanarooj S, et al. 2010. Serotype-specific differences in the risk of dengue hemorrhagic fever: an analysis of data collected in Bangkok, Thailand from 1994 to 2006. *PLoS Negl Trop Dis*. 4:e617.

Grimm NB, Faeth SH, Golubiewski NE, et al. 2008. Global change and the ecology of cities. *Science*. 319:756–760.

Gubler DJ. 2002. Epidemic dengue/dengue hemorrhagic fever as a public health, social and economic problem in the 21st century. *Trends Microbiol*. 10:100–102.

Gubler DJ. 2004. Cities spawn epidemic dengue viruses. 2004. *Nat Med*. 10:129–130.

Gubler DJ, Reiter P, Ebi KL, et al. 2001. Climate variability and change in the United States: potential impacts on vector- and rodent-borne diseases. *Environ Health Perspect*. 109(Suppl 2):S223–S233.

Guernier V, Hochberg ME, Guégan J-F. 2004. Ecology drives the worldwide distribution of human diseases. *PLoS Biol*. 2:740–746.

Guilarde AO, Turchi MD, Siqueira JB Jr, et al. 2008. Dengue and dengue hemorrhagic fever among adults: clinical outcomes related to viremia, serotypes, and antibody response. *J Infect Dis*. 197:817–824.

Hales S, de Wet N, Maindonald J, Woodward A. 2002. Potential effect of population and climate changes on global distribution of dengue fever: an empirical model. *Lancet*. 360:830–834.

Halstead SB. Dengue. 2007. *Lancet*. 370:1644–1652.

Hawley WA, Reiter P, Copeland RS, et al. 1987. *Aedes albopictus* in North America: probable introduction in used tires from northern Asia. *Science*. 1114–1116.

Hemme RR, Thomas CL, Chadee DD, Severson DW. 2010. Influence of urban landscapes on population dynamics in a short-distance migrant mosquito: evidence for the dengue vector *Aedes aegypti. PLoS Negl Trop Dis*. 4:e634.

Honorio NA, Silva WC, Leite PJ, et al. 2003. Dispersal of *Aedes aegypti* and *Aedes albopictus* (Diptera: Culicidae) in an urban endemic dengue area in the state of Rio de Janeiro, Brazil. *Mem Inst Oswaldo Cruz* (Rio de Janeiro). 98:191–198.

International Monetary Fund. 2009. World Economic Outlook Database: Emerging and Developing Economies. Available at: http://www.imf.org/external/pubs/ft/ weo/2009/02/weodata/groups.htm#oem. Accessed September 23, 2010.

Jetten TH, Focks DA. 1997. Potential changes in the distribution of dengue transmission under climate warming. *Am J Trop Med Hyg*. 57:285–297.

Jones KE, Patel N, Levy MA, et al. 2008. Global trends in emerging infectious diseases. *Nature*. 451:990–994.

Knudsen AB. 1995. Global distribution and continuing spread of *Ae. albopictus*. *Parassitologia*. 37:91–97.

Kuno G. 1995. Review of the factors modulating dengue transmission. *Epidemiol Rev*. 17:321–335.

Lafferty KD. 2009. The ecology of climate change and infectious diseases. *Ecology*. 90:888–900.

Lee K-S, Lai Y-L, Lo S, et al. 2010. Dengue virus surveillance for early warning, Singapore. *Emerg Infect Dis*. 16:847–849.

Leo SY, Chow ALP, Tan LK, et al. 2009. Chikungunya outbreak, Singapore, 2008. *Emerg Infect Dis*. 15:836–837.

Li W, Shi Z, Yu M, Ren W, et al. 2005. Bats are natural reservoirs of SARS-like coronaviruses. *Science*. 310:676–679.

Liew C, Curtis CF. 2004. Horizontal and vertical dispersal of dengue vector mosquitoes, *Aedes aegypti* and *Aedes albopictus*, in Singapore. *Med Vet Entomol*. 18:351–360.

Lloyd-Smith JO, George D, Pepin KM, et al. 2009. Epidemic dynamics at the human-animal interface. *Science*. 326:1362–1367.

Lopez AD, Mathers CD, Ezzati J, et al. 2006. Global and regional burden of disease and risk factors, 2001: systematic analysis of population health data. *Lancet*. 367:1747–1756.

Lounibos LP. 2002. Invasions by insect vectors of human disease. *Annu Rev Entomol*. 47:233–266.

Lourenço-de-Oliveira R. 2008. Rio de Janeiro against *Aedes aegypti*: yellow fever in 1908 and dengue in 2008 [editorial]. *Mem Inst Oswaldo Cruz* (Rio de Janeiro). 103:627–628.

Lourenço-de-Oliveira R, Castro MG, Braks MAH, Lounibos LP. 2004. The invasion of urban forest by dengue vectors in Rio de Janeiro. *J Vector Ecol*. 29:94–100.

Luz PM, Mendes BVM, Codeço CT, et al. 2008. Time series analysis of dengue incidence in Rio de Janeiro, Brazil. *Am J Trop Med Hyg*. 79:933–939.

Maciel-de-Freitas R, Codeço CT, Lourenço-de-Oliveira R. 2007. Daily survival rates and dispersal of *Aedes aegypti* females in Rio de Janeiro, Brazil. *Am J Trop Med Hyg*. 76:659–665.

Maciel-de-Freitas R, Neto RB, Gonçalves JM, et al. 2006. Movement of dengue vectors between the human modified environment and an urban forest in Rio de Janeiro. *J Med Entomol*. 43:1112–1120.

Martin JLS, Brathwaite OB, Zambrano B, et al. 2010. The epidemiology of dengue in the Americas over the last three decades: a worrisome reality. *Am J Trop Med Hyg*. 82:128–135.

Massad E, Burattini MN, Coutinho FAB, Lopez LF. 2003. Dengue and the risk of urban yellow fever reintroduction in São Paulo, Brazil. *Rev Saude Publica*. 37:477–484.

Massad E, Coutinho FAB, Burattini MN, Lopez LF. 2001. The risk of yellow fever in a dengue infested area. *Trans R Soc Trop Med Hyg*. 95:370–374.

Massad E, Ma S, Burattini MN, et al. 2008. The risk of chikungunya fever in a dengue-endemic area. *J Travel Med*. 15:147–155.

Medronho RA, Macrini L, Novellino DM, et al. 2009. *Aedes aegypti* immature forms distribution according to type of breeding site. *Am J Trop Med Hyg*. 80:401–404.

Mocellin MG, Simões TC, Nascimento TFS, et al. 2009. Bromeliad-inhabiting mosquitoes in an urban botanical garden of dengue endemic Rio de Janeiro. Are bromeliads productive habitats for the invasive vectors *Aedes aegypti* and *Aedes albopictus*? *Mem Inst Oswaldo Cruz* (Rio de Janeiro). 104:1171–1176.

Monath TP. 1999. Facing up to the re-emergence of urban yellow fever. *Lancet*. 353:1541.

Montgomery MR. 2008. The urban transformation of the developing world. *Science*. 319:761–764.

Nguyen TPL, Kikuchi M, Huong VTQ, et al. 2008. Protective and enhancing HLA alleles, HLA-DRB1*0901 and HLA-A*24, for severe forms of dengue virus infection, dengue hemorrhagic fever and dengue shock syndrome. *PLoS Negl Trop Dis*. 2:e304.

Pascual M, Bouma MJ. 2009. Do rising temperatures matter? *Ecology*. 90:906–912.

Patel RB, Burke TF. 2009. Urbanization–an emerging humanitarian disaster. *N Engl J Med*. 361:741–743.

Reiter P. 2007. Oviposition, dispersal, and survival in *Aedes aegypti*: implications for the efficacy of control strategies. *Vector Borne Zoonotic Dis*. 7:261–273.

Reiter P. 2010. A mollusc on the leg of a beetle: human activities and the global dispersal of vectors and vector-borne pathogens. In: *Infectious Disease Movement in a Borderless World*. Workshop Summary. Microbial Threats Forum, Institute of Medicine. Washington, DC: National Academies:150–165, 175–178.

Reiter P, Amador MA, Anderson RA, Clark GG. 1995. Short report: dispersal of *Aedes aegypti* in an urban area after blood feeding as demonstrated by rubidium-marked eggs. *Am J Trop Med Hyg*. 52:177–179.

Reiter P, Darsie R. 1984. *Aedes albopictus* in Memphis, Tennessee (USA): an achievement of modern transportation? *Mosq News*. 44:396–399.

Reiter P, Fontenille D, Paupy C. 2003. *Aedes albopictus* as an epidemic vector of chikungunya virus: another emerging problem? *Lancet Infect Dis*. 3:463.

Rezza G, Nicoletti L, Angelini R, et al. 2007. Infection with chikungunya virus in Italy: an outbreak in a temperate regions. *Lancet*. 370:1840–1846.

Roy CJ, Milton DK. 2004. Airborne transmission of communicable infection–the elusive pathway. *N Engl J Med*. 350:1710–1712.

Sampaio AMM, Kligerman DC, Júnior SF. 2009. Dengue, related to rubble and building construction in Brazil. *Waste Manag*. 29:2867–2873.

Schneider J, Droll D. 2001. A Timeline for Dengue in the Americas to December 31, 2000 and Noted First Occurrences. Washington, DC: Pan American Health Organization. Available at: www.paho.org/english/hcp/hct/vbd/dengue_finaltime. doc. Accessed September 20, 2010.

Schuffenecker I, Iteman I, Michault A, et al. 2006. Genome microevolution of chikungunya viruses causing the Indian Ocean outbreak. *PLoS Med*. 3:e263.

Sierra BC, Koury G, Guzman MG. 2007. Race: a risk factor for dengue hemorrhagic fever. *Arch Virol.* 152:533–542.

Simon F, Savini H, Parola P. 2008. Chikungunya: a paradigm of emergence and globalization of vector-borne diseases. *Med Clin North Am.* 92:1323–1434.

Siqueira JB Jr, Martelli CMT, Coelho GEC, et al. 2005. Dengue and dengue hemorrhagic fever, Brazil, 1981–2002. *Emerg Infect Dis.* 11:48–53.

Smolinski MS, Hamburg MA, Lederberg J, editors. 2003. *Microbial Threats to Health: Emergence, Detection, and Response.* Washington, DC: National Academies. Available at: http://www.nap.edu/openbook.php?isbn=030908864X. Accessed September 20, 2010.

Suwonkerd W, Mongkalangoon P, Parbaripai A, et al. 2006. The effect of host type on movement patterns of *Aedes aegypti* (Diptera: Culicidae) into and out of experimental huts in Thailand. *J Vector Ecol.* 31:311–318.

Tatem AJ, Hay SI, Rogers DJ. 2006. Global traffic and disease vector dispersal. *Proc Natl Acad Sci U S A.* 103:6242–6247.

Teixeira MG, Barreto ML, Costa MCN, et al. 2002. Dynamics of dengue virus circulation: a silent epidemic in a complex urban area. *Trop Med Int Health.* 7:757–762.

Teixeira MG, Costa MCN, Barreto F, Barreto ML. 2009. Dengue: twenty-five years since reemergence in Brazil. *Cad Saude Publica* (Rio de Janeiro). 25(Suppl 1):S7–S18.

Teixeira MG, Costa MCN, Coelho G, Barreto ML. 2008. Recent shift in age pattern of dengue hemorrhagic fever, Brazil. *Emerg Infect Dis.* 14:1663.

Teixeira TRA, Medronho RA. 2008. Socio-demographic factors and the dengue fever epidemic in 2002 in the Sate of Rio de Janeiro. *Cad Saude Publica* (Rio de Janeiro). 24:2160–2170.

Tsetsarkin KA, Vanlandingham DL, McGee CE, Higgs S. 2007. A single mutation in chikungunya virus affects vector specificity and epidemic potential. *PLoS Pathog.* 3:e201.

United Nations World Tourism Organization. 2009. Tourism Highlights, 2008 Edition. Available at: http://www.unwto.org/facts/eng/pdf/highlights/UNWTO_Highlights09_en_LR.pdf. Accessed September 20, 2010.

Vaughn DW, Green S, Kalayanarooj S, et al. 2000. Dengue viremia titer, antibody response pattern, and virus serotype correlate with disease severity. *J Infect Dis.* 181:2–9.

Watts DM, Burke DS, Harrison BA, et al. 1987. Effect of temperature on the vector efficiency of *Aedes aegypti* for dengue 2 virus. *Am J Trop Med Hyg*. 36:143–152.

Webby R, Hoffman E, Webster R. 2004. Molecular constraints to interspecies transmission of viral pathogens. *Nat Med*. 10(Suppl 12):S77–S81.

Webster RG, Govorkava EA. 2006. H5N1 influenza-continuing evolution and spread. *N Engl J Med*. 355:2174–2177.

Wikipedia. 2010. List of cities by latitude. Available at: http://en.wikipedia.org/wiki/List_of_cities_by_latitude. Accessed September 20, 2010.

Wilder-Smith A, Gubler DJ. 2008. Geographic expansion of dengue: the impact of international travel. *Med Clin North Am*. 92:1377–1390.

Wilson ME. 1995a. Infectious diseases: an ecological perspective. *BMJ*. 311:1681–1684.

Wilson ME. 1995b. Travel and the emergence of infectious diseases. *Emerg Infect Dis*. 1:39–46.

Wilson ME. 2003. The traveller and emerging infections: sentinel, courier, transmitter. *J Appl Microbiol*. 94:1S–11S.

Wilson ME. 2010a. Geography of infectious diseases. In: Cohen J, Powderly WG, editors. *Infectious Diseases*. 3rd ed. New York, NY: Mosby.

Wilson ME. 2010b. Global travel and emerging infections. In: *Infectious Disease Movement in a Borderless World*. Workshop Summary. Microbial Threats Forum, Institute of Medicine. Washington, DC: National Academies: 90–104;126–129.

Yu ITS, Li Y, Wong TW, et al. 2004. Evidence of airborne transmission of the severe acute respiratory syndrome virus. *N Engl J Med*. 355:1731–1739.

Zanotto PM, Gould EA, Gao DF, et al. 1996. Population dynamics of flaviviruses revealed by molecular phylogenies. *Proc Natl Acad Sci U S A*. 93:548–553.

Megacity Metrics:
Current Systems and Developing
a Conceptual Framework

Arpana Verma, MBChB, MPH, MFPH

MEGACITIES ARE INCREASING IN number, with the greatest growth occurring in the developing world. These cities are regarded as areas of innovation, but they are also subject to high concentrations of factors which result in negative health effects—for example, social isolation or exclusion, disease outbreaks, and new diseases. There are many initiatives for frameworks and metrics for the measurement of health, illness and socioeconomic status that are pertinent to specific continents, countries, regions, and cities. The conceptual framework proposed in this chapter is a synthesis of other projects and relies on researchers, policymakers, and civil society working together to determine needs and future resources needed to collect metrics for the advancement of health and well-being in megacities.

In 1978, the United Nations identified the phenomenon of urbanization and created the Human Settlements Programme (UN-HABITAT), for sustainable settlement development and adequate shelter for all (United Nations Human Settlements Programme 2004). At that time, the majority of the world's population lived in rural areas, but by 2008, the escalation in urbanization meant that for the first time, the majority of the world's population lived in cities (United Nations Population Division 2008). Furthermore, almost 10% of the world's population now reside in megacities, which UN-HABITAT defines as a city with a population of at least 10 million people. (United Nations Human Settlements Programme 2010a).

Why has there been such a trend, when the move from rural areas into cities introduces disparities in health and health care, social isolation and exclusion, areas of disease and poverty, and poor environmental and housing conditions (Vlahov et al. 2005)? The answer lies within the effectors of the wider determinants of health as characterized by the Dahlgren and Whitehead model (Dahlgren and Whitehead 1991). The movement of populations into cities is caused in part by the desire to achieve better general socioeconomic, cultural, and environmental conditions.

In addition to the movement of people from rural into urban environments, there is also the phenomenon of a static population who are overtaken by the expansion of an urban environment, known as "urban sprawl." Urbanization is therefore a dynamic process, which describes the extent to which a particular area becomes urban over time (Vlahov and Galea 2003).

Because urbanization is most rapidly occurring in developing countries, it follows that new megacity formation will also be in these countries. According to Rodwin and Gusmano, by 2015, most megacities will be in developing nations (Rodwin and Gusmano 2002). Megacities affect global health and can be seen as "instruments of social and economic development" (Bugliarello 1999; Rodwin and Gusmano 2002). The disparities and inequalities in health outcomes within a megacity can be compared with the differences observed between the developed and developing world, as in the case of life expectancy (Whiteis 1998).

In summary, megacities are rising in number, with the expansion occurring predominantly in the developing world. Megacities and cities are regarded as areas of innovation (e.g., positive initiatives such as development grants for improving housing and green space) but also possess negative aspects such as social isolation and exclusion, disease outbreaks, and new diseases (Galea, Vlahov, and Sisco 2003; Richards et al. 2009).

The Rationale for Good Metrics

The World Health Organization (WHO), European Commission, and Organisation for Economic Co-operation and Development (OECD) all produce statistics for a variety of indicators including wealth, health, and well-being. The statistics include historical data and attempt to facilitate transnational comparisons. With the growth of urbanization, the national data obscure what may be occurring at a subnational level, that is, between cities, within cities, and between urban and rural areas (Rodwin and Gusmano 2002; Riva et al. 2008).

Domains for health and well-being metrics should include the wider determinants as well as the usual metrics associated with health (Daniels 2010). Before assessing the domains best used to measure health and well-being in megacities, it is important to know the reasons behind collecting data (i.e., monitoring, benchmarking, policymaking, investment, and development) and what is defined as a "megacity." The purpose for collecting data is to effect health gain of a population. An a priori reasoning for collecting health and well-being data is essential to determine the system of data collection employed, analyses, demonstration, and dissemination of results.

Planning and policymaking for a changing population is a challenge. Decisions rely on instant access to data, reliable interpretation of the data, policy development, and implementation. Citizens require both empowerment and opportunity, to be able to influence local implementation of health and well-being policy. Development of the Internet, social networks, and new technologies are therefore inherent in improving the health and well-being of megacities.

The Challenges Posed by Megacities for Good Metrics

The UN definition of a megacity, or indeed the definition of any other body, can only be used if we know the boundaries of a "city" or "urban area." There are many definitions proposed. A pragmatic response may be to determine what is rural and then classify everything else as urban. There is a wealth of literature reviewing the question of definition (e.g., Galea and Vlahov 2005; Heller 2008; European Environment Agency 2009). Indicators such as population density, geographical boundaries of functionality, and population number may not apply to all megacities.

It is a fundamental first step to define the boundary and population for any metric, that is, the denominator for presenting data and for analysis. The boundary of a megacity will vary over time as the "urban sprawl" engulfs towns and cities which once were distinct functional units. For example, in China, Hong Kong is now confluent with Shenhzen and Guangzhou; Hong Kong-Shenhzen-Guangzhou is described as a megaregion and is home to 120 million people (United Nations Human Settlements Programme 2010). In comparison, Moscow, Russia's only megacity, has a population of 10.4 million. Is it sensible to compare it with Hong Kong-Shenhzen-Guangzhou, whose population is more than ten times greater?

Social and health problems are often magnified in populations living in megacities. The same limitations described in the study of urban health apply to megacities;

these include the complexity of the infrastructure in megacities, disease causation, and health care systems (Galea and Vlahov 2005; Kamal-Chaoui and Robert 2009; Richards et al. 2009). The impact of rapid urbanization places huge demands on the infrastructure of the locality, within a megacity and the region. Poor planning can lead to an increase in the inequality/inequity gap, isolation of communities, and a rise of hidden or nonengaged populations. Migration into and out of cities, including that of student populations, economic migrants, and traveling communities, adds to the difficulty in planning services and infrastructure. Megacities have been classed as global risk areas as a result of population and economic growth, rural land pressure, urbanization, inequality, climate and political change, technological innovation, social expectation, and global interdependence (Kraas 2008). Rural poverty has pushed villagers into cities leading to "squatter populations" with poor housing, sanitation, and access to health care; crime; alcohol abuse; rise of infectious diseases; and increased morbidity and mortality (Mutatkar 1995).

The unique difference in populations living in megacities is the environment. This includes outdoor air pollution, indoor environment (home and workplace), personal environment (smoking, overcrowding), and social capital (Lawrence 2008). McGranahan outlines the links between "urban environment, wealth and health" in relation to water, sanitation, housing, and climate change (McGranahan 2007). Decker et al. suggest we think of "urban metabolism and urban succession as organizing concepts for data collection, analysis, and synthesis on urban systems" (Decker, Elliot, and Smith 2002). The authors compare the city to an organic being requiring energy to do work and then excreting waste products. "Metabolic flows and pathways" of materials and energy need to be considered when developing the framework. Urban succession compares the megacity to an ecosystem, in which a megacity utilizes the resources of a global economy to grow but may never "climax," unlike its biological counterparts (Decker, Elliot, and Smith 2002). A conflicting view is suggested by various authors who have looked at individual case studies (e.g., Mexico City [Ezcurra and Mazari-Hiriart 1996], ten Asian megacities [Brennan and Richardson 1989], and the growth of megacities in areas of high risk of earthquakes [Jackson 2006]). Megacities may be potential drivers for environmental change, which has been demonstrated through case studies for sharing best practice and linking with resources (Alfsen-Norodom et al. 2004). The impact of megacities on air pollution has also been closely studied with the conclusion that strong political power, policy, and public engagement are essential to reduce emissions (Molina and Molina 2004).

The vast array of literature for population metrics reveals the importance, relevance, and complexity of the megacity infrastructure. Epidemiological paradigms for meticulous methodology of data collection, analyses, interpretation, and dissemination are essential for externally validated results, which are comparable.

The sociodemographic status of populations has been measured at a city level in a variety of different projects, initiatives, and comparative studies, but the comparability of such data has also been questioned. How reliable are registers of births, deaths, or even population surveys? Births, migration, mortality, morbidity, disease occurrence of selected diseases pertinent for urban settings, health care, socioeconomic measures, cultural, environmental, healthy workforce, and social ecology are all important metrics.

The Criteria for Good Metrics

UN-HABITAT has stated that for any global indicator program to be successful, it is required to be sustainable, credible, understandable, timely, important, relevant, accessible, and have limited costs (United Nations Human Settlements Programme 2006). Metrics specific for megacities need to be consistent with these parameters. Most of the megacities are, and will continue to be, in developing countries where infrastructure and finances may hinder adequate metric collection, analyses, and monitoring (United Nations Human Settlements Programme 2010b). The current metrics measuring health and well-being in a megacity use the same principles of urban health monitoring and public health/population health metrics (Florey, Galea, and Wilson 2007). To measure health and well-being metrics for megacities, a new conceptual framework needs to be formulated, validated, piloted, evaluated, and applied. This chapter explores some of the key themes from the published literature pertaining to measuring health and well-being in the context of megacities.

The principles for successful metrics highlighted by UN-HABITAT should be realized (United Nations Human Settlements Programme 2006). Further metrics—that is, comparability, validity, and utility for policy—also should be added to the list. Any proposed conceptual framework for megacity metrics involves many stages and is dependent on need.

Current Alternative Frameworks

A possible alternative framework is the Lalonde model, which states that fields of environment, human biology, lifestyle, and health care organization should be included (Lalonde 1981). However, the model does not allow for the effects of social exclusion, social capital, human ecology, and interaction of the fields. The health care organization field may include the interaction of policy, research, and practice pertaining to the political and social situation in the late 1970s in Canada, but is this model applicable to or even relevant for the twenty-first century, in a world with rapid urbanization, globalization, and unparalleled economic growth of the developing world (United Nations Human Settlements Programme 2009)? There has also been development in the role of a health and social care workforce with a paradigm shift to prevention of disease, self-care, and early intervention (Chen, Evans, and Evans 2006). The Dahlgren and Whitehead model describes the possible constructs on which metrics could be based, similar to Lalonde, but with more of the social determinants included (Dahlgren and Whitehead 1991). These public health models reflect the need for not only health systems to be addressed, but also the wider determinants of health, inequalities or disparities in health, disease prevention, promotion of a healthy workforce, and healthy aging (Lawrence 2002; Richard 2008).

It is vital to review current frameworks and metrics for urban areas to determine which indicators are essential or desirable, accessible and reliable, and which need further development. The various domains give rise to different perspectives. Health, economy, and well-being are inextricably linked.

The most recent UN-HABITAT report has shown the economic power of megacities. For example, the world's largest 40 megaregions account for "66% of all economic activity and about 85% of technological and scientific innovation," and "the five largest cities in India and China now account for 50% of those countries' wealth" (United Nations Human Settlements Programme 2010b). Richardson suggests that the "declining rates of megacity growth may reflect declining productivity advantages" so there are "diseconomies of scale" in megacities (Richardson 1989). The conflicting evidence supporting the growth or decline of megacities has stimulated commentaries to improve megacity population estimates and projections (Brockerhoff 2000). This highlights the need for an infrastructure that can collect data on metrics over time to highlight inefficiencies and early warning systems.

Florey et al. investigated the macrosocial determinants of population health in which the interaction of global health with national and community level are eloquently described from an "epidemiological perspective" (Florey, Galea, and Wilson

2007). Interaction between the global issues affecting national infrastructure and then communities is demonstrated through exemplars such as diarrheal mortality rates, maternal mortality rates, and SARS (Florey, Galea, and Wilson 2007).

There are many initiatives for frameworks and metrics that are pertinent to specific continents, countries, regions, and cities. These have not been considered, as they are designed: for example, the European Urban Health Indicator System and Urban Audit project in Europe, (Heller 2008, Urban Audit 2007), the Big Cities project in the United States (Benbow 2007), and a vast number of regional- and city-specific case studies. Many disciplines that are pertinent to urban health also have frameworks and metrics to support data collection or policy analysis; for example, environmental challenges (European Environment Agency 2009), air and water quality (Duh et al. 2008), healthy weights (Raine et al. 2008), and urban planning (International Society of City and Regional Planners 2008).

Transcontinental and multidisciplinary projects have been listed below to summarize the current frameworks and metrics in use or under development.

UN-HABITAT

UN-HABITAT regularly collates metrics as part of its statistics program, urban indicator program, and best practice program. The programs also feed in to the Millennium Goals (United Nations 1990). The definitions used to describe the boundaries are split into three distinct entities:

- Urban agglomeration is defined as the built-up or densely populated area containing the city proper, suburbs, and continuously settled commuter areas.
- Metropolitan area is the set of formal local government areas which are normally taken to comprise the urban area as a whole and its primary commuter areas.
- City proper is the single political jurisdiction which contains the historical city centre. (United Nations Human Settlements Programme 2004, p. 5)

The urban indicators program focuses on the domains of shelter, social development and eradication of poverty, environmental management, economic development, and governance (Table 5.1). There are 20 key indicators relevant for policy, 9 checklists for nonquantitative metrics, and 13 extensive indicators for in-depth analysis. Each indicator has a comprehensive definition and denominator to allow comparable data to be used in any analyses. There is a global, local, and regional urban observatory network to ensure data are collected

Table 5.1 UN-HABITAT List of Urban Indicators, by Domain

	Indicator
Shelter	Key indicator 1: Durable structures
	Key indicator 2: Overcrowding
	Key indicator 3: Secure tenure
	Key indicator 4: Access to safe water
	Key indicator 5: Access to improved sanitation
	Key indicator 6: Connection to services
	Extensive indicator 1: Housing price and rent-to-income
	Extensive indicator 2: Authorized housing
	Extensive indicator 3: Evictions
	Extensive indicator 4: Land price-to-income
	Checklist 1: Right to adequate housing
	Checklist 2: Housing finance
Social development and eradication of poverty	Key indicator 7: Under-five mortality
	Key indicator 8: Homicides
	Key indicator 9: Poor households
	Key indicator 10: Literacy
	Extensive indicator 5: HIV prevalence
	Extensive indicator 6: School enrollment
	Extensive indicator 7: Women counselors
	Checklist 3: Urban violence
	Checklist 4: Gender inclusion
Environmental management	Key indicator 11: Urban population growth
	Key indicator 12: Planned settlements
	Key indicator 13: Price of water
	Key indicator 14: Wastewater treated
	Key indicator 15: Solid waste disposal
	Key indicator 16: Travel time
	Extensive indicator 8: Water consumption
	Extensive indicator 9: Regular solid waste collection
	Extensive indicator 10: Houses in hazardous locations
	Extensive indicator 11: Transport modes
	Checklist 5: Disaster prevention and mitigation instruments
	Checklist 6: Local environmental plans
Economic development	Key indicator 17: Informal employment
	Key indicator 18: City product
	Key indicator 19: Unemployment
Governance	Key indicator 20: Local government revenue
	Checklist 7: Decentralization
	Checklist 8: Citizens' participation
	Extensive indicator 12: Voters' participation
	Extensive indicator 13: Civic associations
	Checklist 9: Transparency and accountability

Source: United Nations Human Settlements Programme 2004.

to the same definitions and reflected into sustainable policy (United Nations Human Settlements Programme 2010a). UN-HABITAT produces a number of reports, databases, and analyses of the statistics which can all be sourced from the Web site (United Nations Human Settlements Programme 2004, 2006, 2009, 2010a,b). The inclusion of these indicators is relevant to the mission and goals of UN-HABITAT for sustainability and adequate shelter for all. The framework is not specific for health or public health and so is limited in terms of what data are captured for megacity metrics. UN-HABITAT does have a robust and generalizable definition for all megacities to determine the boundaries for metrics, and this has been in use for more than 10 years.

Organisation for Economic Co-operation and Development

For over 40 years, the OECD has provided statistics for governments to compare, share, and coordinate policy (Organisation for Economic Co-operation and Development 2010). At present, there are 32 member countries and over 70 nonmember countries in the organization. There are 31 indicators available in 90 metropolitan areas including the megacities of New York, Los Angeles, London, Istanbul, Paris, Osaka, Mexico City, Seoul, and Tokyo (Table 5.2). The Working Party on Territorial Policy in Urban Areas assesses trends to achieve sustainable urban development, increase competitiveness, and to enhance the capacity of urban governments. Nine megacities are located within the member and nonmember states of the OECD, and recently these states have focused on cities and climate change (Organisation for Economic Co-operation and Development 2009).

The OECD also does not solely focus on the health indicators for megacity metrics. They do include economic, population demography, employment, and climate change indicators that are important for the health of megacity populations.

The Global City Indicators Program

The World Bank recognized the need for a "standardized system for data collection" for evidence-based policymaking at a city level. In 2008, the Global City Indicators Program (GCIP) was established and now has 100 cities included in the collaboration. Definitions for each indicator are available to allow cities to input their own data on a web-based platform and make comparisons with other cities. Pilot cities developed and selected the indicators that are listed in "themes" (Table 5.3). There is a web-based membership program to attract

Table 5.2 Organisation for Economic Co-operation and Development Urban Indicator Set 2000–2007, by Domain

	Indicator
Population and density	Total population
	Total aged 0–14 years
	Total aged 15–64 years
	Total aged 65 years and over
	Males/females total
	Males/females aged 0–14 years
	Males/females aged 15–64 years
	Males/females aged 65 years and older
	Regional surface
	Population density
	Annual average population
	Elderly dependency rate
Employment	Labor force
	Employment
	Unemployment
	Unemployment rate
	Participation rate
	Employment rate
Economic development	Gross domestic product (GDP) in millions of current prices
	GDP in millions of US dollars purchasing power parity
	GDP in millions of constant prices (base 2000)
	Per capita GDP in current prices
	Per capita GDP in US dollars purchasing power parity
	Per capita GDP in constant prices (base 2000)
	Percent patent applications per million population

Source: Organisation for Economic Co-operation and Development 2010.

further membership. Data quality and assurance is the responsibility of each city in the program (Daniels 2010). Data are assumed to be comparable by GCIP because each city uses the same definition. However, information on standardized methodologies for each indicator and which boundaries are used for each city are not available for scrutiny. If cities can decide the boundaries then there may be noncomparable results due to some cities entering data as a city proper and others as an agglomeration. However, the list of indicators is comprehensive and standardized methodology is being developed, together with new indicators.

Table 5.3 Global City Indicators Program Indicators Currently in Use and Under Development, by Domain

	Indicator
City services	
Education	Student/teacher ratio
	Percentage of school-aged children enrolled in schools, by gender
	Percentage of children completing primary and secondary education: survival rate
Energy	Percentage of city population with authorized electrical service
	Total electrical use per capita (kilowatt/hour)
	Total residential electrical use per capita
	Average number of electrical interruptions per customer per year
	Average length of electrical interruptions (in hours)
	Total Energy Use Index*
Finance	Debt service ratio (debt service expenditure as a percent of a municipality's own-source revenue)
	Tax collected as percentage of tax billed
	Own-source revenue as a percentage of total revenues
	Capital spending as a percentage of total finance expenditures
Fire and emergency response	Number of firefighters per 100,000 population
	Response time for fire department from initial call
	Number of fire-related deaths per 100,000 population
Solid waste	Percentage of city population with regular solid waste collection
	Percentage of city's solid waste disposed of in an incinerator
	Percentage of city's solid waste recycled
	Percentage of city's solid waste burned openly
	Percentage of city's solid waste disposed of in an open dump
	Percentage of city's solid waste disposed of in a sanitary landfill
	Percentage of city's solid waste disposed of by other means
Transportation	Miles of high-capacity public transit system per 100,000 population
	Number of two-wheel motorized vehicles per capita
	Miles of light passenger transit system per 100,000 population
	Commercial air connectivity (number of nonstop commercial air destinations)
	Number of personal automobiles per capita
	Transportation fatalities per 100,000 population
	Annual number of public transit trips per capita
	Urban Accessibility Index*
Quality of life	
Urban planning	Jobs/housing ratio
	Aerial size of informal settlements as a percent of city area
	Green area (hectares) per 100,000 population
Wastewater	Percentage of city's wastewater receiving primary treatment
	Percentage of city's wastewater that has received no treatment
	Percentage of city's wastewater receiving secondary treatment
	Percentage of city's wastewater receiving tertiary treatment

(continued on next page)

Table 5.3   (continued)

Water	Water percentage of city population with potable water supply service
	Total water consumption per capita
	Domestic water consumption per capita
	Percentage of water loss
	Percentage of city population with sustainable access to an improved water source
	Average annual hours of water service interruption per household
	Water Quality Index*
Governance	Percentage of women employed in the city government workforce
	Governance Index*
Health	Number of in-patient hospital beds per 100,000 population
	Number of nursing and midwifery personnel per 100,000 population
	Number of physicians per 100,000 population
	Average life expectancy
	Under age five mortality per 1,000 live births
Recreation	Square meters of public indoor recreation facility space per capita
	Square meters of public outdoor recreation facility space per capita
	Recreation and Culture Index*
Safety	Number of police officers per 100,000 population
	Violent crime rate per 100,000 population
	Number of homicides per 100,000 population
Civic engagement	Voter participation in last municipal election (as a percent of eligible voters)
	Citizen's representation: number of local officials elected to office per 100,000 population
Culture	Percentage of jobs in the cultural sector
Economy	City product per capita
	Percentage of persons in full-time employment
	City unemployment rate
	Competitiveness Index*
Environment	PM_{10} concentration
	Greenhouse gas emissions measured in tons per capita
	Greenhouse Gas Index*
Shelter	Percentage of city population living in slums
	Number of households that exist without registered legal titles
	Number of homeless people per 100,000 population
Social equity	Percentage of city population living in poverty
	Social Capital Index*
Subjective well-being	Subjective Well-Being Index*
Technology and innovation	Number of Internet connections per 100,000 population
	Number of telephones (landlines and cell phones) per 100,000 population
	Number of new patents per 100,000 per year
	Number of higher education degrees per 100,000
	Technology Creativity Index*

Source: Daniels 2010.

*Under development.

Table 5.4   World Cities Project Indicators for Current and Future Projects, by Domain

	Indicator
Public health infrastructure	Health status
	Public health risks
	Epidemiological surveillance systems, control mechanisms, and emergency response
Aging and long-term care	Health status of those older than 65 years and 85 years
	Housing arrangements
	Institutional care
	Health and social services
Coronary heart disease	Mortality
	Morbidity
	Treatment patterns
	Health insurance coverage
Avoidable hospital conditions	By age, neighborhood, and ethnicity
Patterns of infant mortality	By neighborhood

Source: Rodwin and Gusmano 2002.

World Cities Project

Urban public health metrics have been investigated by the World Cities Project (WCP) using New York, London, Paris, and Tokyo as exemplars for studying public health infrastructure, health status, and quality of life. The aim of the project is to compare the public health infrastructure, indicators for health status, and health system in the four cities (Table 5.4). The WCP uses the boundaries of the "urban core" which equates to the "city proper" for their metrics.

Conceptual Framework for Megacity Metrics

It is important to develop metrics for megacities in the twenty-first century, and it can be done by linking current metrics with the paradigms highlighted by UN-HABITAT. A number of tasks require completion before metrics can be collected:

1. Define the boundary of the megacity
2. Define the population to be investigated
3. Consider which metrics are important for the megacity
4. Assess how accessible data are for metrics
5. Assess the cost for data collection

6. Assess the comparability of any data collected either within or between megacities

7. Assess the reliability of the sources of data

8. Consider the purpose of collecting metrics—that is, for policy, governance, surveillance, benchmarking, or sharing good practice

Any metrics collected for a megacity need to be in the context of megaregional, national, and global metrics. Similar metrics at different levels may help validate the megacity metrics by determining what is required at a megacity level.

Figure 5.1 demonstrates a proposed framework with the initial prerequisites of definition of population and boundary. Each domain is highlighted in the central box. The individual indicator choice is dependent on the questions being asked. The concurrent themes of governance, policy, and surveillance are essential for the utility of the domains and indicators. Each domain needs, if possible, to be contextualized in relation to the megacity, national, and global indicators. Benchmarking and sharing good practices should be encouraged. Data collection, analyses, and

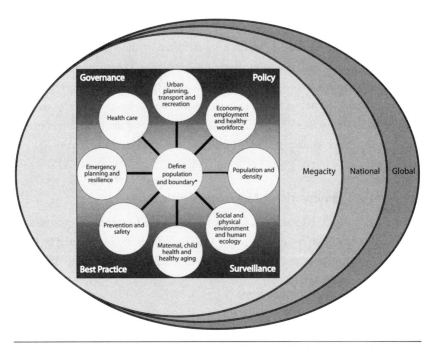

*Assess accessibility and cost of collecting data; assess comparability and validity of data collected and sources accessed.

Figure 5.1 Megacity metric conceptual framework.

dissemination are costly processes and should only be commenced with a clear question and relevance for health and well-being gain. Megacity metrics should hold to this paradigm.

Next Steps

Epidemiological enquiry is increasingly concerned with the impact that the environment has on the health of individuals and populations. Therefore, to prepare for the future, it is vital to focus on the wider determinants of health and social environment in megacities—that is, urban health and well-being. Urban health and well-being relies on multidisciplinary, multiagency, vertical, and horizontal policymaking together with community participation and engagement (Lawrence 2002, 2008; Testi and Ivaldi 2009). This includes all aspects of health but also social care, transport, waste management, crime and disorder, city planning, and communities. It requires partnership working between civil society, industry, health and social care professionals, governments (local, regional, and national), and nongovernmental organizations, including the voluntary sector.

Options for operationalization include:

- Use of existing initiatives, for example, GCIP, UN-HABITAT, and OECD expanded to include all megacities
  - The advantages of this approach would be capitalizing on existing successes and learning from previous challenges. Sustainability and credibility would be maximized. The relevant important, accessible, and timely metrics for each megacity could initially be utilized while the development of new indicators took place.
  - The disadvantages include requiring expansion of the existing structures, magnifying the existing limitations in the structures, and lessening of innovation.
- Developing new initiatives
  - The advantages of this approach would be the opportunity to create tailor-made initiatives, a quicker response to identified needs, new ideas, and innovation.
  - The disadvantages include new funding streams required, competition for funding between new initiatives, less track record leading to difficulty assessing capacity, or resource requirement of new structures.

Collecting data at a megacity level requires commitment of time and resources from governments, nongovernment organizations, and other bodies. Projects may have to rely on various organizations, for example, WHO, UN-HABITAT, the World Bank, research funding bodies, local and national governments, nongovernment organizations, and the voluntary sector for either using current or developing new initiatives. Researchers, politicians, and other professionals need to devise novel and innovative ways of accessing resources in this difficult economic time. Involvement of civil society should be a major contributing factor in establishing metrics, for lobbying, and to help determine need. Above all else, collection of data should only be performed for health gain.

Summary

The majority of the world's population now lives in urban areas, and almost 10% live in megacities, the majority of which are in developing countries. The disparities and inequalities in health outcomes within a megacity are comparable with the differences between the developed and developing world. In order to determine what metrics to collect, it is important to understand the reasons behind the data collection and to have adequately defined the megacity.

The conceptual framework proposed in this chapter relies on researchers, policymakers, and civil society working together to determine needs and future resources to collect metrics for the advancement of health and well-being in megacities. There should always be a need and resources to support any metrics and there should be resultant health gains for the populations who have provided the resources for such endeavours.

Acknowledgments

I would like to thank Annie Harrison, James Higgerson, and Will Morton for their help in the preparation of this manuscript.

References

Alfsen-Norodom C, Boehme SE, Clemants S, et al. 2004. Managing the megacity for global sustainability: the New York metropolitan region as an urban biosphere reserve. *Ann N Y Acad Sci*. 1023:125–141.

Benbow N, editor. 2007. Big Cities Health Inventory: the Health of Urban USA. Washington, DC: U.S. National Association of County and City Health Officials. Available at: http://www.who.or.jp/urbanheart/US_Big_Cities_Healt_Inventory_2007. pdf. Accessed January 11, 2011.

Brennan EM, Richardson HW. 1989. Asian megacity characteristics, problems, and policies. *Int Reg Sci Rev.* 12:117–129.

Brockerhoff M. 2000. The urban demographic revolution. *Popul Today.* 28:1–2.

Bugliarello, G. 1999. Megacities and the developing world. *The Bridge.* 29:19–26.

Chen L, Evans D, Evans T. 2006. *World Health Report 2006: Working Together for Health.* Geneva, Switzerland: World Health Organization. Available at http://www.who.int/ whr/2006/whr06_en.pdf. Accessed January 11, 2011.

Dahlgren G, Whitehead M. 1991. Policies and strategies to promote social equity in health. Geneva, Switzerland: World Health Organization. Available at: http://www. framtidsstudier.se/filebank/files/20080109$110739$fil$mZ8UVQv2wQFShMRF6cuT. pdf. Accessed January 11, 2011.

Daniels J. 2010. Global City Indicators home page. Toronto, Ontario: University of Toronto. Available at: http://www.cityindicators.org. Accessed January 11, 2011.

Decker EH, Elliott S, Smith FA. 2002. Megacities and the environment. *Sci World J.* 374–86.

Duh JD, Shandas V, Chang H, George LA. 2008. Rates of urbanization and the resiliency of air and water quality. *Sci Total Environ.* 400:238–256.

European Environment Agency (EEA). EEA home page. 2010. Copenhagen, Denmark: European Union. Available at: http://www.eea.europa.eu. Accessed January 11, 2011.

Ezcurra E, Mazari-Hiriart M. 1996. Are megacities viable? A cautionary tale from Mexico City. *Environment.* 38:6–35.

Florey LS, Galea S, Wilson ML. 2007. Macrosocial determinants of health in the context of globalization. In: Galea S, editor. *Macrosocial Determinants of Population Health.* New York, NY: Springer:15–51.

Galea S, Vlahov D. 2005. Urban health: evidence, challenges, and directions. *Annu Rev Public Health.* 26:341–365.

Galea S, Vlahov D, Sisco S. 2003. The Second Annual International Conference on Urban Health. October 15–18. *J Urban Health*. 80(3 Suppl 1):II1–II2.

Heller RF, Verma A, Patterson L. 2008. EURO-URHIS Final Report. The EURO-URHIS Project. Available at: http://www.urhis.eu/pdfs/REPORT_Final_01.pdf. Accessed February 11, 2011.

International Society of City and Regional Planners (ISOCARP) Research Team. 2008. Home page. Geneva, Switzerland: World Health Organization. Available at: http://www.isocarp.org. Accessed January 11, 2011.

Jackson J. 2006. Fatal attraction: living with earthquakes, the growth of villages into megacities and earthquake vulnerability in the modern world. *Phil Trans Roy Soc London Ser A*. 364:1911–1925.

Kamal-Chaoui L, Robert A. 2009. Competitive cities and climate change. Paris, France: Organisation for Economic Co-operation and Development. Available at: http://www.oecd-ilibrary.org/content/workingpaper/218830433146. Accessed January 11, 2011.

Kraas F. 2008. Megacities as global risk areas. *Urban Ecology*. 147:6–15.

Lalonde M. 1981. A new perspective on the health of Canadians: a working document. Ottawa, Ontario: Government of Canada. Available at: http://www.phac-aspc.gc.ca/ph-sp/pdf/perspect-eng.pdf. Accessed January 11, 2011.

Lawrence RJ. 2002. Human ecology and its applications. *Landscape Urban Plann*. 987:1–10.

Lawrence RJ. 2008. Urban environmental health indicators: appraisal and policy directives. *Rev Environ Health*. 23:299–326.

McGranhan G. 2007. Urban environments, wealth and health: shifting burdens and possible response in low and middle-income nations. Human Settlements Working Paper Series, Urban Environments No. 1. London, England: International Institute for Environment and Development. Available at: http://www.iied.org/pubs/display.php?o=10553IIED. Accessed January 11, 2011.

Molina MJ, Molina L. 2004. Megacities and atmospheric pollution. *J Air Waste Manag Assoc*. 54:644–680.

Mutatkar RK. 1995. Public health problems of urbanization. *Soc Sci Med*. 41:977–981.

Organisation for Economic Co-operation and Development (OECD). 2010. Home page. Paris, France: OECD. Available at http://www.oecd.org. Accessed January 11, 2011.

Raine K, Spence JC, Church J, et al. 2008. *State of the Evidence Review on Urban Health and Healthy Weights*. Ottawa, Ontario: Canadian Institute for Health Information. Available at: http://secure.cihi.ca/cihiweb/products/Urban%20Health%20and%20 Healthy%20Weights.pdf. Accessed January 11, 2011.

Richards L, Gauvin L, Gosselin C, LaForest S. 2009. Staying connected: neighbourhood correlates of social participation among older adults living in an urban environment in Montreal, Quebec. *Health Promotion International.* 24:46–57.

Richardson HW. 1989. The big, bad city: mega-city myth? *Third World Plann Rev.* 11:355–372.

Riva M, Curtis S, Gauvin L, Fagg J. 2009. Unravelling the extent of inequalities in health across urban and rural areas: evidence from a national sample in England. *Soc Sci Med.* 68:654–663.

Rodwin VG, Gusmano MK. 2002. The World Cities Project: rationale, organization, and design for comparison of megacity health systems. *J Urban Health.* 79:445–463.

Testi A, Ivaldi E. 2009. Material versus social deprivation and health: a case study of an urban area. *Eur J Health Econ.* 10:323–328.

United Nations. 1990. United Nations Millennium Development Goals home page. New York, NY: United Nations. Available at: http://www.un.org/millenniumgoals. Accessed January 11, 2011.

United Nations Human Settlements Programme (UN-HABITAT). 2004. Urban Indicator Guidelines: Monitoring the Habitat Agenda and the Millennium Development Goals. Nairobi, Kenya: UN-HABITAT. Available at: http://ww2.un-habitat.org/programmes/guo/documents/urban_indicators_guidelines.pdf. Accessed September 1, 2010.

United Nations Human Settlements Programme (UN-HABITAT). 2006. Current Status of City Indicators: Part of a Study to Assist Cities in Developing an Integrated Approach for Measuring and Monitoring City Performance. Discussion paper. Nairobi, Kenya: UN-HABITAT. Available at: http://www.cityindicators.org/Deliverables/ Discussion%20Document%20Chapters%201%20to%203_11-28-2007-135233.pdf. Accessed September 1, 2010.

United Nations Human Settlements Programme (UN-HABITAT). 2009. Global Report on Human Settlements 2009: Planning Sustainable Cities. Nairobi, Kenya: UN-HABITAT. Available at: http://www.unchs.org/downloads/docs/GRHS2009/GRHS.2009.pdf. Accessed September 1, 2010.

United Nations Human Settlements Programme (UN-HABITAT). 2010a. State of the World's Cities 2010/2011: Bridging the Urban Divide. Nairobi, Kenya: UN-HABITAT. Available at: http://www.unhabitat.org/pmss/listItemDetails.aspx?publicationID=2917. Accessed September 1, 2010.

United Nations Human Settlements Programme (UN-HABITAT). 2010b. UN-HABITAT home page. UN-HABITAT, Nairobi, Kenya. Available at: http://www.unhabitat.org/categories.asp?catid=9. Accessed September 1, 2010.

United Nations Population Division. 2008. Urban and Rural Areas 2007. New York, NY United Nations. Available at: http://www.un.org/esa/population/publications/wup2007/2007_urban_rural_chart.pdf. Accessed February 16, 2011.

Urban Audit. 2007. Urban Audit home page. Brussels, Belgium: European Commission. Available at: http://www.urbanaudit.org. Accessed January 11, 2011.

Vlahov D, Galea S. 2003. Urban health: a new discipline. *Lancet*. 362:1091–1092.

Vlahov D, Galea S, Gibble E, Freudenberg N. 2005. Perspectives on urban conditions and population health. *Cad Saude Publica*. 21:949–957.

Whiteis DG. 1998. Third-world medicine in first-world cities: capital accumulation, uneven development and public health. *Soc Sci Med*. 47:795–808.

6

Environmental Health and Megacities

Zafar Fatmi, MBBS, FCPS, and Gregory Pappas, MD, PhD

THE GROWTH OF MEGACITIES in the competitive global economy has pushed the limits of what is called the "built environment," with serious consequences for human populations and the natural environment. The recent growth of massive human settlements in response to hyperindustrialization and the rapid expansion of transportation systems is occurring in a context largely devoid of environmental controls. Earlier waves of industrialization in Europe, the United States, and the Soviet Union took place before the development of knowledge, systems, and technology that can limit environmental degradation. However, water and sewage systems and regulation of building construction were eventually adopted in the older megacities in these places, with demonstrated benefits for the health of their populations (Garb 2003; Peterson 1979). Public action to improve housing, sanitation, and working conditions corrected the unsafe living conditions, impure water, and pollution that were common in European and U.S. cities of the nineteenth century (Fairchild et al. 2010). By contrast, the massive scale of current global economic development has had devastating consequences on environments around the world despite the repeated airing of concerns at global summits. Today, the majority of megacities have not benefited from the lessons learned by older megacities. Health care, hospitals, and public health are overwhelmed by the consequences of built environments, characterized by lack of adequate sewage systems, presence of toxins in the air and water, and other health hazards. The seriousness of these problems has raised concerns about the very sustainability of megacities in the future (Saier 2008).

This chapter begins with a discussion of the built environment—an inclusive concept with many links to public health (Renalds, Smith, and Hale 2010). A few megacities, primarily older ones and those with more resources available, have been able to deal successfully with a variety of environmental challenges. Their unique experiences can help guide newer megacities which are struggling with similar issues (McMichael 2000). Megacities have environmental problems related to (1) size and population density, (2) population growth rates, (3) exposure to environmental health hazards, and (4) lack of systems that are able to address environmental and public health hazards.

Health problems caused by environmental hazards in the air and water are major issues in most megacities and are the focus of this chapter. After a review of successful modalities of environmental protection that have been developed for megacities, we describe the barriers to needed reforms. Solutions to problems of environmental hazards in megacities are discussed in the context of the community and social movements needed to make reform possible. Examination of issues of environmental health in megacities has been held back, in part, by the lack of available studies; much of the research in less-developed countries has been focused on rural health issues. With the recent development of megacities around the world, however, the research focus of social science is shifting toward urban populations.

The Built Environment

The term "built environment" refers to products and processes across the entire range of man-made surroundings related to human activities (Bartuska 2007). The built environment has profound direct effects on human health and also influences it indirectly by affecting the natural environment. Public health issues regarding built environments focus on drinking water and sanitation, housing, transportation, the structure of neighborhoods, and the proximity and concentration of industrial sites.

Currently, megacities occupy 2% of the land area of the planet and include 7% of the world's population—approximately 450 million people. However, the ecological footprints of megacities are much bigger areas and include more than just the specified land area of a city; they represent the amount of productive land and sea area needed to regenerate the resources a megacity consumes and to absorb and render harmless the enormous wastes of the megacity. The ecological footprint of London, for example, is roughly 60 times the area of the city itself.

Descriptions of built-up areas—areas with a high density of structures—are an important way to view megacities. For example, some cities have grown vertically, whereas others have grown horizontally. The reasons for the development of these forms vary but are usually related to geographical, political, and macro- or microeconomic influences (Shi et al. 2009). The optimal structural form for megacities is still under consideration and the subject needs fresh inquiry (Gordon and Richardson 1997). The built-up area of Paris is five times that of Cairo; the population in Cairo, on the other hand, is seven times that of Paris. Thus, Cairo has a substantially higher population density. Although data are limited, some exposure to health hazards may be greater in vertical cities (e.g., air and water pollution). On the other hand, the distances traveled in horizontal cities makes them less efficient and are associated with a different pattern of health risks.

The built environment has been associated with the development of sedentary patterns of activity, obesity, and cardiovascular diseases. Patterns of travel, proximity to sources of healthy foods, and availability of recreational spaces are thought to influence these patterns (Commission on Social Determinants of Health 2008; Lovasi et al. 2008). Studies have documented links between the built environment, nonmotorized travel, and physical activity (Handy 2005; Boarnet, Greenwald, and MacMillan 2008); that is, the built environment can either encourage or discourage walking and bicycle use. Proximity to retailers that supply healthy foods is thought to encourage healthy eating, although recent studies are less conclusive (Lovasi et al. 2009). Likewise, proximity to places that sell unhealthy foods (and alcohol) may encourage poor diet and health (Ashley, Mikkelsen, and Cohen 2008). Access to recreation may contribute to greater physical activity and better health. Evidence from the United States suggests that proximity to places appropriate for exercise increases physical activity (Krizek, El-Geneidy, and Thompson 2007). Although most of these studies have been carried out in resource-rich areas where cardiovascular disease has existed at high levels for a long time, rising levels of cardiovascular disease in megacities around the world, particularly Asian megacities, suggests that people living in the new megacities are being adversely affected in similar ways.

Hazards of Population Size, Density, and Growth Rate

In megacities, population size, density, and growth rates, in conjunction with some types of construction, combine to create complex environmental hazards. Although the hazards of specific chemical and physical factors may exist in other settings (both urban and rural), the magnitude of these factors and their multiplier effects in megacities is largely unprecedented. Environmental assessment of risk from one or two factories next to a small town is substantially different from environmental assessment of risk from the presence of hundreds of industrial facilities, vehicular traffic, and other environmental hazards found in megacities. The concentration of large populations themselves poses enormous problems, including adequate supplies of drinking water, management of solid waste, and control of air pollution. As a result, the combined effect of environmental risks on the health of populations in megacities is difficult to assess.

Although the rapid pace of population growth and social change in megacities over the past few decades makes them unique, it has also created substantial environmental and social problems. Between 1950 and 2005, New York City grew by just 5.1%, whereas Lagos grew by 4,761%. Karachi's population, which was half a million in 1947, grew to more than 15 million during the subsequent 50 years. Environmental resources and human and management capacities have lagged far behind the pace of population growth. Most of the new megacities have limited human and organizational resources with which to plan and implement programs to deal with environmental problems. In many cases, this has led to the rapid deterioration of environments. In older megacities, planning was used to solve urban conflicts. Strategic and structural approaches to problems were aimed at integration of regional and city interests through a balance of economic and physical solutions (Clarke 1985). New megacities did not have the benefit of sufficient time to "plan" balanced strategies to deal with environmental problems—they expanded too rapidly. Lack of urban planning has contributed to the forms development has taken in these megacities, as well as the associated environmental and public health problems. Megacities in less-developed countries frequently lack adequate planning and, even when planning is carried out, global market forces often blocked implementation of plans or take control of the planning process.

Changes during the past few decades have resulted not only in increased size of cities, but also in increased industrialization and the development of transportation systems relying on motorized vehicles. The resulting production of hazardous wastes has created concentrations of pollutants that have had a negative impact on health (Kjellstrom et al. 2007). The current pace of technological development is adding increasing numbers of chemicals and substances into the environment, many with unknown hazards. Approximately 1,000 new synthetic chemical substances are invented every year. In 1984, there were 3,350 pesticides, 3,410 cosmetics, 8,627 food additives, and 1,815 therapeutic medicines (National Research Council 1984). The effects on human health of most of these synthetic organic chemicals released into the environment have not been tested. The reason for this is the large cost and time required to carry out these investigations.

Megacities, as the leading edge of economic development, are frequently the first places these chemicals appear. A review of studies of urban ecosystems (i.e., soils in urban areas) published over the past ten years suggests that although lead is still the major concern, other materials with known hazards are copper, zinc, nickel, chromium, arsenic, cadmium, and mercury. New contaminants with unknown toxicities are on the rise in many megacities; these include vehicle-related platinum, rhodium, and palladium (Biasioli, Barberis, and Ajmone-Marsan 2006). Legislation on soil limits for trace metals and their monitoring are a new trend for megacities. The particular combinations of hazards and chemicals that occur in megacities are not well studied, but the potential burden of disease is enormous.

Unequal Hazards

The rapid rate of population growth and social change in megacities has been accompanied by increasing social and economic inequalities. These inequalities have a spatial dimension. Older megacities have been transformed so that unequal distribution of environmental hazards has become part of the urban landscape. Unequal exposure to pollution and other environmental hazards has led to the development of a global literature on "environmental justice" (Sandler and Pezzullo 2007; Redwood et al. 2010). There is a near-consensus that social class and race/ethnicity correlate with the distribution of environmental hazards (Olden 2009; Morrison 2009). Lower-income neighborhoods are more likely to be near environmental hazards (Downey 2007). However, the link between proximity to specific environmental hazards and the occurrence of specific adverse health outcomes is more difficult to establish (Committee on Environmental Justice 1999; Ritz et al. 2002).

The rapid increase in urbanization and poverty has led to development of squatter settlements in the newer megacities. The *favelas* in Brazil, *jhopar patti* in India, *kampungs* in Indonesia, *colonias* in Mexico, *villas miséria* in Argentina, and *katchi abadis* in Pakistan all have similar characteristics. Squatter settlements comprise 20 to 60% of populations in most megacities in less-developed countries. Discussion of the environmental health of megacities cannot be complete without inclusion of squatter settlements; these are unplanned settlements and therefore frequently are without legal status (Srinivas 2007). The environmental and health literature suggests that housing is very poorly constructed in these settlements, creating many health hazards and dangers (Takano et al. 2002).

Orangi, in Karachi, Pakistan, and Dharavi, in Mumbai, India, compete as Asia's largest squatter settlements. In Karachi, *katchi abadis* have no drinking water or sewers; in Mumbai, millions are born, live, and die on the streets, never having a home (Mehta 2004). Yet both Karachi and Mumbai are economic powerhouses, contributing substantially—35 to 60% of revenues—to the economic activity of their respective countries (Rafique 1991). The governance, security, and service issues of squatter settlements associated with these megacities are largely neglected, because land occupancy is frequently illegal and residents have no voting rights or formal rights to services.

The Need for Systems to Respond to Environmental Hazards

Older megacities in resource-rich settings, such as New York City, London, and Tokyo, have developed infrastructures—technologies, bureaucracies, policies, and procedures—to avoid or reverse health problems arising from environmental hazards (Jacobs 1961). The evolution of sewage control in London and other nineteenth-century cities is well documented (Halliday 1999; Burian et al. 2000). Similarly, controls have been implemented in many megacities to reduce the hazards of air pollution. However, the rapid growth of many of the new megacities has outstripped their capacity to deal with environmental hazards. Inadequate and inefficient municipal systems have not been able to keep up with population growth, industrial development, and technological change. Critical infrastructures involved with provision of drinking water and disposal of solid wastes in most megacities are deteriorating because of age and because their burdens exceed designed capacity. Infrastructures associated with transportation suffer from poor planning and lack of planning, which, in the face of population growth, leads to environmental hazards (Amekudzi, Thomas-Mobley, and Ross 2007; Morichi 2009). The spatial restructuring of older megacities and the development of new ones have led to longer transportation routes and increased dependence on motorized vehicles. In many countries, government systems to regulate industrial pollution are poorly developed or have fallen behind the rapid changes in industry over the past few decades. Although these problems also occur in smaller urban settings, the enormous scale of these problems in megacities creates unique challenges.

Neoliberalism, called the "Washington Consensus" by some, has promoted deregulation as a global policy that has impeded municipal governments and national bodies from adopting successful approaches—standards, monitoring, and enforcement programs—that could help control environmental degradation (Besley and Zagha 2005). The adverse effects of open trade policies on environments in less-developed countries was predicted by both economists and environmentalists. The neoliberal assumption behind much of the policy over the past few decades—that economic growth would be accompanied by increasing environmental quality—was more a hope than a reality (Michael 1996). The same companies that successfully controlled pollution in countries with strong regulatory systems are also major polluters in less-developed countries. Global industries are neither the only nor the worst polluters. The huge numbers of microindustries in megacities, along with trash burning in cities that lack adequate systems for solid waste disposal, create pollution on an enormous scale in some megacities. These environmental hazards exist in close proximity to housing areas, particularly slums in which recent migrants to the city reside. Megacities are magnets for the poor and poorly educated populations that have no role in the global economy, and huge slums with major environmental hazards have become the symbol of many megacities.

Water, Megacities, and Health

Water is a useful focus for considering the environmental health issues present in megacities. Increasing demand for water resulting from industrialization and population growth, as well as overall lack of water and poor water quality in many cities, has led to health problems including dehydration, cholera and other diarrheal diseases, parasites, and skin infections. In addition to biological contaminants, there is growing and long-term exposure of residents in megacities to hazardous chemicals in water because of groundwater contamination from industrial and residential areas. Chromium, lead, nickel, arsenic, and salt components in water have serious long-term health effects (Rahman, Lee, and Khan 1997). Poor water management systems for residents create multiple health problems in the complex built environment of megacities. Limited water treatment capacities, lack of political will, and poor governance have led to the drainage of industrial effluents directly into water bodies. Such actions create huge burdens on the environment and adverse health consequences for residents of megacities. In most megacities in less-developed countries, industrial and residential effluent treatment capacity is between 5 and 15%.

The threat of poor quality water and water-borne diseases is not restricted to the populations of developing megacities, but these serve as breeding grounds for emerging and reemerging infectious diseases that can spread globally. Water-borne diseases migrate from developing countries' megacities to industrialized countries through visitors, immigrants, and refugees (Durand 2000).

Size of population has greater importance for water resources in megacities than in smaller urban or rural settlements. Large amounts of water must be diverted from rivers and lakes to meet the needs of megacities. In addition to population size and the limits posed by the availability of water itself, a major factor limiting the availability of water to megacities in less-developed countries is the lack of investment in water supply infrastructure (Van der Bruggen, Borghgraef, and Vinckier 2009). Even middle-income megacities like Istanbul are struggling to maintain drinking water standards and keep pace with population growth (Baykal, Tanik, and Gonenc 2000). In such instances, groundwater often becomes the major source of water for megacities, with the major investment made out of pocket by residents themselves. Groundwater is replenished by rainfall, but heavy use of groundwater by megacity populations and associated large-scale industry overwhelms the system. Extraction of groundwater now often exceeds the recharge rate in aquifers. Water table levels fall, causing increased pumping costs, lower water quality, and eventual exhaustion of the supply. The lessons of ancient cities made extinct by lack of an adequate water supply—for example, Babylon, Persepolis, and Fatehpur Sikr, capital of the Mughal Empire—seem to have gone unheeded. In addition, the dependence on groundwater of many megacities has also led to serious land subsidence (Martin 2000). According to United Nations reports, 80% of the residents of Jakarta, Indonesia, use underground water. In low-lying North Jakarta, groundwater depletion and the resultant land subsidence is making the area more vulnerable to flooding and allowing seawater from the Java Sea to seep 15 kilometers inland into the coastal aquifers. Investment in pipelines to bring water from other sources is expected to exceed US$1 billion. After 30 years of growth, only about 41% of the population of Jakarta receives water through an organized water supply system.

It is well known that Mexico City is sinking because of the withdrawal of underground water. At the same time, only 50% of the residents of Mexico City's squatter settlement have access to piped water. In Bangkok, Thailand, seawater is making incursions into aquifers. In Manila, The Philippines, an astonishing 58% of the water that passes through the city pipes goes unaccounted for and disappears unpaid for (Joint Academies Committee 1995, Martin 2000).

As much as one fourth of the populations of Karachi and Mumbai do not have access to running water. Water scarcity in those cities is exacerbated by inadequate pipes through which as much as one quarter of the water is lost through leakage. Thirty-five percent of the water is "nonrevenue" and it is stolen through illegal connections in Karachi.

A major factor affecting access to water in megacities is the "water-mafias," criminals who control the distribution of drinking water (Hasan 2001). Water-mafias make enormous amounts of money by stealing water—most of which is considered unsafe for drinking purposes—and arranging subsequent informal distribution through water trucks and bottled water. Some of the tankers used by these syndicates are equipped with vacuum equipment and can be seen taking up water from illegal connections; the water is then sold to patrons who depend on water delivery to home tanks. Involvement of water-mafias in the destruction of existing organized water supply systems in megacities is not uncommon.

Water quality is a serious problem in most megacities, along with associated health problems. In many higher-income countries, where past poor waste management practices led to contaminated water sources during the 1980s succeeded in improving water quality. In middle-income countries, water quality did not improve, and in lower-income countries water quality declined (World Bank

1993). In some megacities in less-developed countries, no safe drinking water is delivered through a piped system; drinking water in these cities is either processed at home or purchased from bottling companies. Despite this situation, during the next two decades population growth and migration are expected to add an esti-mated 1.3 billion new urban residents who will need water and sanitation services (Bartone 1995).

The health consequences of unsafe drinking water and inadequate sanita-tion services fall most heavily on the poor. Urban populations in less-developed countries are growing most rapidly in the low-income, high-density districts, including the informal settlements such as squatter areas, *favelas*, shantytowns, and *villas miséria* that can be found in and around most megacities in less-developed countries. Thus, the infant mortality rate in the squatter settlements of Dhaka, Bangladesh, is higher than that in the countryside: 142 per 1,000 live births compared with the national rate of 90 deaths per 1,000, and the rural rate of 93 deaths per 1,000. Many of these infant deaths are associated with diarrheal diseases and infections stemming from poor hygiene. In Manila, diarrhea among the urban poor is twice as common as in the rest of the city (Martin 2000). In these areas, there are few if any facilities for proper disposal of human wastes, water for household use is rarely convenient or sufficient and is often contami-nated, hygiene is poor, and in the event of illness, access to medical treatment is difficult. Diarrheal diseases from gastrointestinal and parasitic infections and acute respiratory illnesses resulting from these conditions are among the leading causes of sickness and death among infants and young children in the developing world (World Bank 1993). It is estimated that in developing countries, 1.5 million children under the age of 5 years die each year from diarrheal diseases (United Nations Children's Fund and World Health Organization 2009). Infectious and parasitic diseases linked to poor sanitation are the third leading cause of poor worker productivity in the developing world.

Children in squatter settlements have death rates 2 to 10 times those of chil-dren in areas with adequate drinking water, systems for disposal of human wastes, and available medical services (Stephens 1995). Even those who can af-ford to boil water or buy bottled water for drinking are affected. A study of chil-dren in a middle-class neighborhood of Karachi showed that half of school-age children have intestinal parasites, which can be related to poor hygiene and lack of water (M. Kadir, Aga Khan University, personal communication, 2010). The problem of lack of drinking water and systems for disposal of human wastes has been the subject of numerous international forums and reviews. A declaration and plan of action to improve health, including safe water, wastewater removal, and other aspects of sanitation, was adopted in 1990 at the United Nations World Summit for Children, and had been joined by 174 countries as of July 1995. Progress has been slow in reaching goals in megacities, a problem compounded by high rates of growth (United Nations Children's Fund 1989).

Water quality is closely related to problems of sewage treatment. In a worst-case scenario, leaky water pipes traverse a sewage system and sporadic flow in water pipes leads to mixing of sewage with drinking water, spreading disease and death to large numbers of people; this is a routine occurrence in some megacities (e.g., Karachi, Mumbai). Treatment of sewage, disposal of human wastes, and management of storm water are poorly developed in rapidly growing megacities, particularly those in Asia and Africa. Of the approximately 1.3 million cubic meters of sewage generated each day in Jakarta, less than 3% is treated (Corcoran et al. 2010). More than one third of people living in Delhi, India, have no toilet facilities in their dwellings. At least 3 million residents on the edge of Mexico City do not have sewers; untreated waste is discharged into local water bodies, contaminating the groundwater, in addition, most of municipal and industrial wastewater are untreated in Mexico City (Stephens 1995). Illegal dumping, both industrial and residential, of toxic chemicals into watershed areas has led to catastrophic health problems in many megacities.

In tropical settings, vector-borne diseases like dengue hemorrhagic fever have been associated with the growth of megacities and their water management systems (World Health Organization 2007). Dengue, which is spread by the *Aedes aegypti* mosquito, was a rare disease until megacities in the tropics grew to their current size. Inadequate water management systems—home storage, open sewers, standing water—have created breeding sites for mosquitoes, with resulting seasonal epidemics (and some deaths) caused by dengue.

Despite serious environmental problems in the majority of Chinese megacities, strong civic action had been successful in meeting the water needs of the country's largest cities. Successful strategies have included saving water, recycling water, reusing brackish water, and implementing economic pricing for water. According to data collected by the Chinese government, almost all drinking water in Guangzhou met quality standards in 2008, and the majority of wastewater is treated (Guongdong Environmental Information Center 2002). However, serious problems remain in the Pearl River Delta, the world's largest population amalgamation, with the merging of different river segments into a single category potentially masking localized high levels of pollutant discharge (Ediger and Hwang 2009). For example, one study related heavy metals in drinking water to behavioral problems among school children in a study of three villages in the Hengshihe area (Bao et al. 2009).

Lessons learned from older megacities point to the wastefulness of polluting watersheds and rivers that must be cleaned up afterward at great expense. Exemplary watershed management and water treatment is seen in New York City, one of the few cities in the United States with safe drinking water that does not require purification water treatment plants. Tokyo and Osaka also have highly efficient water and sewer management systems.

Air Pollution—a Challenge and an Opportunity for Megacities

Air pollution is a major concern for all megacities, but also has regional implications. Airborne emissions from megacities affect air quality and climate change at regional, continental, and global levels. Megacities, which function as *mega-point source plumes*—small areas with heavy emission—provide an opportunity to exert control over air pollution in these few concentrated areas, where most of the air pollution is occurring, and to affect climate change globally. An estimated 20% to 30% of all respiratory diseases in Asian megacities such as Beijing, Jakarta, Karachi, Kolkata, and Delhi are caused by air pollution, which generates a significant health burden for the large populations in these cities (Molina and Molina 2004).

Despite global efforts to examine all aspects of the problem, air pollution remains one of the most difficult environmental issues to address. Air pollution control is not only scientifically difficult to understand but also economically and politically challenging to achieve. Megacities in developing countries, such as Beijing and Jakarta, have to deal with the pressures of rapid economic growth and industrialization at the same time they are competing with megacities in developed countries. The challenge for these cities is to avoid air pollution problems similar to those encountered by older megacities (e.g., the London smog disaster of 1952); simultaneously, they are witnessing the effects of pollution on global climate change.

Against a background of increasing awareness of the environmental hazards associated with rapidly growing cities in less-developed countries, several works have been published focusing on air pollution in megacities (Gurjar et al. 2004, 2008; Baldasano, Valera, and Jimenez 2003). However, knowledge of the specific scope and consequences of air pollution in these population centers remains limited. First, comprehensive and reliable inventories of emissions are a prerequisite to monitoring air quality, and most megacities in less-developed countries are limited in their air quality data. Second, because there is no scientific consensus on which uniform criteria to use for comparing air pollution in megacities, simple comparison may be misleading. It is especially problematic to apply uniform criteria for air quality to megacities across developing and developed countries. Using single indexes of a criteria pollutant does not provide sufficient information to rate and compare megacities.

One approach to comparing air pollution across megacities that is not without difficulties is the multipollutant index, based on the combined level of three criteria pollutants: total suspended particles (TSP), sulfur dioxide (SO_2), and nitrogen dioxide (NO_2) (Gurjar et al. 2008). Using this index, Dhaka was rated the most polluted megacity in the world; using just TSP, an individual criteria pollutant, Karachi was ranked number one. The impact of air pollution must consider both human health and damage to resources such as buildings, cultural heritage, and vegetation. Currently, no single measure captures all dimensions of the consequences of air pollution.

Air quality monitoring has been performed for some megacities since the 1970s. The World Health Organization (WHO) and the United Nations Environment Program (UNEP) created a network for monitoring air pollution as a component of the global environment monitoring system (GEMS) urban air pollution monitoring network (GEMS/Air) in 1974 (Bennett et al. 1985). However, this program used crude indicators of air pollution. Information on TSP, SO_2, and lead (Pb) was collected from major urban areas, including most of the megacities. Air pollution control programs in many megacities were prioritized and guided by this program (World Health Organization 1992). TSP was seen as a problem in most of the megacities in less-developed countries (Baldasano, Valera, and Jimenez 2003). Ambient TSP is a multisource indicator contributed by natural and human activities or photochemical processes. Emissions from combustion of fossil fuels in industry are more toxic than are those from natural sources;

however, simple measures such as TSP cannot distinguish between them. Also, desert areas can show high TSP levels in some megacities, such as Cairo, but these may be nontoxic, related to desert dust. The contribution of sulfur oxide and nitrogen oxide remains low in megacities in less-developed countries compared with levels in developed countries. However, at the least, the program provided guidance on air quality monitoring, analysis of data, and methods of measuring human exposure.

In 1992, the WHO and UNEP began studying air quality, taking more specific measures, in 20 cities projected to have populations exceeding 10 million by the year 2000. Particulate matter of less than 10 microns (PM_{10}) was measured and NO_2, carbon monoxide (CO), and ozone (O_3) were included as additional air quality parameters. Some megacities, including Los Angeles, Mexico City, New York City, Osaka, São Paulo, Seoul, and Tokyo continue to report real-time air quality information for all major pollutants. As a result, area residents can make decisions to avoid exposure based on the air quality for the day. Other megacities, such as Bangkok, Beijing, Delhi, Kolkata, Mumbai, London, and Rio de Janeiro, report air quality data for a more limited group of pollutants. Still other megacities, such as Buenos Aires, Cairo, Karachi, Manila, Moscow, and Tehran, report inadequate information on air quality. The remainder report little or no air quality data and are not discussed here. The results of the studies of air quality in megacities suggest that megacities are not necessarily the most polluted areas of the world, but the exposure of populations in megacities continues to be a concern. Each of the 20 cities considered exceeded the limit for health protection on at least one major pollutant, and most crossed the limit for at least two pollutants. Megacities like Beijing, Cairo, Jakarta, Los Angeles, Mexico City, Moscow, and São Paulo were the worst air pollution offenders, with multiple pollutants exceeding recommended health limits.

The Environmental Kuznets Curve (EKC; Yandle, Vijayaraghavan, and Bhattarai 2002) suggested three phase relations between economic development and air pollution levels: (1) low level of economic development with low air pollution, (2) developing economies with high air pollution levels, and finally (3) a higher developmental stage in which air pollution levels are controlled. Globally, much of manufacturing has shifted to megacities in less-developed countries, including Beijing, Mumbai, and Karachi, which have experienced a deterioration in air quality as a consequence. Specific chemicals, such as SO_2

and Pb, were successfully reduced in developed megacities and, later, in developing megacities, and largely controlled. However, suspended particulate matter is still the main concern overall and—more importantly—for megacities in developing countries.

Sources of air pollution in most megacities have changed over time. Moreover, several commonalities, more recently among megacities, deviate from the proposed EKC pattern. An estimated 75 million people travel an average of 10 kilometers each day in megacities. These distances increase as the size of the city increases and result in traffic congestion, leading to inefficiency and increased transit time. The result is economic loss to individuals and society. The economy of Bangkok is estimated to be 2.1% smaller as a result of time lost in traffic jams. By contrast, New York City's population density, low automobile use, and high transit utility make it among the most energy efficient cities in the United States. Overall, the contribution of traffic-related air pollution emissions to overall emissions has increased in all megacities during the past 30 years (Mage et al. 1996). For example, in Delhi the source of air pollution has reversed from 1970 to 2001. In 1970 and 1971, industries accounted for 56%, vehicles 23%, and domestic sources 21% of pollution. In 2000 and 2001, estimated contribution by industries was 20%, vehicles 72%, and domestic sources 8%. Put simply, the cause of pollution is related more to large populations and transport patterns than to industry in many megacities.

As expected, because of rapid motorization, emissions of NO_2 and fine particulate matter are a concern in all Asian cities. Traffic is responsible for 70% of TSP and NO_2 emitted in the city of Jakarta, and Karachi has seen a rapid increase in vehicle count in the past decade. Concentrations of SO_2 are stable at a relatively low level in Asian megacities. Ground-level O_3, though not comprehensively studied, is assumed to increase from photochemical smog associated with motor vehicle emissions.

Trash burning contributes heavily to air pollution in megacities of developing countries, leading to exposures to several thousand hazardous chemicals called "air toxics." One of the biggest environmental myths—and a prevailing belief in developing megacities—is that "burning cleans the trash." Large amounts of plastics are burned in many of the cities in less-developed countries, releasing very dangerous dioxins. A similar misconception is that the release of waste in larger water bodies leads to dilution and thus less adverse consequences for those who use that water source. Both myths are killing people.

Role of Megacities in Global Climate Change

Global climate change and its future effects are closely linked with levels of emissions as well as control efforts in megacities, particularly those in Asia, as most of the ten largest megacities are located. The size of these megacities will continue to increase, as will the levels of emissions they produce. Asian emissions will increasingly affect hemispheric background O_3, undoing the progress made by regional control measures in Europe and the United States. Since 1990, control efforts in Bangkok, Beijing, Dhaka, Jakarta, Kolkata, Manila, Mumbai, Delhi, Seoul, and Tokyo have led to reductions in air pollution but in the majority of megacities including Dhaka, Manila, Mumbai, and Karachi, air pollution guideline values for certain pollutants are still exceeded. For example, Delhi is experiencing a relatively cleaner environment after switching to compressed natural gas to fuel its public transport system. Mexico City introduced catalytic converters in vehicles and spent money on improving fuel quality. Iran recently adopted regulations and laws for controlling air pollution in Tehran. Jakarta officials have taken action against automobile congestion. The Blue Sky Program (Program Langit Biru) was initiated in 1991 and 1992 to improve air quality in the five largest cities of Indonesia, including its capital, Jakarta. The program's goal was revamping the transportation sector and controlling emissions from idle sources (e.g., residential, commercial, and industrial sectors). It has been fairly successful in bringing about an increase in the percentage of vehicles meeting pollution standards, the phasing out of leaded gasoline, and the introduction of natural gas-fueled public transportation in Jakarta (National Communication to the United Nations Framework Convention on Climate Change [UNFCCC]).

Environmental Policies That Work

Although the magnitude of environmental hazards and the potential threat from the introduction of new chemicals with unknown consequences are continuing challenges for health in megacities, much has been learned. Environmental disaster is not the natural course of urbanization or development, even though current development in many ways repeats history in the United States, Europe, and the former Soviet Union. For the period between 1980 and 2000, more than 15% of the improvement in overall life expectancy in the United States was contributed through improvement in ambient air pollution (Pope, Ezzati, and Dockery

2009). Similar examples can be provided for water pollution and solid waste management solutions.

Toxicological and epidemiological science has informed regulatory systems that have improved air quality in many places. During the 1940s and 1950s, coal burning led to SO_2 exposure, which was later identified as the cause of increased sickness and death during London's "killer smog" of 1952 (Stone 2002). Switching to low-sulfur fuels improved this situation.

It is not just the presence of a particular chemical in the air (e.g., SO_2), but the concentrations and combined pollution of all hazardous chemicals (such as carbon compounds) that cause health problems. Multisource, multichemical, and multimedia contexts need to be considered to deal effectively with the impacts of air pollution generated by megacities. One approach is to look at the macroenvironment of megacities—that is, the indoor and outdoor environment as well as the overall urban ecosystem and the built environment. This requires bringing together environmental engineers and public health specialists to develop a favorable environment for human needs. This coexistence and collaboration is a dire need for the future of public health and the health of megacities.

Four stages of development of air quality management have been formulated for megacities: problem recognition, policy formation, implementation, and monitoring (Winsemius 1986). Lessons from megacities have added the importance of well-developed communication strategies to ensure the public is informed through various stages of the development. The specifics of the complex combinations of pollutants in particular megacities require approaches which a national strategy or smaller city strategy would overlook. Focuses on single pollutants, isolated problems, or national compilations of data cannot the solve problems of megacities. It is the local complexities which must be included in modeling solutions. Although air quality monitoring technology and emission inventories available in resource-rich megacities may not be perfectly matched to the needs of all megacities, development of these approaches is certainly within their reach.

Accurate air quality control models require data on emissions (what chemicals are in the air and which sources contribute most—i.e., an emissions inventory) and data on weather conditions (e.g., wind speed and amount of sunshine) over time. Availability of real-time air quality data and increased awareness of air conditions by resident populations can lead to reduced exposure to air pollution.

Real-time air quality data are available in only a few megacities. Special studies have been designed to understand the causes of emissions and to measure progress in limiting them.

Mexico City provides an example of the success and limitations of the application of science, regulatory efforts, and social mobilization to improve air quality. More than a decade ago, Mexico City, with more than 18 million people, was considered by many to be the most polluted city in the world; it experienced an estimated 6,400 deaths per year attributed to the air breathed by its residents (Loomis et al. 1999), including associations with childhood asthma and infant mortality (Romieu et al. 1992). Air pollution increased school absenteeism and the use of hospital emergency rooms, placing a heavy burden on primary health care clinics (Romieu et al. 1996).

Mexico City has applied the beneficial results of studies and programs implemented in other megacities and adopted corrective actions iteratively since the mid-1980s. Early studies identified the types and percentage of vehicles found to be the source of problem emissions, and so one of the first policy changes regarding air pollution was to enforce replacement of old vehicles, increase the number of tuned engines, and remove heavy-emission vehicles, such as trucks, from the roads (at least from main city roads). This led to initial air quality improvements. Later, the introduction of catalytic converters continued the trend toward better air. Additional focused local data led to the discovery that low-income communities had low levels of air quality compared with higher-income areas. Community action in poor areas further improved air quality in those neighborhoods. Further study led to an understanding that oil refineries, power plants, forest fires, and cooking were also sources of emissions that were dangerous to health. Over a decade of careful study and action, air improved in Mexico City.

Barriers to Policy Reform

Policymaking regarding environmental issues is more likely to be complicated by social and political factors than by scientific knowledge, and nowhere is this more evident than in megacities. Models exist for policies and systems on environmental management in megacities, but many cities are constrained by municipal and global policies that prevent movement in this direction. Good urban planning is needed to improve megacity air quality by encouraging people to live closer to where they work, developing cost-effective and convenient mass transit networks, creating economic activities outside of megacities to reduce long commutes, and strategically locating industries.

Urban planning is embedded in governance issues affecting megacities. Megacities are typically spread over a number of independent jurisdictions, even across international borders. This adds to the complexity of environmental management. Planning and reform to deal with environmental issues may require a decade of effort—which is difficult to achieve given the limited terms of most political offices. Independently funded metropolitan institutions have been a successful solution to these dimensions but are sometimes unpopular with the public. In a series of case studies including six megacities, Molina and Molina have shown that municipal environmental management is closely linked to financial capacity (Molina and Molina 2004). Environmental planning agencies often find themselves with inadequate budgets and problems that have low political priority. Conflicts between different government agencies are usually resolved through political means that may not address environmental problems. When economic development and environmental issues come in conflict, economic development usually prevails.

Barriers to environmental management in megacities can be better understood within the broader issues of neoliberal policy (Liverman and Vilas 2006). Despite the clear and present danger of environmental hazards that have developed over decades in megacities, neoliberal policies that promote free trade and less government interference have weakened environmental management structures in many countries. Privatization and pricing of environmental services and common property resources, the environmental impacts of free trade, and the transfer of environmental management to local or nongovernmental organizations have had negative consequences on the environment and the health of the general population. Although some cities have adapted to and benefited from neoliberal policies, urban environments overall have suffered more than they have benefited.

Reconciliation between the political pressures exerted by environmental and neoliberal forces has been attempted with little success (Hartwick and Peet 2003). Economic growth and environmental protection are commonly presented as irreconcilable. The notion of sustainable development has rarely succeeded in the face of neoliberalism that continues to thrive despite the massive poverty in megacities, denying sustainable development as a clear alternative (Heynen et al. 2007). The economic needs of the poor are pitted against the health needs of the population.

The Potential for Community Action

The causes and consequences of environmental hazards have been well known, as are the means of controlling them. Regulatory solutions can be effective in making the increasingly unsustainable and unhealthy environments of megacities more livable. The social and political problems that occur in megacities, however, have limited what regulatory efforts can accomplish (Megacities Project 2010).

Community action in Mexico City as a means of dealing with environmental hazards has been an illustrative case, both in terms of highlighting the potential of social movements to effect change and the limits in their ability to do so. Although the magnitude of the health consequences of air pollution in Mexico City is generally agreed upon, the relative importance of the problem has seen less agreement. The poor and minorities suffer most from air pollution in Mexico City, but they have not been at the forefront of efforts to combat the problem. New migrants to the city, who tend to be poor, are more concerned with issues of home ownership and economic opportunity than air quality (Izazola, Martinez, and Marquette 1998). Thus, the response to air pollution in Mexico City has come primarily from more affluent residents.

During the past decade, grassroots activists in Mexico City have attempted to change the way the government implements environmental controls, framing the movement in terms of social justice and civil rights. Community health and environmental activists have joined with professionals and academics to form a powerful coalition. In 1995, chemists Luisa and Mario Molina received the Nobel Prize for their work on air pollution in Mexico City. A broad coalition in Mexico City has demonstrated the relationship between pollution in the city, the health of the population, and climate change. In the process, they have built strong links to other environmental organizations in Latin America and across the globe (Pulver 2007).

The government of Mexico has responded to the pollution problem in a variety of ways, but continues to emphasize the need for external funding for pollution control. The success of these environmental reforms depends heavily on economic recovery. Environmental policy in Mexico still suffers from underfunding, bureaucratic fragmentation, and heavy reliance on voluntary enforcement mechanisms (Mumme and Sanchez 1992; DuPuis 2004).

Besides air pollution, megacities have taken action on comprehensive environmental safety. The "Healthy Town" initiative in Japan created a vision for sustaining a healthy environment through community participation. The Healthy Town initiative depended on scientific study and monitoring data to which communities respond (Takano and Nakamura 2004). The involvement of communities in future planning could be considered a way forward for megacities (Reichow 1968).

Summary

Pollution and its health consequences are not the natural outcome of megacity development, despite the prevalence of serious pollution problems in many of the world's growing megacities. The built environment and processes associated with these areas—rapid growth, industrialization, automobile proliferation, amalgamation, and inequalities—have led to a complex combination of exposures, with equally complex health consequences. Environmental problems have been addressed and improved through a application of science, use of data, and regulatory efforts. Barriers to these reforms embedded in neoliberal economic policy have been countered by community mobilization. Future improvements will require continued scientific study of these problems and strengthening of regulatory frameworks globally. Community mobilization and global political response to environmental degradation are needed to support both the science and the policy needed for improving environmental conditions and health.

References

Amekudzi AA, Thomas-Mobley L, Ross C. 2007. Transportation planning and infrastructure delivery in major cities and megacities. *Transp Res Rec.* 1997:17–23.

Ashley L, Mikkelsen L, Cohen L. 2008. *Restructuring Government to Address Social Determinants of Health.* Oakland, CA: Prevention Institute and Trust for America's Health. Available at: http://www.preventioninstitute.org/component/jlibrary/article/id-77/127.html. Accessed June 21, 2010.

Baldasano JM, Valera E, Jimenez P. 2003. Air quality data from large cities. *Sci Total Environ.* 307:141–165.

Bao Q-S, Lu C-Y, Song H, et al. 2009. Behavioural development of school-aged children who live around a multi-metal sulphide mine in Guangdong province, China: a cross-sectional study. *BMC Public Health.* 9:217.

Bartone C. 1995. Urban sanitation, sewerage, and waste-water management: responding to growing household and community demand. Presented at: Second Annual Conference on Environmentally Sustainable Development: The Human Face of the Urban Environment; September 19–21; Washington, DC.

Bartuska TJ. 2007. The built environment: definition and scope. In: McClure WR, Bartuska TJ, editors. *The Built Environment: A Collaborative Inquiry Into Design and Planning.* 2nd ed. Hoboken, NJ: Wiley:3–14.

Baykal BB, Tanik A, Gonenc IE. 2000. Water quality in drinking water reservoirs of a megacity, Istanbul. *Environ Manage.* 26:607–614.

Bennett B, Kretzchmar JG, Akland GG, De Koning HW. 1985. Urban air pollution worldwide. *Environ Sci Technol.* 19:298–304.

Besley T, Zagha R, editors. 2005. *Development Challenges in the 1990s: Leading Policymakers Speak From Experience.* New York, NY: World Bank and Oxford University.

Biasioli M, Barberis R, Ajmone-Marsan F. 2006. The influence of a large city on some soil properties and metals content. *Sci Total Environ.* 356:154–164.

Boarnet MG, Greenwald M, MacMillan TE. 2008. Walking, urban design, and health: toward a cost-benefit analysis framework. *J Plann Educ Res.* 27:341–358.

Burian SJ, Nix SJ, Pitt RE, Durrans SR. 2000. Urban wastewater management in the United States: past, present, and future. *J Urban Technol.* 7:33–62.

Caryana YK. 2004. Blue Sky Program for Transportation Sector in Indonesia: Greater Jakarta Pilot Project. Paper presented at the Second Asian Petroleum Technology Symposium. Available at: http://igs.nigc.ir/igs/standard/cd-cng/STATION/INDONESIA.pdf. Accessed June 28, 2010.

Clarke G. 1985. Jakarta, Indonesia: planning to solve urban conflicts. In: Lea JP, Courtney JM, editors. *Cities in Conflict: Studies in the Planning and Management of Asian Cities.* Washington, DC: World Bank: 34–58.

Commission on Social Determinants of Health. 2008. *Closing the Gap in a Generation: Health Equity Through Action on the Social Determinants of Health.* Final Report. Geneva, Switzerland: World Health Organization.

Committee on Environmental Justice. 1999. *Toward Environmental Justice: Research, Education, and Health Policy Needs.* Washington, DC: Institute of Medicine.

Corcoran E, Nellemann C, Baker E, et al., editors. 2010. *Sick Water? The Central Role of Wastewater Management in Sustainable Development.* A Rapid Response Assessment. Nairobi, Kenya: United Nations Environment Programme and UN-HABITAT. Available at: http://www.grida.no/_res/site/file/publications/sickwater/SickWater_screen.pdf. Accessed August 11, 2010.

Davis M. 2008. *Planet of Slums.* New York, NY: Verso.

Downey L. 2007. US metropolitan-area variation in environmental inequality outcomes. *Urban Stud.* 44:953–977.

DuPuis EM, editor. 2004. *Smoke and Mirrors: The Politics and Culture of Air Pollution.* New York, NY: Verso: New York University.

Durand S. 2000. *Globalization of Infectious Diseases.* Washington, DC: Population Resource Center. Available at: http://www.prcdc.org/files/Infectious_Disease.pdf. Accessed June 29, 2010.

Ediger L, Hwang L. 2009. Water quality and environmental health in Southern China. Report from the First BSR Environmental Health Forum. Guangzhou, China. May 15, 2009. Hong Kong, China: BSR. Available at: http://www.bsr.org/reports/BSR_Southern_China_Water_Quality_Environmental_Health_Forum.pdf. Accessed November 13, 2010.

Fairchild A, Rosner D, Colgrove J, et al. 2010. The exodus of public health: what history can tell us about its future. *Am J Public Health.* 100:54–63.

Garb M. 2003. Health, morality, and housing: the "tenement problem" in Chicago. *Am J Public Health.* 93:1420–1430.

Gordon P, Richardson HW. 1997. Are compact cities a desirable planning goal? *J Am Plann Assoc.* 63:95–106.

Guongdong Environmental Information Center. [2002.] 2001 Guangdong Environmental Status Report. Guangzhou, China: Guangdong Environmental

Protection Bureau. Available at: http://www.gdep.gov.cn/eng/2001/es/index.html. Accessed November 13, 2010.

Gurjar BR, Butler TM, Lawrence MG, Lelieveld J. 2008. Evaluation of emissions and air quality in megacities. *Atmos Environ.* 42:1593–1606.

Gurjar BR, van Aardenne JA, Lelieveld J, Mohan M. 2004. Emission estimates and trends (1990–2000) for megacity Delhi and implications. *Atmos Environ.* 38:5663–5681.

Halliday S. 1999. *The Great Stink of London: Sir Joseph Bazalgette and the Cleansing of the Victorian Metropolis.* Stroud, England: Sutton.

Handy S. 2005. Critical assessment of the literature on the relationships among transportation, land use, and physical activity. Resource paper for *Does the Built Environment Influence Physical Activity? Examining the Evidence.* Transportation Research Board Special Report 282. Washington, DC: Transportation Research Board and Institute of Medicine.

Hartwick E, Peet R. 2003. Neoliberalism and nature: the case of the WTO. *Ann Am Acad Pol Soc Sci.* 590:188–211.

Hasan A. *Working With Community.* 2001. Karachi, Pakistan: City.

Heynen N, McCarthy J, Prudham S, Robbins P, editors. 2007. *Neoliberal Environments: False Promises and Unnatural Consequences.* New York, NY: Routledge.

Izazola H, Martínez C, Marquette C. 1998. Environmental perceptions, social class and demographic change in Mexico City: a comparative approach. *Environ Urban.* 10:107–118.

Jacobs J. 1961. *The Death and Life of Great American Cities.* New York, NY: Random House.

Joint Academies Committee on the Mexico City Water Supply; Water Science and Technology Board; Commission on Geosciences, Environment, and Resources, et al. 1995. *Mexico City's Water Supply: Improving the Outlook for Sustainability.* Washington, DC: National Academies.

Kjellstrom T, Friel S, Dixon J, et al. 2007. Urban environmental health and health equity. *J Urban Health.* 84(3 Suppl):i86–i97.

Krizek K, El-Geneidy A, Thompson K. 2007. A detailed analysis of how an urban trail system affects the travel of cyclists. *Transportation.* 34:611–624.

Liverman DM, Vilas S. 2006. Neoliberalism and the environment in Latin America. *Annu Rev Environ Resour.* 31:327–363.

Loomis D, Castillejos M, Gold DR, et al. 1999. Air pollution and infant mortality in Mexico City. *Epidemiology.* 10:118–123.

Lovasi G, Bader M, Quinn J, et al. 2008. Neighborhood safety, aesthetics and body mass index in New York City. *Obesity.* 16:S249.

Lovasi GS, Hutson MA, Guerra M, Neckerman KM. 2009. Built environments and obesity in disadvantaged populations. *Epidemiol Rev.* 31:7–20.

Mage D, Ozolins G, Peterson P, et al. 1996. Urban air pollution in megacities of the world. *Atmos Environ.* 30:681–686.

Martin T, editor. 2000. *ITT Industries Guidebook to Water Management Issues.* White Plains, NY: ITT Corporation. Available at: http://www.itt.com/waterbook. Accessed June 20, 2010.

McMichael AJ. 2000. The urban environment and health in a world of increasing globalization: issues for developing countries. *Bull WHO.* 78: 68–78.

Megacities Project. 2010. Home page. Available at: http://www.megacitiesproject.org. Accessed June 28, 2010.

Mehta S. 2004. *Maximum City: Bombay Lost and Found.* New York, NY: Random House.

Michael T. 1996. Rock pollution intensity of GDP and trade policy: can the World Bank be wrong? *World Dev.* 24:471–479.

Molina MJ, Molina LT. 2004. Critical review: megacities and atmospheric pollution. *J Air Waste Manage Assoc.* 54:644–680.

Morichi S. 2009. Sustainable transport development in East Asian megacities. *IJESD.* 8:229–246.

Morrison DS. 2009. Rallying point: Charles Lee's long-standing career in environmental justice. *Am J Public Health.* 99:S508–S510.

Mumme SP, Sanchez RA. 1992. New directions in Mexican environmental policy. *Earth Environ Sci.* 16:465–474.

National Research Council. 1984. *Toxicity Testing: Strategies to Determine Needs and Priorities*. Washington, DC: National Academy.

Olden K. 2009. Impact of environmental justice investments. *Am J Public Health*. 99:S484.

Peterson JA. 1979. The impact of sanitary reform upon American urban planning, 1840–1890. *J Soc Hist*. 13:83–103.

Pope CA, Ezzati M, Dockery DW. 2009. Fine-particulate air pollution and life expectancy in the United States. *New Engl J Med*. 360:376–386.

Pulver S. 2007. Climate politics in Mexico in a North American perspective. Encyclopedia of Earth. Available at: http://www.eoearth.org/article/Climate_politics_in_Mexico_in_a_North_American_perspective. Accessed June 21, 2010.

Rafique J. 1991. Role of Karachi Stock Exchange in capital formation (market capitalisation in Pakistan). *Econ Rev*. June 1, 1991.

Rahman A, Lee HK, Khan MA. 1997. Domestic water contamination in rapidly growing megacities of Asia: case of Karachi, Pakistan. *Environ Monit Assess*. 44:339–360.

Redwood Y, Schulz AJ, Israel BA, et al. 2010. Social, economic, and political processes that create built environment inequities: perspectives from urban African Americans in Atlanta. *Fam Community Health*. 33:53–67.

Reichow HB. 1968. Healthy environment in the town landscape—the city of tomorrow. *Offentl Gesundheitswes*. 30:386–397.

Renalds A, Smith T, Hale PJ. 2010. A systematic review of built environment and health. *Fam Community Health*. 33:68–78.

Ritz B, Yu F, Fruin S, et al. 2002. Ambient air pollution and risk of birth defects in southern California. *Am J Epidemiol*. 155:17–25.

Romieu I, Lugo MC, Velasco SR, Sanchez S. 1992. Air pollution and school absenteeism among children in Mexico City. *Am J Epidemiol*. 136:1524–1531.

Romieu I, Meneses F, Ruiz S, et al. 1996. Effects of air pollution on the respiratory health of asthmatic children living in Mexico City. *Am J Respir Crit Care Med*. 154:300–307.

Saier MH. 2008. Are megacities sustainable? *Water Air Soil Pollut*. 19:1–3.

Sandler R, Pezzullo PC, editors. 2007. *Environmental Justice and Environmentalism: The Social Justice Challenge to the Environmental Movement*. Cambridge, MA: MIT Press.

Shi L, Shao GS, Cui X, et al. 2009. Urban three-dimensional expansion and its driving forces—a case study of Shanghai, China. *Chin Geogr Sci.* 19:291–298.

Srinivas H. 2007. Defining squatter settlements. Global Development Research Center. Available at: http://www.gdrc.org/uem/define-squatter.html. Accessed June 20, 2010.

Stephens C. 1995. The urban environment, poverty, and health in developing countries. *Health Policy Plan.* 10:109–121.

Stone R. 2002. Counting the cost of London's killer smog. *Science.* 298:2106–2107.

Sugandhy A, Bey A, Gunardi, Boer R, et al, editors. 1999. Indonesia: The First National Communication on Climate Change Convention. Jakarta, Indonesia: Government of Indonesia. Available at: http://unfccc.int/resource/docs/natc/indonc1.pdf. Accessed December 18, 2010.

Takano T, Fu J, Nakamura K, et al. 2002. Age-adjusted mortality and its association to variations in urban conditions in Shanghai. *Health Policy.* 61:239–253.

Takano T, Nakamura K. 2004. Participatory research to enhance vision sharing for Healthy Town initiatives in Japan. *Health Promot Int.* 19:299–307.

United Nations Children's Fund. 1989. *Convention on the Rights of the Child.* New York, NY: United Nations. Available at: http://www.unicef.org/crc. Accessed June 29, 2010.

United Nations Children's Fund and World Health Organization (WHO). 2009. *Diarrhoea: Why Children Are Still Dying and What Can Be Done.* Geneva, Switzerland: WHO.

Van der Bruggen B, Borghgraef K, Vinckier C. 2009. Causes of water supply problems in urbanized regions in developing countries. *Water Resour Manag.* 24:1885–1902.

Wheeler D, Shome S. 2010. Less smoke, more mirrors: where India really stands on solar power and other renewables. Working Paper 204. Washington, DC: Center for Global Development. Available at: http://www.cgdev.org/content/publications/detail/1423937. Accessed May 31, 2010.

Winsemius P. 1986. *Guest at Home: Reflections on Environmental Management.* Alphen aan den Rijn, Netherlands: HD Samsom, Tjeenk Willink.

World Bank. 1993. *Development and the Environment: World Development Report 1992*. New York, NY: Oxford University.

World Health Organization. 2007. Defeating dengue: a difficult task ahead. *Bull WHO*. 85:737–738.

World Health Organization and United Nations Environment Programme. 1992. *Urban Air Pollution in Megacities of the World*. Oxford, England: Blackwell.

Yandle B, Vijayaraghavan M, Bhattarai M. 2002. *The Environmental Kuznets Curve: A Primer*. Bozeman, MT: Property and Environment Research Center. Available at: http://www.perc.org/articles/article688.php. Accessed May 31, 2010.

Scenes from Karachi, Pakistan
May 2010

Photos by Imran Khan

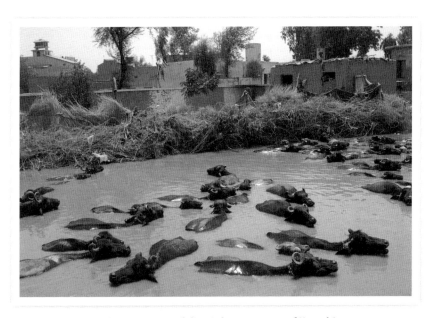

**Malir Town: one of the eighteen towns of Karachi,
near Jinnah International Airport**

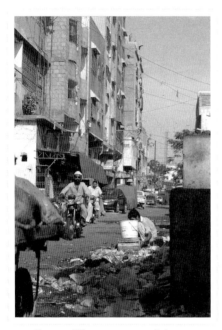

Keamari Town: commercial area

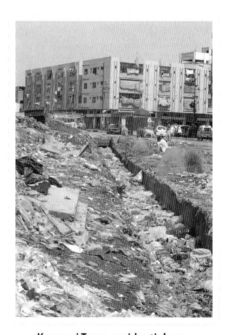

Keamari Town: residential area

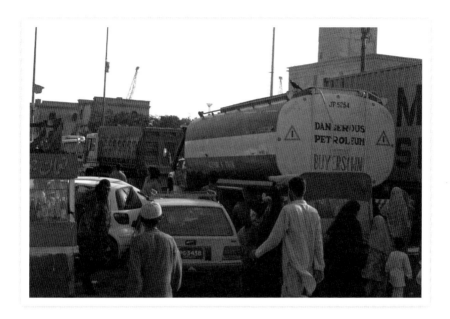

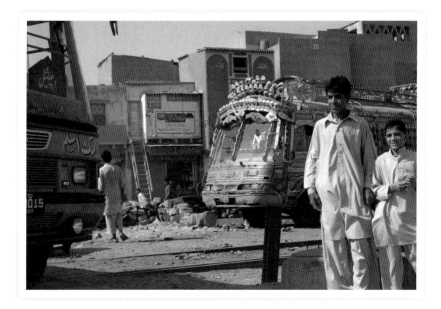

Major industrial areas are also home to millions

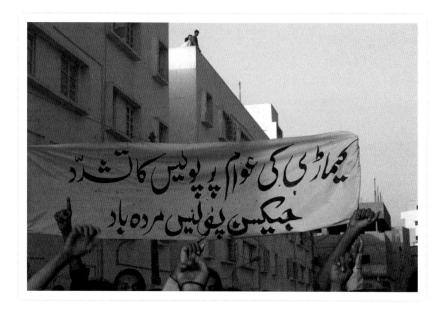

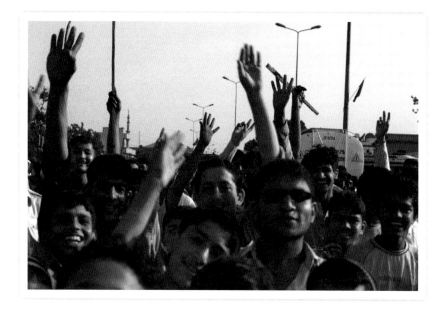

Electricity outage protest and police defiance

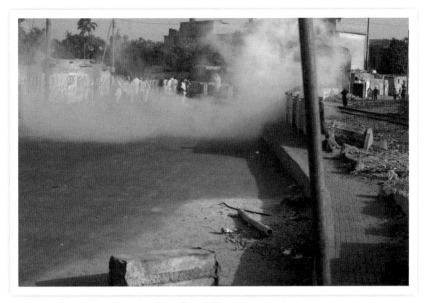

Tear gassing electricity outage protestors

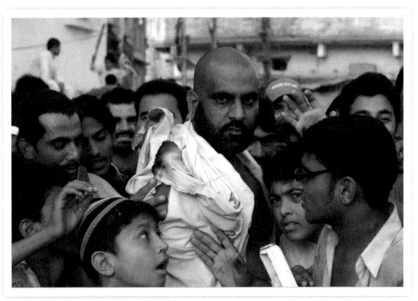

Police brutality victim displays his wounds

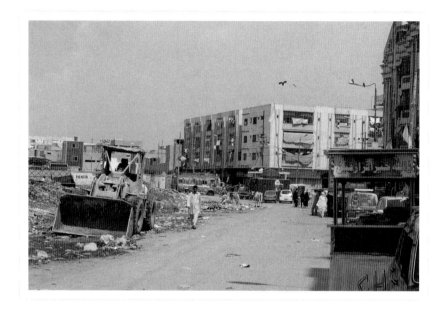

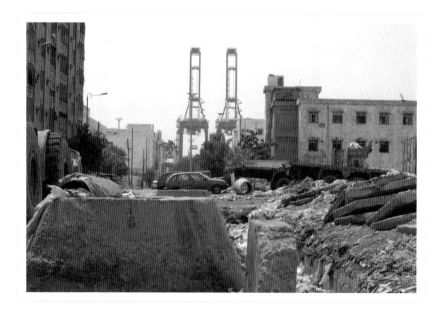

Port Karachi and adjacent neighbor

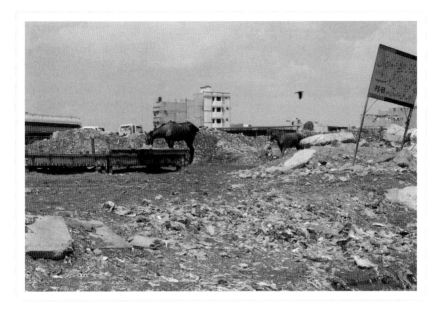

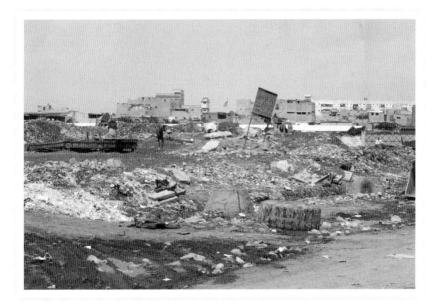

Failed school building program that has become a garbage dump

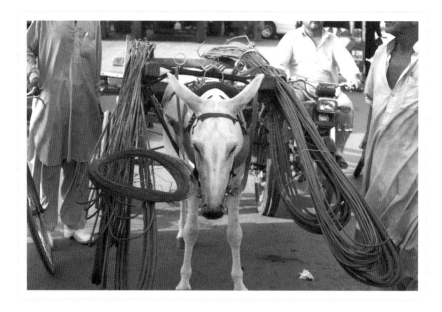

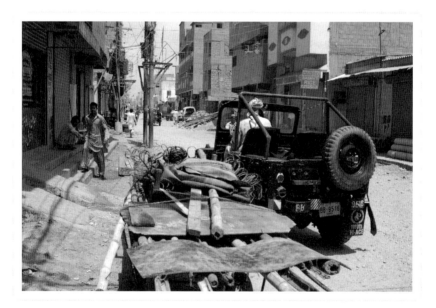

Saddar Town: main commercial areas of Karachi

7

Forced Displacement of African Americans in New York City and the International Diffusion of Multiple-Drug-Resistant HIV

Rodrick Wallace, PhD

THE WORLD CONFERENCE ON Human Rights, held in Vienna in 1993 by the United Nations, described forced displacement in these terms:

> The practice of forced displacement involves involuntary removal of persons from their homes or land, directly or indirectly attributable to the State . . . The causes of forced evictions are very diverse. The practice can be carried out in connection with development and infrastructure projects . . . housing or land reclamation measures, prestigious international events, unrestrained land or housing speculation, housing renovation, urban redevelopment or city beautification initiatives, and mass relocation or resettlement programmes . . .

> The practice of forced displacement shares many characteristics with related phenomena such as population transfer, internal displacement of persons, forced removals during or as a result or object of armed conflict, "ethnic cleansing," mass exodus, refugee movements, etc. . . . (OHCHR 1996, p. 3)

In this chapter, we examine a decades-long process of forced displacement affecting African Americans in New York City, focusing particularly on the Harlem section of the Borough of Manhattan. We explore the likely impacts of continued displacement on the emerging scourge of multiple-drug-resistant (MDR) or other evolutionarily transformed variants of HIV, the etiological agent of AIDS.

A well-known report by Freeman and McCord (1990) examined excess mortality in Harlem, finding that, at the time, men in Bangladesh had a higher probability of survival after age 35 years than did men in Harlem. They noted, almost in passing, that Harlem's population had declined from 233,000 in 1960 to only 122,000 by 1980, with most of the population loss concentrated in people living in substandard housing, much of it abandoned or partially occupied buildings. During that period, the death rate from homicide increased from 25.3 to 90.8 per 100,000, with cirrhosis and homicide together accounting for some 33% of Harlem's excess deaths between 1979 and 1981. By 1990, AIDS became the most common cause of death for persons between 25 and 44 years of age in Harlem.

The policy-driven process inducing that depopulation has been described in some detail elsewhere (e.g., R. Wallace 1990; R. Wallace and D. Wallace 1997a; D. Wallace and R. Wallace 1998, 2003; D. Wallace 2001, and references therein). Withdrawal of essential housing-related municipal services, including fire extinguishment resources, from minority voting blocs in the 1970s triggered processes of large-scale contagious urban decay and forced migration involving a devastating synergism of fire, housing abandonment, and pathology (R. Wallace 1988). The process was described by the New York State Assembly Republican Task Force on Urban Fire Protection as follows:

> There is mounting evidence that the lack of fire protection which has plagued communities in the South Bronx, Central Harlem, Brownsville and Bushwick is assuming city-wide dimensions as it spreads to [other neighborhoods] . . . there are indications the City Planning Commission and other agencies condoned [fire service] reductions in the context of a "planned shrinkage" policy . . . there is strong evidence that these actions have resulted in unwarranted loss of life and destruction of city neighborhoods . . . (Task Force on Urban Fire Protection 1978, p. 1)

After examining the consequences, R. Wallace wrote:

> . . . [T]he . . . origins of public health and public order are much the same and deeply embedded in the security and stability of personal, domestic and community social networks and other institutions . . . [D]isruptions of such networks, from any cause, will express themselves in exacerbation of a nexus of behavior, including violence, substance abuse and general criminality. These in turn have the most severe implications for . . . [many pathologies including the] evolution and spread of AIDS. (R. Wallace 1990, p. 801)

The policy-driven displacement of population affecting Harlem between 1970 and 1980 created a massive de facto refugee camp environment for emerging and reemerging infection. The withdrawal of fire service and other social services were protested by poor neighborhoods during this period, to little avail, and predictions of uncontrolled fires and forced relocations were made by poor residents (Susser 1982). By 1990, Harlem was an epicenter of both AIDS and tuberculosis and of their interaction (D. Wallace and R. Wallace 1998, 2003; R. Wallace and D. Wallace 1997b; D. Wallace 2001).

By 2005, Harlem and East Harlem rivaled the gay center of New York City, Manhattan's Chelsea-Clinton neighborhood, in rates of HIV diagnoses per 100,000 population, at, respectively, 132.4 and 108.2 versus 135.0. Age-adjusted death rates per 1,000 persons with AIDS were, however, quite different: 31.9 and 32.6 versus 11.4 (New York City Department of Health 2006). This divergence represents not only a contrast in the effective availability of antiretroviral drugs, but also obvious population differences in patterns of burden and affordance between African Americans, other minorities, and middle-class Whites, in spite of similarly draconian pressures enforcing the social and spatial segregation of ethnic and sexual minorities in the United States (R. G. Wallace 2003; Massey and Denton 1992).

The planned shrinkage depopulation of Harlem between 1970 and 1980 that exacerbated the spread of AIDS and tuberculosis (D. Wallace and R. Wallace 1998) had, by 1990, enabled a subsequent round of displacement. The loss of economic, social, and political capital consequent on the induced contagious urban decay of the 1970s left Harlem without effective means of resisting gentrification by majority populations—that is, the ongoing reduction of Harlem to a largely White "Central Park North." An essential context for this process has been the pattern of massive U.S. deindustrialization consequent on diversion of national technical resources from civilian to military enterprise during the Cold War that left New York City, by default, economically dependent on a preexisting elite already highly networked into the global financial network (e.g., R. Wallace et al. 1999; Ullmann 1998). Displacement of poor African Americans in Harlem was part of the city's policy response to new economic arrangements—deindustrialization—and essentially simply another implementation of longstanding policies of serial forced displacement that have affected U.S. minorities since the 1930s (R. Wallace and Fullilove 2008). Newman and Wyly describe this process as follows:

> Central Harlem received an influx of middle-class residents throughout the 1970s and 1980s but the changes during the late 1990s and early 2000s are different. Harlem's residents report a solid flow of SUV's (sport utility vehicles) of people driving through the neighborhood scouting for homes. One resident described the housing demand: "People

are coming up while you're on the street asking who owns the building. It's a daily thing." The neighborhood also appeals to renters seeking livable space with manageable commutes. In less than 15 minutes, residents are whisked to midtown on a 2 or A train; in 30 minutes, they can reach jobs on Wall Street. A 20-minute cab ride gets you to LaGuardia Airport and every highway intersects with Harlem. Rents for floor-through apartments in brownstones are capturing [US]$1,700 a month. (Newman and Wyly 2006, p. 53)

They conclude:

According to neighborhood informants, many [of those displaced by the rise in rents] are moving out of the city to upstate New York, New Jersey and Long Island . . . Those who are forced to leave gentrifying neighborhoods are torn from rich local social networks of information and cooperation (the "social capital" much beloved by policymakers); they are thrown into an ever more competitive housing market shaped by increasingly difficult trade-offs between affordability, overcrowding and commuting accessibility to jobs and services. All of the pressures of gentrification are deeply enmeshed with broader inequalities of class, race and ethnicity, and gender . . . As affordable housing protections are dismantled in the current wave of neo-liberal policymaking, we are likely to see the end-game of gentrification as the last remaining barriers to complete neighborhood transformation are torn down . . . Low-income residents who manage to resist displacement may enjoy a few benefits from the changes brought by gentrification, but these bittersweet fruits are quickly rotting as the supports for low-income renters are steadily dismantled. (Newman and Wyly 2006, p. 53)

The forced displacement of New York City's African American population to a suburban/exurban ring around New York City has created conditions analogous to those in the Black townships surrounding Cape Town, South Africa. This circumstance can be expected to induce a new round of patterns of behavior like those in refugee camps, and will further exacerbate the spread of HIV among African Americans, who, at present, account for only 15% of the U.S. population but constitute more than half of new HIV infections.

Hurricane Katrina–like dispersal of New York City's communities of color can be expected to fatally compromise:

(1) Ongoing antiretroviral drug treatment of those already infected with HIV,
(2) The effectiveness of treating new cases with antiretrovirals, and
(3) Virtually all possible infection prevention strategies.

This will markedly accelerate the development and spread of drug-resistant viral strains.

Mathematical analysis of a contagious process in a commuting field (R. Wallace et al. 1997, 1999; R. Wallace 1999) suggests that for national diffusion, metropolitan regions are the systems of fundamental interest. From that perspective, a disease epicenter has much the same large-scale force of infection whether it is concentrated in the center or dispersed around the periphery of a particular large city: urban-suburban linkages are strong enough to create a functional equivalence (R. Wallace and D. Wallace 1993).

Given the powerful central role of New York City and its metropolitan region in the economic and political function of the global economic system, larger-scale—that is, international—hierarchical diffusion of infection from it can be expected. Recent elegant, and very disturbing, phylogeographic analysis by Gilbert et al. (2007) clearly confirms that the first wave of the international spread of HIV was driven by incubation within the United States. Their work demonstrates convincingly that for HIV-1 group M subtype B, the predominant variant in most countries outside of sub-Saharan Africa, while the virus had an initial transfer event from Africa to Haiti around 1966, the key to subsequent geographic diffusion was what then happened in the United States:

> . . . [A]ll . . . subtype B infections from across the world emanated from a single founder event linked to Haiti. This most likely occurred when the ancestral pandemic clade virus crossed from the Haitian community in the United States to the non-Haitian population there. . . . HIV-1 was circulating in one of the most medically sophisticated settings in the world for more than a decade before AIDS was recognized . . . [That is], [o]ur results suggest that HIV-1 circulated cryptically in the United States for approximately 12 years before the recognition of AIDS in 1981. (Gilbert et al. 2007, p. 18569)

The essential inference is not that AIDS originated in Haiti but rather that HIV-1 group M subtype B became entrained into the U.S. social and spatial system, strongly dominated by New York City and its metropolitan region, where it circulated for over a decade, and then spread hierarchically from the United States to its trading partners. This is the pattern which may be expected for drug-resistant or other evolutionarily transformed variants of the virus which are now incubating in the vast marginalized subpopulations of the United States.

A recent comprehensive review by Jones et al. (2008), which examined the pattern of emerging infections from 1940 to 2004, broadly confirms this analysis. They found that two developed regions strongly dominated the expression of all new diseases in that period: the northeast corridor of the United States, including Boston, New York, Philadelphia, Baltimore, and Washington, DC, each of which has a vast marginalized subpopulation, and the Greater London Metro Region.

We recapitulate something of the evolutionary biology of HIV and of the canonical pattern of hierarchical disease diffusion within the United States, and end with the implications of African American forced displacement for both the national and international spread of evolutionarily transformed HIV.

The Evolutionary Biology of HIV

Affluent subpopulations in the United States have, at least over the short term, benefited greatly from the introduction of highly active antiretroviral therapy (HAART) from 1995 to 1997, for example, HIV/AIDS deaths declined 63% in New York City, primarily among middle-class, and highly organized, gay males (Chiasson et al. 1999). Declines in AIDS deaths have otherwise been quite heterogeneous, depending critically on both the economic resources and community stability of affected populations. R. G. Wallace (2003), for example, found that AIDS declines differed greatly by ethnicity within New York City zip codes: White populations tended to have greater declines in AIDS incidences than did Latino populations, which in turn had greater declines than did Black populations.

Thus, at present, AIDS deaths in the United States are largely another marker of longstanding patterns of racism and socioeconomic inequity (e.g., R. Wallace and McCarthy 2007; R. Wallace et al. 2007). Those who have economic resources, or reside in stable communities not subject to various forms of "redlining" or de facto ethnic cleansing, have effective access to HAART; others do not.

HIV is, however, as indeed are most retroviruses, an evolution machine (e.g., Rambaut et al. 2004) which, at the individual level, almost always develops multiple-drug resistance, resulting in overt AIDS and subsequent premature fatality. Such response to chemical pesticides, as has been the case with myriad other biological pests, is now becoming manifest at the population level. By 2001, in the United States some 50% of patients receiving antiretroviral therapy were infected with viruses that express resistance to at least one of the available retroviral drugs,

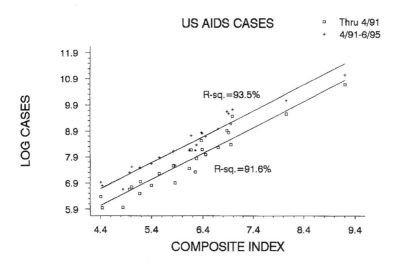

Figure 7.1 Log number of AIDS cases in the 25 largest U.S. metropolitan regions, through April 1991 and April 1991 through June 1995. The composite index is X = .764 Log(USVC91) + .827 Log(USME87/USME72) + .299 Log(Prob. NY). USVC91 is the number of violent crimes, USMEnm the number of manufacturing jobs in year *nm*, and (Prob. NY) the probability of contact with New York City according to U.S. Census migration data for 1985–1990. Applying multivariate analysis of covariance, the two lines are parallel with different intercepts: The second is obtained simply by raising the first. The NYMR is at the upper right of Figure 7.1. The pattern is consistent with the assumption that NYMR drives the hierarchical diffusion of HIV nationally. This suggests a powerful, coherent, national-scale, spatiotemporal hierarchical diffusion strongly linking marginalized communities in NYMR, the apartheid policies which marginalize them, and the epidemic outbreak within them, to the rest of the country.

and transmission of drug-resistant strains is a growing concern (Clavel and Hance 2004; Grant et al. 2002). MDR HIV is, in fact, rapidly becoming the norm, and the virus may even develop a far more virulent life history strategy in response to the evolutionary challenges presented by HAART, its successor microbicide strategies, or planned vaccines (R. G. Wallace 2004; R. Wallace and R. G. Wallace 2004), a circumstance which may have already been observed (e.g., Simon et al. 2003).

The review by Rambaut et al. puts the matter thus:

> HIV shows stronger positive selection than any other organism studied so far . . . [its viral] recombination rate . . . is one of the highest of all organisms . . . Within individual hosts, recombination interacts with selection and drift to produce complex population dynamics, and perhaps provide an efficient mechanism for the virus to escape

from the accumulation of deleterious mutations or to jump between adaptive peaks. Specifically, recombination might accelerate progression to AIDS and provide an effective mechanism (coupled with mutation) to evade drug therapy, vaccine treatment or immune pressure . . . More worryingly, there is evidence that some drug-resistant mutants show a greater infectivity, and in some cases a higher replication rate, compared with viruses without drug resistant mutations. (Rambaut et al. 2004, p, 52)

R. G. Wallace finds that

. . . HAART may select for . . . an HIV with a semelparous life history and a precocious senescence . . . [which] may be embodied by an accelerated time to AIDS or related pathogenesis . . . Because infection survivorship is physiologically enmeshed with host survivorship the asymptomatic stage becomes under HAART a demographic shield against epidemiological intervention. The results appear to exemplify how pathogens use processes at one level of biological organization to defend themselves against impediments directed at them at another. (R. G. Wallace 2004, p. 250)

R. Wallace and R. G. Wallace suggest that

As population-level structured stress appears a fundamental part of the biology of disease [including AIDS], we raise the possibility that simplistic individual-oriented magic bullet drug treatments, vaccines, and risk-reduction programs that do not address the fundamental living and working conditions which underlie disease ecology will fail to control many current epidemics. In addition, such reductionist interventions may go so far as to select for more holistic pathogens characterized by processes operating at multiple levels of biocultural organization. (R. Wallace and R. G. Wallace 2004, p. 105)

MDR-HIV is already emerging in the very epicenters and epicenter populations where HIV itself first appeared (Clavel and Hance 2004), since these were the first to benefit from HAART, and thus seems likely to follow diffusion patterns similar to those of the earlier stage of the AIDS epidemic. More general environmentally transformed (ET)-HIVs can be expected to follow a similar pattern.

The New York Metro Region Drives the Hierarchical Diffusion of HIV

Infectious disease is often seen as a marker for underlying urban structure. For example, Gould and Tornqvist write:

As the urban lattice hardens, and the links between the major centers strengthen, the dominant process is apt to change from a [spatially] contagious to a hierarchical one. (Gould and Tornqvist 1971, p. 160)

We have few examples of this dramatic change in innovation diffusion, but a particularly striking one comes from the early history of the United States (Pyle 1969). The disease of cholera is hardly an innovation we would like to spread around, but it does form a useful geographical tracer in a spatial system, rather like a radioactive isotope for many systems studied by the biological sciences. The first great epidemic struck in 1832 in New York City and Montreal and then diffused slowly along the river systems of the Ohio and Great Lakes. A graphical plot of the time the disease was first reported against distance shows a clear distance effect, indicating that processes of spatial contagion were operating. A plot of time against city size shows no relation whatsoever. However, by 1849, the rudimentary urban hierarchy of the United States was just beginning to emerge. The second epidemic struck in New York City and New Orleans, and a plot of first reporting times against city size indicates that a hierarchical effect was beginning to structure innovation flows at this time. Finally, in 1865, when the third epidemic struck, the railways were already strengthening the structure of America's urban space. The disease jumped rapidly down the urban hierarchy, and a plot of reporting time against city size shows that a clear hierarchical process was at work.

The first stages of the AIDS pandemic in the United States provide a modern example. The cover of Gould's 1993 book *The Slow Plague*, with more detail in Gould's work *Becoming a Geographer* (1999), presents a time sequence of maps showing the number of AIDS cases in the United States on a logarithmic scale. Cases first appear in the largest U.S. port cities: New York, Los Angeles, San Francisco, Miami, and Washington, DC. Subsequent spread is by hierarchical hopscotch to smaller urban centers, followed by a spatially contagious wine-stain-on-a-tablecloth diffusion from city center into the surrounding suburban counties.

Geography has provided public health with concepts including spatial and hierarchical contagion that have been useful to understand the spread and distribution of both infectious and chronic diseases (Cromley and McLafferty 2002; Christakis and Fowler 2007). Spatial distribution is most usually associated with infectious disease in which human contact plays a role and diseases travel with humans across landscapes. Hierarchical diffusion occurs when a phenomenon spreads through an ordered sequence of classes or places. This geographic and social spread is strongly associated with progression of the HIV epidemic.

Figure 7.1, from R. Wallace et al. (1999), gives a detailed analytic treatment of the hierarchical hopscotch. Using multivariate analysis of covariance, it shows the log of the number of AIDS cases in each of the 25 largest U.S. metropolitan regions for two periods, (1) through April 1991 and (2) from April 1991 through June 1995, as functions of a composite index defined in terms of a region's local pattern of susceptibility and its position in the U.S. urban hierarchy. The local indices are (1) the log of the number of violent crimes in the region for 1991, and (2) an index of "rust belt" deindustrialization, the log of the ratio of manufacturing employment in 1987 to that in 1972. The global index, of position on the U.S. urban hierarchy, is the log of the probability of contact with the New York City metro region, the nation's largest, determined from a county-by-county analysis of migration carried out by the U.S. Census for 1985 to 1990.

Locally, high levels of violence and industrial displacement represent bust-town and boomtown social dynamics leading to the loosening of social control. Nationally, the probability of contact with New York City represents inverse socio-spatial distance from the principal epicenter of the U.S. AIDS epidemic. Multivariate analysis of covariance finds the lines for the two time periods are parallel and each accounts for more than 90% of the variance in the dependent variable. Thus, later times are obtained from the earlier simply by raising the graph in parallel. This means that processes within the New York metropolitan region (NYMR), the upper right point of Figure 7.1, drive the national hierarchical diffusion of AIDS during this time span, the pre-HAART period of AIDS spread. We take this as representing a propagating, spatiotemporally coherent epidemic process which has linked disparate, marginalized "core group" neighborhoods of gay males, intravenous drug users, and ethnic minority populations across time and space with the rest of the urbanized United States, ultimately placing some three quarters of the nation's population at increasing risk: as go the NYMR's segregated communities, so goes the nation. See R. Wallace et al. (1999) for details, and Abler, Adams, and Gould (1971) or Gould (1993, 1999) for more general background.

The results of Gilbert et al. (2007) prove conclusively that a similar pattern characterizes the hierarchical spread of HIV variants from the United States to its principal trading partners, and the work of Jones et al. (2008) confirms the northeast corridor of the United States as a hotbed of all emerging infections from 1940 to 2004. New York City hit megacity levels, over 10 million in 1950, an important factor driving the creation of these hierarchies of disease spread, in addition to its centrality in the global economic system.

Recent work by R. G. Wallace et al. (2007) and R. G. Wallace and Fitch (2008) using phylogeographic techniques much like those of Gilbert et al. (2007) shows clearly that China's Guangdong Province serves as the primary international source for incubation and spread of avian influenza H5N1. The work of Gilbert et al. can be interpreted as demonstrating that the United States, and by inference its dominant conurbation, NYMR, served the same role for diffusion of HIV-1 group M subtype B to the industrialized world, and will almost certainly continue to do so for its evolutionary transformed variants.

Discussion and Conclusions

The social and geographic spread of infectious disease within a polity is constrained by, and must be consistent with, an underlying sociogeography in which segregated and oppressed subgroups traditionally constitute ecological keystone populations. Acutely marginalized communities within and surrounding the largest cities are particularly central. There is, then, a blood-simple synergism determining the diffusion of HIV and similar diseases out of the globalized megacities across the world:

(1) All roads lead to Rome, and
(2) All roads lead from Rome.

First, de facto colonial exploitation of economically peripheral zones by global economic networks in which New York City functions as a very important hub has created circumstances ripe for the emergence of new infectious disease by a variety of mechanisms. These pathogens are then entrained by economically determined travel patterns into the largest urban centers of the United States and its allies (in particular the northeast corridor of the United States, and the London Metro Region), which serve as one of the major hubs of the "New Rome" of the current global imperial system. This amalgam, which now functions as an integrated unit, exceeds a population of 55 million.

Second, the U.S. domestic version of the global neoliberal enterprise—in particular, the fatal legacy of slavery that developed into the present system of American apartheid—has created vast marginalized populations within the nation's largest metropolitan regions, particularly the northeast corridor. Newly imported emerging infections then incubate largely unnoticed within these huge permanent de facto refugee camps, and subsequently blow back down the U.S. urban hierarchy, and across to its more developed client states, in particular the European Union.

There are several implications of this model for HIV. Most simply, the find-the-cure "treatment culture," which has dominated both official and nongovernmental organizations' AIDS policy in the United States for some time, and particularly since the development of HAART, is ending as HIV inevitably evolves resistance to drug regimens or alters its life history. An alternative evolutionary strategy for the virus would be to develop greater virulence, that is, higher infectivity and a shortened or absent asymptomatic period (R. G. Wallace 2004; Simon et al. 2003; R. Wallace and R. G. Wallace 2004). Possible vaccines seem similarly challenged by HIV's protean evolutionary nature that allows the virus to rapidly evolve out from under immune suppression. Indeed, a consensus recently emerged that the 20-year search for a vaccine against HIV has made no progress, with little hope for future results (Baltimore 2008).

As the current "test and treat" experiment disintegrates under the relentless pressure of pathogen evolution—as the American God of the Quick Technical Fix fails—new social organizations must emerge to confront the disease. Traditional public health approaches that address underlying structural factors responsible for disease incubation and spread at the population level—primarily the power relations between groups—have largely been abandoned in the United States for obvious political reasons (Garrett 1995). The field is now dominated by the kind of neoliberal, rightist intellectuals who have failed so uniformly on social outcomes and increasingly on economic performance as well. The religious adherence to neoliberal doctrines of disinvestments by governments in basic human needs and deregulation of increasing segments of the social economy is an analog to the sterile Marxism–Leninism studies of the fallen Soviet Union, effectively a center-right Lysenkoism strongly driven by funding patterns.

Controlling MDR, vaccine-resistant, and other evolutionarily transformed HIVs will require resurrection of traditional public health, but this will be difficult because, in the United States, so much of the discipline's history has been lost in favor of the blame-the-victim, medicalized, and individual-oriented perspectives now popular with the current crop of major AIDS funding agencies and their client organizations. Many resulting projects are characterized as fundable trivialities or planting a tree in a desert by even those providing financial support.

ET-HIVs are poised to spread from traditional AIDS epicenters to the rest of the United States in much the same manner the pre-HAART pandemic spread nationally. By contrast, evidence exists that for at least one more egalitarian social system—Amsterdam—there is a declining trend in transmission of drug-resistant HIV (Bezemer et al. 2004).

What is also clear, at least in the New York metropolitan area, which drives the hierarchical diffusion of all emerging infection (Gould 1993, 1999) and is thus a keystone in the international spread of HIV variants from the United States to its trading partners (Gilbert et al. 2007; Jones et al. 2008), is that rebuilding of housing lost to prior policies of ethnic cleansing, and stabilization of remaining low-income housing, is necessary for both regional and national control of ET-HIVs. The current gentrification of Central Harlem and other communities of color, given the region's recent history, will simply further tighten the contact probability field which links metropolitan counties (e.g., R. Wallace and McCarthy 2007 and references therein), and thus hasten the diffusion of the new virus within NYMR, and, from that most central and dominant human ecosystem, throughout the rest of the nation, and by the mechanisms traced by Gilbert et al. (2007), to the rest of the developed world.

In sum, displacing African American and other poor populations from Harlem and East Harlem into the lower-rent suburban periphery, while these communities have among the highest infection and death rates from HIV, will create refugee camp conditions in the outlying NYMR for the development and both national and international spread of evolutionarily transformed HIVs, including MDR strains of the virus, by a number of obvious mechanisms. Urban-suburban linkages are strong in and near New York City and can be expected to link periphery and center in a new, virulent, ecology of ET-HIV that will then diffuse down the urban hierarchy and from city center to suburban ring, effectively placing at increased risk, as stated earlier, some three quarters of the U.S. population. Subsequent spread of ET-HIVs to other industrialized countries will follow the pattern uncovered by Gilbert et al. (2007).

Before the recent economic collapse, condominiums in Manhattan were selling for an average well above US$1 million each. Thus, at that time, assembling a package of only a dozen or so 100-unit apartment houses in Harlem represented a potential profit of over US$1 billion. For a billion dollars, most developers, and their clients among public officials and the leaders of nongovernmental organizations, are unlikely to give much thought to the national and international diffusion of MDR HIV.

Since the economic collapse, although these prices have declined somewhat, the underlying economic incentive remains, and future development of Central Harlem seems aimed at clearcutting existing tenements and building enormous high-rise apartment buildings, increasing unit density fivefold or more, with more than proportionate increase of profit from economies of scale.

Early in 2010, the Bloomberg administration announced plans to close some 25 fire companies (Baker 2010), using the same flawed mathematical models that were responsible for the first wave of large-scale urban burnout in the 1970s, since these both provide a shield against legal accusations of "arbitrary and capricious" action and serve to shelter the city from U.S. civil rights laws that require proof of intent in matters of racial discrimination, rather than proof of effect. It is as if the city chose to save money by decreasing chlorination of the water supply: at some point a cholera epidemic would become inevitable. Given the realities of contagious urban decay driven by increasing signs of fire damage, erosion of fire extinguishment services will, at some point, inevitably trigger a recurrence of the fulminating South Bronx process of the 1970s, destroying the housing of the poor and accelerating the "Cape Town–ization" of NYMR, with all the implications for public health and public order.

Although the initial plans for company closings were successfully opposed by the city council after a considerable battle, as of early 2011 New York City plans to close some 20 fire companies at night, when the demand for fire service declines but when fires that do occur tend to be discovered at a late stage and thus grow rapidly, with greater potential for property damage and injury.

The results of these processes seem likely to establish NYMR as the global source of MDR- and extensively-drug resistant (XDR)-HIV, in much the same manner for deep structural reasons that China's Guangdong Province—a megalopolis topping New York City in population—for deep structural reasons has become the epicenter for the worldwide transmission of avian influenza.

Summary

HIV displays the strongest positive selection of any known animal organism, and easily adapts to selection pressures generated by antiretrovirals, other microbicides, and vaccines. HIV can respond not only by developing multiple-drug resistance, but also through significant alterations in life history strategy, that is, increased virulence. Thus, effective control requires sophisticated multifactorial ecosystem intervention, including a return to traditional public health approaches aimed squarely at improving living and working conditions among marginalized populations that are the ecological keystones of pandemic infection.

We have examined a precise counterstrategy, a systematic program of forced displacement affecting poor African Americans living in New York City's most heavily infected neighborhoods, given that the city is both the principal driving epicenter for the hierarchical spatial diffusion of emerging infections in the U.S. and its economic partners and is a central focus of HIV itself. Thus, the NYMR appears to play a similar central role for the spread of MDR- and other ET-HIVs to the rest of the industrialized world as does China's Guangdong Province for the international dispersal of avian influenza.

References

Abler R, Adams J, Gould P. 1971. *Spatial Organization: The Geographer's View of the World*. Engelwood, NJ: Prentice-Hall.

Baker A. 2010. City Fire Department Braces for Cuts. *New York Times*. February 2, 2010:19.

Baltimore D. 2008. Speech given at the Annual Meeting of the American Association for the Advancement of Science, Boston, MA, February 2008.

Bezemer D, Jurriaans S, Prins M, et al. 2004. Declining trend in transmission of drug-resistant HIV-1 in Amsterdam. *AIDS*. 18:1571–1577.

Chiasson M, Berenson L, Li W, et al. 1999. Declining HIV/AIDS mortality in New York City. *J Acquir Immune Defic Syndr*. 21:59–64.

Christakis N, Fowler J. 2007. The spread of obesity in a large social network over 32 years. *New Engl J Med*. 357:370–379.

Clavel F, Hance A. 2004. HIV drug resistance. *New Engl J Med*. 350:1023–1035.

Cromley EK, McLafferty SL. 2002. *GIS and Public Health*. New York, NY: Guilford.

Freeman H, McCord C. 1990. Excess mortality in Harlem. *New Engl J Med.* 322:173–180.

Garrett L. 1995. *The Coming Plague: Newly Emerging Diseases in a World Out of Balance*. New York, NY: Penguin.

Gilbert M, Rambaut A, Wlasiuk G, et al. 2007. The emergence of HIV/AIDS in the Americas and beyond. *Proc Natl Acad Sci U S A.* 104:18566–18570.

Gould P. 1993. *The Slow Plague*. Oxford, England: Blackwell.

Gould P. 1999. *Becoming a Geographer*. New York, NY: Syracuse University.

Gould P, Tornqvist G. 1971. Information, innovation, and acceptance. In: Hägerstrand T, Kuklinski R, editors. *Information Systems for Regional Development—A Seminar*. Lund Series in Geography. Ser. B, Human Geography No. 37. Lund, Sweden: Gleerup:148–168.

Grant R, Hecht F, Warmerdam M, et al. 2002. Time trends in primary HIV-1 drug resistance among recently infected persons. *JAMA.* 288:181–188.

Jones K, Patel N, Levy MA, et al. 2008. Global trends in emerging infection. *Nature.* 451:990–993.

Massey D, Denton NA. 1993. *American Apartheid: Segregation and the Making of the Underclass*. Cambridge, MA: Harvard University.

New York City Department of Health and Mental Hygiene. 2006. *HIV Epidemiology Program, 2nd Semiannual Report*. Vol. 1, no. 2. Available at: http://www.nyc.gov/html/doh/html/dires/hivepi.shtml. Accessed February 17, 2011.

Newman K, Wyly E. 2006. The right to stay put, revisited: gentrification and resistance to displacement in New York City. *Urban Stud.* 43:23–57.

Pyle G. 1969. Diffusion of cholera in the United States. *Geogr Anal.* 1:59–75.

Office of the High Commissioner on Human Rights (OHCHR). 1996. Fact Sheet 25, Forced Evictions and Human Rights. Geneva, Switzerland: OHCHR. Available at: http://www.ohchr.org/Documents/Publications/FactSheet25en.pdf. Accessed March 28, 2011.

Rambaut A, Posada D, Crandall K, Holmes E. 2004. The causes and consequences of HIV evolution. *Nat Rev Genet.* 5:52–61.

Simon V, Padte N, Murray D, et al. 2003. Infectivity and replication capacity of drug-resistant human immunodeficiency virus type 1 variants isolated during primary infection. *J Virol.* 77:7736–7745.

Susser I. 1982. *Normal Street: Poverty and Politics in an Urban Neighborhood.* New York, NY: Oxford University.

Task Force on Urban Fire Protection. 1978. Report of Assembly Republican Task Force on Urban Fire Protection [press release, January 27, 1978]. New York, NY: Office of the Republican Leader of the New York State Assembly.

Ullmann JE. 1988. *The Anatomy of Industrial Decline: Productivity, Investment, and Location in U.S. Manufacturing.* Westport, CT: Greenwood-Quorum Books.

Wallace D. 2001. Discriminatory public policies and the New York City tuberculosis epidemic, 1975–1993. *Microbes Infect.* 3:515–524.

Wallace D, Wallace R. 1998. *A Plague on Your Houses.* New York, NY: Verso.

Wallace D, Wallace R. 2003. The recent tuberculosis epidemic in New York City: warning from the de-developing world. In: Gandy M, Zumla A, editors. *The Return of the White Plague: Global Poverty and the 'New' Tuberculosis.* New York, NY: Verso:125–146.

Wallace R. 1988. A synergism of plagues: "planned shrinkage," contagious housing destruction, and AIDS in the Bronx. *Environ Res.* 47:1–33.

Wallace R. 1990. Urban desertification, public health and public order: "planned shrinkage," violent death, substance abuse and AIDS in the Bronx. *Soc Sci Med.* 31:801–813.

Wallace R. 1999. Emerging infections and nested Martingales: the entrainment of affluent populations into the disease ecology of marginalization. *Environ Plan A.* 31:1787–1803.

Wallace R, Fullilove MT. 2008. *Collective Consciousness and Its Discontents: Institutional Distributed Cognition, Racial Policy and Public Health in the United States.* New York, NY: Springer.

Wallace R, Huang Y, Gould P, Wallace D. 1997. The hierarchical diffusion of AIDS and violent crime among U.S. metropolitan regions: inner-city decay, stochastic resonance and reversal of the mortality transition. *Soc Sci Med.* 44:935–947.

Wallace R, McCarthy K. 2007. The unstable public health ecology of the New York metropolitan region: implications for accelerated national spread of emerging infection. *Environ Plan A.* 39:1181–1192.

Wallace R, Wallace D. 1993. Inner city disease and the public health of the suburbs: the sociogeographic dispersion of point-source infection. *Environ Plan A*. 25:1701–1723.

Wallace R, Wallace D. 1997a. Community marginalization and the diffusion of disease and disorder in the United States. *BMJ*. 314:1341–1347.

Wallace R, Wallace D. 1997b. The destruction of U.S. minority urban communities and the resurgence of tuberculosis: ecosystem dynamics of the white plague in the de-developing world. *Environ Plan A*. 29:269–291.

Wallace R, Wallace D, Ahern J, Galea S. 2007. A failure of resilience: estimating response of New York City's public health ecosystem to sudden disaster. *Health Place*. 13:545–550.

Wallace R, Wallace D, Ullmann JE, Andrews H. 1999. Deindustrialization, inner-city decay, and the hierarchical diffusion of AIDS in the USA: how neoliberal and cold war policies magnified the ecological niche for emerging infections and created a national security crisis. *Environ Plan A*. 31:113–139.

Wallace R, Wallace RG. 2004. Adaptive chronic infection, structured stress, and medical magic bullets: do reductionist cures select for holistic diseases? *BioSystems*. 77:93–108.

Wallace RG. 2003. AIDS in the HAART era: New York's heterogeneous geography. *Soc Sci Med*. 56:1155–1171.

Wallace RG. 2004. Projecting the impact of HAART on the evolution of HIV's life history. *Ecol Modell*. 176:227–253.

Wallace RG, Fitch W. 2008. Influenza A H5N1 immigration is filtered out at some international borders. *PLoS One*. 3:e1697.

Wallace RG, HoDac H, Lathrop R, Fitch W. 2007. A statistical phylogeography of influenza A H5N1. *Proc Natl Acad Sci U S A*. 104:4473–4478.

8

Megacities and Disaster Preparedness

Irshad Shaikh, MD, PhD, MPH, and Gregory Pappas, MD, PhD

ALL BUT THREE OR four of the world's 25 megacities are located in regions where disastrous seismic or weather-related events are largely inevitable (Revkin 2010; Bell et al. 2009; Pacific Disaster Center and Earthquake and Megacities Initiative 2010). Millions of deaths could result from a single earthquake in a megacity such as Mexico City, Karachi, or Tehran (Bilham 1999). More than half of the almost 12 million people in Lagos live in a flood plain (Oyebande 1990).

Megacities face risks from both natural disasters and industrial accidents; they are frequently located in proximity to nuclear power plants and other major industrial facilities. Human conflict (e.g., wars, terrorism) in or near megacities raises similar concerns. Additionally, the potential for social and political violence arising from the living conditions experienced by slum populations in megacities is well documented (Susser 2002).

Concern over the preparedness of megacities for disaster has been raised within a general framework, but has not yet addressed the unique social and structural vulnerabilities of such cities (Fernandez et al. 2006; Pacific Disaster Center and Earthquake and Megacities Initiative 2010). This chapter addresses three questions related to megacities and disasters: What is unique about disasters in megacities? Why should megacities be given priority in disaster preparedness efforts? What directions should disaster preparedness efforts in megacities take? To answer these critical policy and program questions, we drew on the extensive social science literature on megacities—in the areas of demography, sociology, anthropology, political science, and others—which provides useful perspectives on disaster preparedness efforts.

In 2007, for the first time in human history, more than half of the world's population was living in urban areas (United Nations Population Division 2008). This figure is expected to increase to 70% by 2025. The growth of megacities is relatively recent, with New York City being the first to reach ten million in 1950. By 1990, there were 12 megacities; 57 cities are projected to reach populations of ten million by 2015 (Brinkhoff 2010). Many of these urban centers are huge amalgamations, continuous urban landscapes in which a number of cities have grown together; they are also called "megalopolises." Most importantly, almost three quarters of megacities (19 of 25) are located in less-developed countries. Not surprisingly, disaster preparedness in these cities is weak. A study of disaster preparedness in four megacities—Manila, Mumbai, Tehran, and Istanbul—pointed out strengths and weaknesses of disaster preparedness for large municipal areas. Although these megacities had performed risk analysis and evaluation, particularly in regards to earthquakes, other areas were not well developed. Governance and knowledge management for disasters preparedness were identified as areas which needed improvement in these megacities. Lack of preparedness in informal settlements was noted as a serious problem for megacities (Fernandez et al. 2006).

The Implication of Megacity Growth and Inequalities for Disaster Preparedness

Megacities have unique characteristics beyond their huge size that must be understood to fully consider disaster preparedness for megacities. As a group, megacities are both on the cutting edge of globalization and attract large and increasingly marginalized populations (Castells 1998). They are hubs for global banking and politics; they are innovation and media centers; and they are sites of military activity, global gangsterism, and potential pandemics. Through megacities, the interconnectedness of global institutions—economic, political, social, and military—encourages further networking, growth, and development (Pappas, Hyder, and Akhter 2003).

The same forces that have led to the growth of megacities as economic hubs have also led to growing inequalities within urban populations and the growth of slums. During the past few decades, megacities have been influenced by two global trends in policy: deregulation and disinvestment in basic human needs.

This trend, alternatively called "neoliberalism" or the "Washington Consensus," has led to rapid urban growth accompanied by increasing social inequality (Held 2004). Older megacities such as New York City were transformed from industrial centers into financial centers, changing the social composition of the city and creating new mosaics of class and ethnicity and new vulnerable populations (Susser 2002).

Because of rapid unplanned growth and the social and spatial transformation of megacities, the needs of these cities' populations often exceed the ability of administrative structures to meet those needs. Megacities have acted like magnets, drawing populations from surrounding regions and around the world, creating huge slums in the process. Widening disparities in the human condition are a defining feature of megacities (Baer, Singer, and Susser 2003). Daily life in many megacities is characterized by problems of access to basic services (e.g., electricity, water, sewage, solid waste management, security). In megacities throughout the less-developed world, even minor disruptions of daily life (traffic jams, storms, strikes) pose serious problems for entire metropolitan areas. Should these populations experience an environmental disaster on the scale of a flood, earthquake, or hurricane without sufficient disaster preparedness, the result can only be enormous loss of life.

What Is Unique About Disasters In Megacities?

The features of megacities are associated with a unique set of risks and resiliencies for disaster preparedness. The clearest risk is the potential for large numbers of human casualties in a disaster. Mass casualties are predictable in densely populated areas after a major disaster; additionally, communicable diseases spread more rapidly in densely populated urban areas (Bell et al. 2009).

Fragile infrastructures such as water and sewer systems in many megacities—risks for human health on a daily basis—create serious vulnerabilities and challenges for disaster preparedness. In earthquake-prone cities, the death rate is a function of the quality of construction; the difference between life and death can be as simple as how much sand went into the concrete and how much steel went into supporting columns. As one source put it, "In recent earthquakes, buildings have acted as weapons of mass destruction" (Bilham 2010, p. 1). Even a relatively small earthquake or storm in a megacity like Karachi, Cairo, or Jakarta would have a devastating impact on the water, sewer, and solid waste management systems on which millions of people depend. The majority of megacities have potentially vulnerable nuclear power facilities nearby that pose enormous secondary hazards. Security systems (fire/rescue and police), which in many megacities are currently ill prepared and inadequate for daily needs, are equally at risk of disruption and loss in the event of a disaster. Social disruption in megacities takes on its own dynamics because of sheer numbers of people as well as population density; for example, lack of infrastructure for adequate crowd control (e.g., political gatherings, sporting events) frequently leads to deaths.

The underlying vulnerability of poor people in megacities to the secondary and tertiary consequences of a disaster is clear when the enormous numbers of people affected are taken into account. The potential for a mass exodus from a city or for a surge of people into a city from surrounding areas has been predicted in the event of megacity disasters (Axworthy, Fallick, and Ross 2005). The literature on mob psychology and descriptions of recent disasters in megacities offer bleak narratives for the response and reconstruction phases of disasters. Disruption of water, electricity, and solid waste management creates conditions that quickly overwhelm whatever medical capacity is available after a disaster. Megacities have highly vulnerable supply lines for food, fuel, medicine, and other necessities that also would be disrupted in the event of a major disaster. Millions of poor people without access to food, water, and shelter become the secondary and tertiary consequences of the initial disaster event. Unless sufficient human and physical resources can be brought to bear to deal with these secondary and tertiary consequences, various complex and negative scenarios may result that have worldwide implications.

While low levels of infrastructure development in some megacities are major obstacles to disaster preparedness, poor communities have some resilience that should be considered in disaster planning. Home electrical generators and storage of water are common strategies for people in megacities, where the services provided by the municipal infrastructure are not dependable. The quality and extent of backup systems in megacities vary greatly, and wealthy residents have better systems in place than do poor residents (Ugaz and Price 2003).

As hubs of economic, political, and media attention, megacities are of particular interest to terrorists, and the transportation systems of these cities have been the site of a number of terrorist attacks. Releasing a hazardous material into a public transportation system in a megacity, as occurred in Tokyo in 1995, exploits the size and density of megacity populations. As the center of a regional media industry, Mumbai also has been a predictable target of terrorism.

The unique and emerging nature of sprawling megacities, and resultant hazards and risks, have not been fully integrated into disaster risk reduction and emergency preparedness planning (Wisner 2003). Priorities and practices in disaster management have historically focused on the response to the disaster and on spending substantial resources to mitigate consequences and aid recovery. Significantly fewer resources been spent on identifying and reducing vulnerability of slums to disaster and on general preparedness for disaster. The need to improve disaster risk reduction and emergency preparedness has tended to fall through the cracks of development cooperation and emergency relief.

Regardless of any resiliency, the most vulnerable populations in megacities are least prepared for disaster (Musani and Shaikh 2006). Historical political patterns and long-standing neglect have often led to distrust between neighborhoods and the municipal bodies responsible for disaster preparedness. Nongovernmental organizations (NGOs) and community-based organizations (CBOs) working in the poorer areas of megacities have grown up around the problems of vulnerable populations. These organizations are often part of social and political organizations and movements, and their relationships with governments have been complex and often confrontational.

Should Megacities Be Given Priority in Disaster Preparedness Efforts?

The rationale for giving megacities priority in disaster preparedness efforts flows from (1) the acknowledged size of vulnerable populations in these urban centers, (2) the unique role they play in the global order, and (3) the unique opportunities they present for successful disaster preparedness efforts. Increased funding and a refocusing of efforts in megacities are needed both to prevent and to mitigate disasters.

Massive loss of human life at the time of the initial crisis is predictable in large, densely populated cities. The challenge presented to rescue workers will be insurmountable in most megacities, even with the best-organized and immediate global response. In addition, the high connectivity of international transport systems based in megacities increases the risk of spreading influenza and other highly contagious diseases globally (Horton 1996). Pandemics in a megacity are predicted to lead to rapid and high rates of morbidity and mortality (Lee et al. 2007).

The highly predictable secondary consequences of the breakdown of basic infrastructure and health systems in megacities would also be severe and leave large numbers of people at risk. Provision of basic services (e.g., water, sewage, utilities, security, and health care) after disasters creates enormous problems. Finally, the overwhelmed traffic conditions that are a daily occurrence in many megacities can easily be projected to block transport of medical emergency services during a major disaster.

Because of the presence of global economic, social, and military institutions in megacities, the occurrence of a disaster would have major global implications. Many of these cities are either capitals or major population centers critical to a national government, and a large-scale disaster in such a place could lead to national and regional political instability. Exacerbation of regional tensions and increases in military conflicts also are predictable (Brancati 2007). Because megacities are hubs for economic production, coordination, and distribution, disasters have serious consequences for disruption of the fragile economies of many countries and regions (Noji 1997). The collapse of megacity-controlled markets would have devastating effects on global financial markets. These scenarios of social and economic deterioration highlight the importance of megacities in the world today and emphasize the need to give priority to megacity disaster preparedness.

Another reason to give priority to disaster preparedness in megacities is that some features of megacities contribute to the success of disaster preparedness efforts. Although megacities harbor unique disaster risks for poorer segments of the population, they also contribute to effective disaster preparedness as a result of other unique megacity characteristics. The critical mass of human resources in megacities—government agencies, organizations, industry, and institutions of research and higher learning—can be mobilized in planning efforts to deal with disasters, and the fact that most national and global agencies responsible for disaster preparedness are located in megacities makes coordinated planning more feasible. Preparedness capacity in megacities is also more likely to be sustainable, because of the concentrated human resources in those places.

In addition, investment in capacity-building for disaster preparedness in megacities creates resources that can be used to respond to future regional, national, and global disasters. The improved capacity for community development in the NGO and CBO sector, many of which work in the area of disaster preparedness, is another resource that can be built upon in megacities.

What Directions Should Disaster Preparedness Efforts in Megacities Take?

The unique vulnerabilities and potentials of megacities should give direction to preparedness efforts. We identified four strategies to improve disaster preparedness in megacities: (1) twinning of megacities in preparedness, (2) megacity simulations exercises, (3) investments in information technologies, and (4) development of public-private partnerships including vulnerable communities (Table 8.1).

Twinning of Cities

Creating links between megacities to build capacity is an attractive direction for programming and funding. Some megacities have developed unique systems to prevent, mitigate, and respond to disasters, and others can learn from these cities' knowledge and experiences. The megacity of Osaka, Japan, an amalgamation of more than 16 million people, has developed a sophisticated capacity for dealing with earthquakes and related disasters. Kobe (part of the Osaka amalgamation) maintains an earthquake museum that is a global resource for information on earthquakes in megacities (Goldstein 1998). Pairing Osaka with Tehran (which also experiences severe earthquakes), for example, could lead to a constructive dialogue between city officials about earthquake preparedness. The unique problems and potential in each of these cities can help build Tehran's programs and

Table 8.1   Four Strategies for Development of Megacity Disaster Preparedness

1	Twinning of sister cities for preparedness
2	Disaster simulation exercises
3	Investment in information technology
4	Development of public-private partnerships including vulnerable communities

refine those in Osaka. Differences between megacities in terms of infrastructure, available resources, and age of population must be given careful consideration when twinning is considered, however.

Cities such as Tokyo and New York, with extensive experience with disasters, have developed mechanisms unique to their largescale networks of government and private sector institutions, universities, and foundations. Megacities in resource-poor settings could benefit from access to these information networks that would strengthen disaster preparedness in their regions.

Simulations of Disasters

Conducting disaster simulations in megacities can provide important information on which to base disaster preparedness programs. Most disaster simulations have been designed for national and regional settings; other specially designed simulations have been used to promote the understanding of disaster risks for megacities. These exercises point the way toward implementation of effective programs for prevention, mitigation, and response to environmental and other types of disasters in large cities. A series of simulation exercises for megacities that include observers from twinned and neighboring cities would be useful for sharing information. Such an exercise should be supported by global or regional agencies charged with disaster preparedness.

Technological Innovations

Technological innovations that address disaster preparedness are more likely to be developed in megacities and can have dramatic life-saving potential. This recommendation takes advantage of a technological capacity already present in megacities: mobile phones. The digital, networked nature of megacities (even in less-developed countries) provides a basis for development of an early warning system and a citizen's information network utilizing mobile phones to supplement or complement broadcast communications (Teich et al. 2002). The fact that these technological innovations are now in the hands of many urban residents creates enormous potential for disaster preparedness. However, such broad access must be managed; misinformation also flows through networks of cell phone users. The use of cell phones has been documented as a useful tool in disaster response and can be further developed in megacities. In one study, the high capacity of Tokyo for use of geographic information systems

(GIS) has led to a detailed proposal for expansion of humanitarian response systems (Kwan and Lee 2005). The potential for sharing hospital information during disasters via network technology has also been discussed (Arnold et al. 2004).

One of the most frustrating and common problems encountered in coordination of disaster response efforts is the lack of information. The problems created by a lack of timely information about conditions during a disaster have been likened to the "fog of war." Perhaps one of the most interesting potential developments in disaster preparedness technology is the use of satellite visual imaging to quickly estimate damage and to project secondary consequences. Satellite images have become an effective tool for collecting information before, during, and after a disaster. Images can be analyzed by software that detects changes and projects consequences, including estimation of numbers dead and injured, numbers of displaced persons, destruction of key infrastructures, and other critical information. Population estimates developed from satellite imaging also have been developed (Sutton et al. 2001).

Technological advances could speed information flow from days or weeks to mere hours. Advanced systems could collect and analyze data to estimate the consequences of disasters and to direct response. In the near future, software may be able to compare images collected before and after a disaster to detect changes and estimate numbers of dead and injured, numbers of displaced, destruction of key infrastructures, and other critical information.

Disaster management in the past has been based more on conventional wisdom than on scientific evidence. Prevention and preparedness strategies based on science and evidence could save billions of dollars and lives by improving the efficiency of disaster response operations (Laxminarayan et al. 2006). Within existing systems (economic, military, and political), communication, decision-making, and deployment of resources for disasters can be strengthened through the existing template of networks between megacities.

Public–Private Partnerships

Perhaps the most important direction for disaster risk reduction and emergency preparedness in megacities is community involvement. The Hyogo Framework, a globally adopted document that provides guidance for building disaster preparedness, strongly recommends systematic inclusion of communities in planning and development of public–private partnerships (International Strategy for Disaster Reduction 2005). Megacities provide an impressive set of human resources even in resource-poor settings, but the massive size of their populations make it difficult for civil authorities to meet disaster preparedness needs. The rise of NGOs and CBOs, now a strong presence in most megacities, presents an opportunity for governments charged with disaster risk reduction and emergency preparedness to move forward with new forms of engagement to meet the special needs of megacities.

New partnerships are needed to address the problems and challenges that confront disaster management in megacities. Community response has long been emphasized as an important component of disaster response, but conditions in megacities make it increasingly difficult to mobilize human resources for effective response. Focused programming to overcome existing divisions between municipal bodies and community groups, especially in vulnerable poor communities, must be planned, funded, and implemented. A new model based on a Tokyo study suggests ways to carry out socially sensitive vulnerability assessments (Uitto 1998).

A number of problems have been identified regarding the community-response model of disaster preparedness. Poor individuals lack resources to respond to disasters and poor neighborhoods lack institutions and infrastructure to respond. However, investment in CBOs encourages collaboration with government plans for disaster preparedness and is essential. Neoliberal policies have slowed efforts to incorporate civil-society groups in preparedness efforts (Gunewardena and Schuller 2008).

Summary

This chapter presents the unique problems of disaster preparedness in megacities and a rationale for giving megacities priority for support to improve disaster preparedness. It also provides direction for investment in disaster preparedness by megacities, emphasizing the twinning of megacities to help them learn from each another, creating simulations of megacity disasters that focus attention on the unique problems in particular cities, working through public-private partnerships, and the implementation of technological innovations that can be used in planning for and responding to disasters.

The literature on megacities has helped frame the special issues of disaster risk reduction and emergency preparedness in megacities. Megacities are different from other large population centers in terms of population size and density, and the enormous scale of these differences has in addition shaped the ways megacities function. The unique problems faced by megacities should lead to disaster risk reduction strategies tailored to their special needs.

Finally, the increased human risk and fragility of megacities during disasters should be considered a feature of megacities. The appearance of H1N1 infection in Mexico City and New York revealed serious issues for emergency preparedness in those two megacities (Bell et al. 2009). Megacities are for now a permanent feature of life on the planet, and all indications are that they are becoming both more complex and more common.

Acknowledgments

The authors would like to acknowledge Kayla Street, who provided some of the bibliographic citations as part of a graduate studies project. Thanks to Linda Landesman for sharing a manuscript on disaster preparedness in New York City, which helped inform this report, and to Omar Khan for his helpful comments on the manuscript.

References

Arnold JL, Levine BN, Manmatha R, et al. 2004. Information-sharing in out-of-hospital disaster response: the future role of information technology. *Prehosp Disaster Med.* 19:201–207.

Axworthy L, Fallick AL, Ross K. 2005. The secure city. Vancouver Working Group Discussion Papers for the World Urban Forum 2006, Oberlander HP, editor. Vancouver, BC: Liu Institute for Global Issues, University of British Columbia. Available at: http://www.ahva.ubc.ca/WUF/pdf/e_the_secure_city_eng.pdf. Accessed September 10, 2010.

Baer HA, Singer M, Susser I. 2003. *Medical Anthropology and the World System.* Westport, CT: Praeger.

Bell DM, Weisfuse IB, Hernandez-Avila M, et al. 2009. Pandemic influenza as 21st century urban public health crisis. *Emerg Infect Dis.* 15 [serial online].

Bilham R. 1999. Millions at risk as big cities grow apace in earthquake zones. *Nature*. 401:738.

Bilham R. 2010. Lessons from the Haiti earthquake. *Nature*. 463:878–879. Available at: http://www.nature.com/nature/journal/v463/n7283/full/463878a.html. Accessed July 25, 2010.

Brancati D. 2007. Political aftershocks: the impact of earthquakes on intrastate conflict. *J Conflict Resolut*. 51:715–743.

Brinkhoff T. 2010. *The Principal Agglomerations of the World*. Available at: http://www.citypopulation.de/world/Agglomerations.html. Accessed June 24, 2010.

Castells M. 1998. *Why the Megacities Focus? Megacities in the New World Disorder*. Piermont, NY: The Megacities Project. Publication MCP-018. Available at: http://www.megacities.net/pdf/publications_pdf_mcp018intro.pdf. Accessed June 25, 2010.

Fernandez J, Bendimerad F, Mattingly S, Buika J. 2006. *Comparative Analysis of Disaster Risk Management Practices in Seven Megacities*. Quezon City, Philippines: Earthquakes and Megacities Initiative. Available at: http://emi.pdc.org/DRMlibrary/General/Comparative-analysis-DRM-in-7-megacities.pdf. Accessed June 25, 2010.

Goldstein D. 1998. 1995 Kobe Earthquake. The Earthquake Museum. Available at: http://www.olympus.net/personal/gofamily/quake/famous/kobe.html. Accessed July 25, 2010.

Gunewardena N, Schuller M. 2008. *Capitalizing on Catastrophe: Neoliberal Strategies in Disaster Reconstruction*. Lanham, MD: AltaMira.

Hasan A. 2001. *Working With Community*. Karachi, Pakistan: City.

Held D. 2004. *Global Covenant: The Social Democratic Alternative to the Washington Consensus*. Malden, MA: Polity.

Horton R. 1996. The infected metropolis. *Lancet*. 347:134–136.

International Strategy for Disaster Reduction. 2005. *Hyogo Framework for Action 2005–2010: Building the Resilience of Nations and Communities to Disasters*. Geneva, Switzerland: United Nations Inter-Agency Secretariat of the International Strategy for Disaster Reduction.

Kwan M-P, Lee J. 2005. Emergency response after 9/11: the potential of real-time 3D GIS for quick emergency response in micro-spatial environments. *Comput Environ Urban Syst*. 29:93–113.

Laxminarayan R, Mills AJ, Breman JG, et al. 2006. Advancement of global health: key messages from the Disease Control Priorities Project. *Lancet*. 367:1193–1208.

Lee VJ, Chen MI, Chan SP, et al. 2007. Influenza pandemics in Singapore, a tropical, globally connected city. *Emerg Infect Dis*. 13:1025–1065.

Musani A, Shaikh I. 2006. Preparing for and responding to conflict and disaster in the Eastern Mediterranean Region (EMR): a case for research capacity strengthening (RCS). Presented at: Global Forum for Health Research; October 29–November 2; Cairo, Egypt. Available at: http://www.emro.who.int/eha/pdf/GF10_paper.pdf. Accessed June 25, 2010.

Noji EK, editor. 1997. *The Public Health Consequences of Disasters*. New York, NY: Oxford University.

Oyebande L. 1990. Aspects of urban hydrology and the challenges for African urban environments. *Afr Urban Q*. 5:39–68.

Pacific Disaster Center and Earthquake and Megacities Initiative. 2008. Home page. Available at: http://www.pdc.org/emi/emihome.html. Accessed June 1, 2010.

Pappas G, Hyder AA, Akhter N. 2003. Globalization and health: toward a new framework for public health. *Social Theory Health*. 1:91–107.

Revkin AC. 2010. Disaster awaits cities in earthquake zone. *New York Times*. February 25.

Susser I, editor. 2002. *The Castells Reader on Cities and Social Theory*. Malden, MA: Blackwell.

Sutton P, Roberts D, Elvidge C, Baugh K. 2001. Census from heaven: an estimate of the global human population using night-time satellite imagery. *Int. J Remote Sens*. 22:3061–3076.

Teich JM, Wagner MM, Mackenzie CF, Schafer KO. 2002. The informatics response in disaster, terrorism, and war. *J Am Med Inform Assoc*. 9:97–104.

Ugaz C, Waddams Price C, editors. 2003. *Utility Privatization and Regulation: A Fair Deal for Consumers?* Cheltenham, England: Edward Elgar.

Uitto JI. 1998. The geography of disaster vulnerability in megacities: a theoretical framework. *Appl Geogr*. 18:7–16.

United Nations Population Division. 2008. *An Overview of Urbanization, Internal Migration, Population Distribution and Development in the World*. New York, NY: Department of Economic and Social Affairs United Nations Secretariat.

Wisner B. 2003. Disaster risk reduction in megacities: making the most of human and social capital. In: Kreimer A, Arnold M, Carlin A, editors. *Building Safer Cities: The Future of Disaster Risk*. Disaster Risk Management Series No. 3. Washington, DC: World Bank:181–196.

9

Emergency Management in a Megacity: The 2003 Niagara Mohawk Blackout and the Impact on New York City

Linda Young Landesman, DrPH, MSW, and
Isaac B. Weisfuse, MD, MPH

PREPARING FOR AND RESPONDING to emergencies is a key challenge for megacities—even those as rich in resources as New York City (NYC) and its surrounding areas. This case study provides a look at NYC's medical and public health response when the region lost power for up to 30 hours in 2003.

NYC, with 27,000 people per square mile, is the most densely populated city in the United States. Almost 8.4 million residents, in addition to scores of tourists and commuters, live and work in a vertical world of skyscrapers spread across five boroughs. The key business center, Manhattan, is an island separated from the other boroughs by water, bridges, and tunnels. Nine different transit systems bring more than 9.3 million passengers into NYC on an average weekday (U.S. Department of Transportation 2004). With the largest rapid transit system in the world, NYC faces a daily challenge of moving people. Life in NYC is so dependent on the subway that the city is home to one of only three 24-hour subway systems in the world.

NYC has the largest local Department of Health and Mental Hygiene (DOHMH) in the country and is home to six major medical schools. It has more than 60 acute care hospitals and over 180 nursing homes, with over 23,000 hospital and 45,000 nursing home beds in service daily (NYC Emergency Response Task Force 2003). In addition, hundreds of continuing care facilities and ambulatory care centers provide preventive services, care for chronic disease, and state-of-the-art care for the most complicated health problems. This extensive capacity facilitates the provision of medical and public health services on a regular basis and is organized to be quickly activated in emergencies. Providing emergency services is complicated, because NYC is an international city, with approximately 170 languages spoken within its limits.

Electrical Power Distribution

Electrical power is essential to modern life in a megacity. It is used for heating, cooling, lighting, refrigeration and cooking, computing and entertainment, and keeping life-saving medical equipment operational. Unlike fuels such as coal or natural gas, electricity is difficult to store, so power is only generated as it is used.

In the United States, the plants where electricity is generated and the locations where power is used are interconnected through a system of planned distribution. Electrical power is sent from the plant where it is produced to our homes and workplaces through a state-to-state network of wires called a "grid." When running smoothly, this distribution system provides for continuous power, even when one of the power plants or transmission towers is taken out of service.

Unexpected demands for power can upset the distribution of electricity in a grid; therefore, these power demands are monitored by control centers. A loss of power in one section can ripple through the entire grid. During major blackouts, when one part of the system fails, the electrical load is shifted onto the neighboring systems. As neighboring grids become overloaded, adjoining parts also become overburdened. Where the adjoining grid is already at capacity, the wires shut down or fail sequentially, shutting down one section after another. When power is restored, it is done in stages, so that restoration does not cause a sudden surge in demand beyond what the system can handle.

Blackout Events

It had been more than 25 years since the New York City blackout of 1977 when NYC lost all power on a hot and sunny August afternoon in 2003. A massive electrical shutdown began in Ohio and affected the Niagara Mohawk power grid, which covered most of the northeastern United States and parts of eastern Canada. The grid failed as a result of a chain reaction of mistakes compounding other mistakes, including transmission lines that needed maintenance, careless system operators, and critical monitoring software that had been turned off (Belson and Wald 2003).

The chain of events began when power lines in Ohio hung down onto overgrown trees and caught on fire, shutting off nearby electricity. The software used to monitor that section of the grid was not working because a technician had turned it off when he went to lunch. As a result, those controlling the system did not know of the failures quickly enough to redirect the power. With the problem not addressed, the remaining power lines became overloaded and shut themselves down, one by one. By the time this sequential shutdown was about to affect NYC, operators at the Consolidated Edison Electric Company (Con Ed) control center in New York had an impossible 8 seconds to react before their electrical grid started shutting down. Figure 9.1 shows the states and provinces affected by the blackout.

Impacts on New York City

The operators who controlled the electrical grid could not move fast enough to stop the shutdown of the grid powering NYC. As a result, most of NYC was

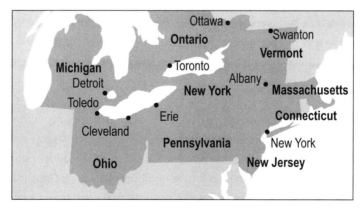

Figure 9.1 States and provinces affected by the 2003 Niagara Mohawk blackout.

without power for more than a day. Computers did not operate. Traffic signals failed. Elevators stopped in between floors. Four hundred thousand passengers were stuck on subways (U.S. Department of Transportation 2004). Water systems shut down. The elderly and disabled were trapped in high-rise apartments without air conditioning and water. Communication networks were disrupted, including cell phones, as cellular towers lost power. Even the ability to call 911 was affected when service went down in three of Verizon's central offices. Moving around the city became difficult; the streets filled with office workers who couldn't get home by subway or train, and some stranded passengers camped out rather than walk home. Most businesses closed, though sales of flashlights, candles, and bottled water soared.

NYC became a large community of volunteers who helped one another throughout the city. Neighbors checked on the elderly and held impromptu picnics to use up the food in their refrigerators. On the streets, strangers gathered around operating boom boxes to get news. Although the overall crime index was lower than during the same period in the previous year, the number of serious fires increased more than sixfold as a result of people using candles for light (NYC Emergency Response Task Force 2003).

Emergency Response

The NYC public health system is one of the best prepared in the United States. The emergency response system has instituted many enhancements in the past decade. Both DOHMH and the hospitals use an all-hazards approach for preparedness which facilitates response for the broadest range of emergencies. Their response system has a predefined chain of command, with responders knowing their assignments in advance so that the system works in emergencies large and small.

A secure Web-based data collection system called *HERDS* (Health Emergency Response Data System) captures daily bed capacity information across New York State. For accreditation, hospitals engage in regular drills and review and improve their response plans. A dedicated radio channel, established before 2000, now requires daily roll calls of all hospitals in the city, including numbers of full and empty beds. Regular drills using the radio were conducted before the blackout. Despite extensive preparations, a total loss of power stressed the public health and medical care system and required the activation of many resources.

NYC coordinates its response to emergencies through a centralized emergency operations center (EOC). At NYC's EOC, the mayor and key decision-makers convene in event of an emergency to provide policy and overall management of the city's response. The EOC is staffed by city agencies, which also activate separately located tactical command centers to oversee each agency's operations. Hospitals and DOHMH each implement an EOC for their own agency functions. Although local and state transportation agencies had response plans in place, no one was prepared for the scope and duration of this blackout. Decision-makers had to decide where to allocate resources such as personnel, equipment, emergency power, and lighting (U.S. Department of Transportation 2004).

The NYC Health and Hospitals Corporation (HHC) and DOHMH are key members of the team that coordinates activities from the citywide EOC. In addition, the Greater New York Hospital Association, a trade organization representing all of the hospitals in the region, participates in coordination at the citywide EOC. Being represented at the EOC facilitates the ability to obtain resources (e.g., generators or fuel) for one's organization.

The citywide EOC began to operate less than 10 minutes after the blackout affected the NYC region and remained staffed around the clock from August 14 to August 17. HHC and DOHMH set up command centers at their respective administrative offices to coordinate emergency services, including gathering and distributing information.

Emergency Medical Services

There is no state requirement that emergency medical services (EMS) have a disaster plan (State of New York Public Health Law 2001). The regulations assume that EMS will be able to continue providing services, including staffing, backup radio, and vehicles. But, lacking its own disaster plan, EMS had difficulty meeting the challenges of the blackout. The volume of calls during the blackout was overwhelming, resulting in increased times to get to those in need. Response was complicated, as EMS units either lost their communication systems and had no backup or relied on commercial vendors who could not provide service themselves (S. Benson, NYC Office of Emergency Management, personal communication, March 11, 2009).

Despite these problems, NYC EMS served 133% more patients during the blackout than in a typical 24-hour period (NYC Emergency Response Task Force 2003). Typically, 3000 ambulance runs are made per day in NYC. The emergency 911 telephone system received 80,000 calls and logged in more than 800 elevator rescues. The NYC Fire Department responded to more than 5000 calls—twice the normal daily amount (U.S. Department of Transportation 2004).

Hospitals and Public Health

A large number of individuals had health care issues that were acutely affected by the blackout. Fifteen thousand seniors were homebound, and 68,000 received homecare services from city agencies (NYC Emergency Response Task Force 2003). Of the 1 million New Yorkers who are disabled, 60,000 use wheelchairs or other mobility aides. Once these battery-powered mobility aids lost their electrical charges, they did not work. Caring for the needs of the disabled was complicated by the fact that many mentally or physically disabled individuals did not make their own emergency preparations, such as arranging for emergency contacts or a buddy to check on them, and having backup food, water, or medical supplies on hand. All of these individuals face daily obstacles to caring for themselves when there is adequate power. The blackout left many in desperate conditions.

Public Health Response: Organizational Activities

Once the blackout occurred, the DOHMH EOC was activated. This center helped coordinate the agency's response using the incident command system created at DOHMH before the attacks of September 11, 2001, and extensively revised afterward. Many key agency staff had been trained in the incident command system between 2002 and August 2003 (Beatty et al. 2006).

The DOHMH EOC was operational for 90 continuous hours. When the blackout began, DOHMH immediately dispatched a representative to the citywide NYC Office of Emergency Management's EOC, which coordinated the entire NYC response. Once darkness fell on August 14, the DOHMH EOC was outfitted with flashlights, 800-MHz radios, and battery-powered emergency lamps previously stored for such an emergency. Emergency generators at the Public Health Laboratory building (a separate facility from the EOC) were checked, and the amount of fuel remaining was routinely reported to the EOC.

Surveillance

An immediate concern was that the blackout may have been part of a larger terrorist attack. Therefore, it was imperative to keep normal surveillance activities running so that NYC could detect whether people were falling ill unexpectedly. One of the systems used in NYC is syndromic surveillance through the hospitals' emergency departments. This refers to a daily system that electronically collates data sent from most NYC hospitals which track the reason people are seeking medical care from emergency departments across the city. Since many bioterrorism agents initially present with flulike illness, a sudden increase in visits as a result of fever and respiratory complaints (especially in August) would trigger immediate investigation by DOHMH. The critical part of the system is the electronic download of data that are sent from participating hospitals to DOHMH every day just after midnight. In the absence of the ability to transmit these data, the agency sent public health personnel to hospital emergency departments to collect the data manually. Only analysis of these data could confirm that a large-scale release of a bioterrorism agent had not occurred. However, an increase in patients presenting to NYC emergency departments complaining of diarrheal illness was detected through syndromic surveillance.

A second surveillance system, the U.S. Department of Homeland Security's BioWatch program, detects the release of a bioterrorism agent. As part of BioWatch, air monitors are deployed across NYC. Each day, the filters from these monitors are tested for bioterrorism agents by the Public Health Laboratory of DOHMH. As with syndromic surveillance, this is a crucial part of the surveillance approach that needed to be continued during the course of the blackout.

Before the blackout, the need for agreements between DOHMH and other laboratory facilities in NYC to ensure operations at the proper level of security and safety (biosafety level 3 [BSL-3]), and their accommodating BioWatch filter testing if additional capacity were needed, was anticipated. When the secondary generator at the Public Health Laboratory could not power all DOHMH facilities needed to conduct this testing, the testing location was shifted to another NYC BSL-3 laboratory that had sufficient electrical coverage. This testing was done by DOHMH personnel and with DOHMH equipment during the blackout, enabling the department to maintain BioWatch testing.

Environmental Activities

The safety of both drinking and beach water became immediate concerns during the blackout. There was concern about both the quantity and the quality of NYC's drinking water. DOHMH Public Health Laboratory continued its routine tap water testing and found no problems with water purity. Tall buildings in NYC rely on electrical pumps in getting water to the higher floors, which became a problem without power. Lack of water, especially given the heat, could have led to dehydration among the elderly and others. Fortunately, electricity was restored before the onset of serious dehydration problems for many people.

Failure of several backup generators supplying wastewater treatment plants resulted in the discharge of 500 million gallons of untreated water into NYC waterways. Beaches were immediately closed—an enormous inconvenience on a hot summer weekend when beaches are crowded, even when electricity is available. They were reopened three days after the blackout, when testing from the Public Health Laboratory showed that the water was safe to bathe in.

Food spoilage in restaurants, with the potential for resultant food poisoning, was also a concern, so restaurant inspectors conducted 500 inspections during daylight hours of the blackout. Normally, spoiled food is carted away by private contractors, who during the blackout were not able to meet the demand. DOHMH issued an emergency order allowing the NYC Department of Sanitation to collect this refuse. Further, concern over rodent infestation due to increased garbage on the street resulted in continued rodent abatement activities.

Communication

Communicating with NYC residents to prevent adverse events from the blackout was a critical activity. Health alerts on a variety of issues, such as the need for beach closures, how to prevent heat-related health effects, and the hazards and proper disposal of spoiled food were created. Avenues of distribution included press conferences, radio, and newspapers.

Communication with physicians also occurred. Immediately after the blackout, a health alert was sent to NYC physicians by e-mail and fax to inform them of the need to discard any vaccine that was compromised by prolonged lack of refrigeration.

Ongoing Activities

Most routine activities of DOHMH continued during the blackout. DOHMH's sexually transmitted disease and tuberculosis clinics remained open. Larvicide was applied in key water areas to combat mosquitoes that may carry West Nile Virus. An animal brain was tested for rabies at the laboratory. The DOHMH-run poison control center responded to 1,000 calls. Approximately 400 death certificates were issued. Security for DOHMH facilities and personnel was provided by DOHMH police. Finally, LIFENET, a mental health emergency hotline, was able to continue providing crisis mental health counseling. While these activities were typical, the processes for conducting these activities frequently changed because of the blackout. With no computers available, personnel used manual processes to collect and record information. Additionally, DOHMH provided transportation for personnel who normally would rely on mass transit to come to work.

Aftermath and Lessons Learned

A case-control study of patients who presented to NYC emergency departments was conducted following the blackout (Marx et al. 2006). The objective was to understand better the risk factors for acquisition of diarrhea during this period. Controls were randomly selected from patients who attended emergency departments during the blackout for other reasons. The results showed that diarrhea cases were more likely to have eaten meat or seafood in the period between the blackout and symptom onset. The conclusion was that consumption of spoiled food was probably the reason for the increase in documented cases of diarrhea, which highlights the need for enhanced communication to the public about food safety during and following a power outage.

Staff who worked in the EOC were asked to participate in a lessons-learned exercise. Several themes emerged: communication problems, supply of the EOC with electricity, facility management, and adequacy of emergency supplies. DOHMH staff had difficulty calling DOHMH to determine where they needed to report, because most agency telephones required electrical power to function. The 800-MHz radios were valuable, but they too eventually lost power because they couldn't be recharged. It was also difficult to generate the many press releases and substantial public guidance needed during the emergency. Many inefficiencies were introduced, because protocols and supporting documents were on computers without accessible hard-copy backups. Facility access was a problem when there were no building staff on hand to open locked doors. Finally, there was a lack of available emergency supplies to support EOC work.

Since the blackout, many improvements have been made to incorporate the lessons learned. A new DOHMH EOC was built, with its own heating and ventilation system and the ability to accept an emergency generator to keep the entire room, including computers, functional. Many template press releases and information sheets have been written and stockpiled on a variety of subjects. A hard-copy library of key documents has been created so that if computers are inaccessible, access to important plans is available. A larger number of 800-MHz radios have been stockpiled, with an ample charging station where they are kept charged up and ready for use. DOHMH has worked hard to train all staff in advance of an emergency to know their roles, thus reducing the need to issue new instructions to staff during a crisis. Finally, DOHMH, like all city agencies, has been asked to create a continuity-of-operations plan to allow NYC government to function in the face of a crisis.

Hospital Response

Hospitals use emergency generators, which should turn on automatically, to support their critical functions during power outages. Generators are tested at regular intervals, and hospitals develop contingency plans for equipment that is not powered. During the blackout, most, but not all, generators functioned as anticipated (New York City Council Committee on Health. 2003; New York City Health and Hospitals Corp. 2003). Some did not switch on, some overheated, and others had mechanical difficulties. In addition, because of the duration of the blackout, some hospital generators stopped operating because they ran out of fuel. Keeping the generators functioning was complicated by transportation difficulties in the delivery of backup fuel. Everyone at the citywide EOC pitched in to help solve this problem. The NYC Office of Emergency Management secured replacement generators, delivered fuel, and repaired equipment. HHC provided backup generators to hospitals within its system. The Greater New York Hospital Association provided fuel to hospitals in need.

Without functioning generators, electrically powered equipment failed, endangering patients dependent on the equipment. Hospitals whose generators failed transferred ventilator-dependent patients to neighboring facilities. Some hospitals were able to move generator-dependent services internally, where the physical plant made it possible to do so. Other generator difficulties occurred. At a hospital in Brooklyn, a generator damaged insulation when it shorted out and failed. In northern Manhattan, generators ran at a high temperature; personnel watched them carefully so they didn't stall. The generators were turned off, and Con Ed, once notified, increased the exhaust capability in the generator room to prevent overheating.

Some key areas of hospitals are not equipped with backup power. Loss of power caused the failure of life safety systems and loss of internal communication for a significant number of hospitals (New York City Council Committee on Health 2003; New York City Health and Hospitals Corp. 2003). The internal phone system lost power and stopped working, so there was no way to communicate internally. Communication was sporadic without long-range pagers. Elevators didn't work, and air conditioning, critical during the very hot weather, was lost.

The delivery of health care was severely affected. Although two shifts of staff were working at the time of the blackout, some hospitals had incomplete contact lists, which made it difficult to notify other staff. Hospitals could not sterilize equipment, because steam was not being generated and steam pressure needed for sterilization did not return to normal for several days. As a result, elective surgeries were canceled. Because the blackout occurred before the end of the workday, hospitals did not have a chance to back up their computers and lost lab results. Without functioning electronic medical records, providers could not retrieve data and had to "go back" to a paper system (S. Benson, NYC Office of Emergency Management, personal communication, March 11, 2009). Vaccines spoiled when refrigeration stopped. Radiology capability was lost, because equipment was not connected to a generator. Twenty patients with psychiatric symptoms needed to be seen in one hospital network, forcing it to recredential physicians so they could practice in other hospitals in their network. The morgue refrigeration failed. Furthermore, surveillance was hampered when electronic data could not be entered into the citywide syndromic surveillance system.

Feeding hospitalized patients was a challenge. At one Manhattan hospital, the food service supplies were located in the basement, the kitchen for preparing the food was located on the 12th floor, and patients were hospitalized on every floor. The staff formed a human assembly line to carry patient trays up and down the stairs.

Many who required medical care came to hospital emergency departments when their usual source of care was unavailable. Because noncritical health care facilities, such as community clinics, are not required to have backup power, patients who normally would have been seen in these clinics came to hospital emergency departments. The increased demand included patients needing dialysis, patients needing prescriptions filled, patients dependent on electrically powered medical devices, and seniors seeking shelter or whose apartments had no water or air conditioning. In addition, six deaths in NYC from carbon monoxide, fire, and a fall during a robbery were attributed to the lack of power.

Lacking functioning radiology equipment, emergency departments could not perform x-ray imaging. When power to waiting rooms was lost, some hospitals retriaged patients. During the blackout, there was a high demand on hospital laboratories, which performed numerous critical lab tests for both patients in the emergency department and for governmental partners.

Finally, there were difficulties discharging patients. A standard practice during an emergency is to discharge patients to free up beds for the sicker patients who may need to be admitted during the emergency. Hospitals could not send patients home who lived in high-rise buildings, because elevators there were not working. Because phones lost power, personnel could not arrange for follow-up postdischarge by communicating with home care agencies or providers of durable medical equipment. This inability to discharge patients resulted in a backlog and further overcrowding of emergency departments.

Follow-Up

Blackouts of this magnitude can happen again, but are less likely to occur in the future in the United States because of both regulatory and technical improvements. Previously, standards for maintaining reliable electrical service were voluntary. These standards became mandatory through the National Energy Policy Act of 2005. The National Energy Policy Act included approximately 100 requirements, including rules for trimming trees. The Federal Energy Regulatory Commission strengthened the penalties for not meeting the tougher guidelines. Further, utilities now audit their neighbors to identify flaws that need fixing.

Finally, grids were improved by strengthening the relays that act as circuit breakers, and power lines, transformers, and power plants will be taken out of service if they are overloaded. For the future, as part of their standard emergency prevention activities, communities should prepare for blackouts by planning for the interruption of the entire infrastructure, including transportation.

Summary

Emergency preparedness for the modern megacity is a complicated task because of the extensive infrastructure, diversity of population, and traffic congestion that is common to these massive metropolitan areas. The modern megacity is dependent on technology driven by electrical power. Much of public health surveillance is achieved through data transmission and analysis, making this monitoring function more manual during emergencies in which electrical power is affected. The lesson for emergency preparedness is to be prepared to carry out normally-computerized tasks by use of pencil and paper and generator-aided methods during times of emergency in the megacity.

The blackout highlighted many important events that can complicate response to an emergency in a large urban setting. Timely public communication in multiple languages was a challenge during the blackout and is a typical problem in megacities because of their large and diverse populations. The coordination of resources (in this case, emergency generators), was performed by the city's Office of Emergency Management, and was necessary to keep critical operations functioning. This coordination is especially critical in large cities, where considerable demand and competing interests may complicate an already difficult situation.

Quickly assuring residents that there is clean water, both to drink and at the beaches, was important. Lack of potable water might have been catastrophic to elderly persons, many of whom live in retirement communities or nursing homes in large cities. Other vulnerable populations may also live in large numbers in megacities, and specific plans may be needed to accommodate their needs during an emergency.

Cities may be targets of terrorist attacks, and so at the outset of an emergency, authorities need to assure the public that there are no other concomitant public health threats. The unique features of cities that make a public health response so complicated have recently been documented (World Health Organization 2009), and are worthy of further collaborations among megacities to share best practices and to mitigate the public health consequences of blackouts or other crises.

References

Beatty ME, Phelps S, Rohner C, Weisfuse I. 2006. Blackout of 2003: public health effects and emergency response. *Public Health Rep*. 121:36–44.

Belson K, Wald M. 2003. Blackout Is Recalled Amid Lessons Learned. *New York Times*. August 14:B3.

Marx MA, Rodriguez CV, Greenko J, et al. 2006. Diarrheal illness detected through syndromic surveillance after a massive power outage: New York City, August 2003. *Am J Public Health*. 96:547–553.

New York City Council Committee on Health. 2003. Testimony of the Greater New York Hospital Association on New York City Hospitals in the Blackout of 2003: Lessons Learned Public Hearing. September 29.

New York City Emergency Response Task Force. 2003. *Enhancing New York City's Emergency Preparedness: A Report to Mayor Michael R. Bloomberg*. October 28.

New York City Health and Hospitals Corporation. 2003. Internal After-Action Report on Response During Blackout of 2003.

State of New York Public Health Law, Article 30 and Article 30a, Emergency Medical Services Revisions as provided for by Chapter 190 of the Laws of 2001, Chapter 349 of the Laws of 2001, and Chapter 463 of the Laws of 2001.

U.S. Department of Transportation. Intelligence Transportation Systems (ITS) Joint Program Office and Federal Highway Administration Office of Transportation Operations. 2004. *Effects of Catastrophic Events on Transportation System Management and Operations: August 2003 Northeast Blackout–New York City*. Final Report. Cambridge, MA: U.S. Department of Transportation. ITS Joint Program Office and Federal Highway Administration Office of Transportation Operations. DOT-VNTSC-FHWA-04-04.

World Health Organization. 2009. *Cities and Public Health Crises*. Report of the International Technical Consultation; October 29–30; Lyon, France:1–32. Available at: http://www.who.int/ihr/lyon/FRWHO_HSE_IHR_LYON_2009.5.pdf. Accessed July 26, 2010.

10

Spatial Planning, Noncommunicable Disease, and Health at the Strategic Level in London

Neil Blackshaw, BA (Hons), MA

The major urban challenges of the 21st century include the rapid growth of many cities and the decline of others, the expansion of the informal sector and the role of cities in creating and mitigating climate change. Evidence from around the world suggests that contemporary urban planning has largely failed to address these challenges.

Ban Ki-moon, United Nations Secretary General
(United Nations Human Settlement Programme 2009)

THE BURDEN OF NONCOMMUNICABLE disease is growing inexorably. It contributes 60% of global deaths; 80% of these are in low- and middle-income countries (United Nations Economic and Social Council 2009). Noncommunicable diseases have been characterized as diseases of affluence caused in large part by lifestyle factors. But, in truth, a large proportion of noncommunicable diseases are attributable to structural and upstream factors. This chapter will examine some aspects of this phenomenon and the public health response it has generated in the context of London.

The Role of Spatial Planning in Addressing Health

Although both have a long history, public health and town planning became almost synonymous 150 years ago and developed rapidly in parallel as part of the response to the intolerable burden of infectious disease. The nineteenth-century Public Health Acts and the Housing and Town Planning Act of 1909 in the United Kingdom were explicitly directed at creating more salubrious and healthy places and provided the means, however inadequate, to mitigate existing problems and to avoid emerging problems. However, as the struggle to contain infectious disease met with increasing success, and the role of medicine burgeoned in the twentieth century, the links between public health and urban planning weakened.

Increasingly, and explicitly after 1948, public health was seen as the domain of the health service, and town planning first returned to its roots in town design and then became increasingly technocratic, bureaucratized, and politicized in the complex world of urban development. In this paradigm, health was either a contingent or implicit outcome or was simply ignored. Thus, the increasing significance of noncommunicable disease went largely unrecognized in the wider public policy field outside the health service. One of the outcomes of this approach is the emergence of what has now become known as the obesogenic environment (Swinburne and Egger 2002). The combination of increased personal mobility and dispersed land uses has radically discouraged physical activity and undermined a sense of community. At the same time, the relative decline of infectious disease and the gradual increase in life expectancy disguised the fact that inequalities in health were reproducing themselves. To an extent, this problem was recognized, and the slum clearance drive, underpinned by the Public Health Acts, persisted until it reached its limits in the early 1970s. The slum problem was, however, defined largely in terms of its physical manifestation. The solutions, mediated through the town planning system, were overtly physical. Ironically, this movement to led to a disillusionment with urban planning.

Currently, there is no common frame of reference between health and urban planning, and despite the growth of the discipline of urban health, most theories of planning continue to exclude health as an issue of concern. However, the emergence of the "social determinants of health" model can be said to provide the basis for such a common agenda. The model makes clear that the most significant influences on an individual's—and hence a community's—health status are the social, economic, and environmental circumstances in which they find themselves. The Dahlgren and Whitehead model (1991) graphically illustrates these influences, distal to proximal, as a series of concentric arcs. Diderichsen et al. attempted to explain how these spheres of influence give rise to inequities (Diderichsen, Evans, and Whitehead 1991). Social structure, defined by economic, legal, fiscal, and social policies, determines social position. Social position is the fulcrum at which differential circumstances interact with personal characteristics and result in diverse outcomes. This diversity in health outcomes is reproduced geographically as well as in social groupings.

In general, the focus of spatial planning in the United Kingdom is sustainable development. The definition of sustainable development remains contested and problematic, but health is an explicit, if essentially secondary or contingent, element of the current U.K. government sustainable development plan (Department for Environment, Food, and Rural Affairs 2005). Furthermore, the statutory scope of spatial planning is defined to transcend the limited notion of "land use" that characterized postwar planning up to 2004. It now includes all those activities that make up a sustainable community (Communities and Local Government 2005). In practice, plans will typically address employment, education, housing, transport, social infrastructure, and of course environment—all of those factors that populate the social determinants of health model.

The interpretation of the determinants of health model therefore provides a common framework and agenda for reconnecting population health and town planning, and the scope of spatial planning has provided the tools for this to happen. This chapter examines to what extent, and to what effect, spatial planning at a strategic level has been exploited to address the health challenges in contemporary London; whether the determinants of health model is useful in analyzing such interventions; and whether the London experience provides lessons for the rest of the United Kingdom and for other megacities. Is the spatial planning system indeed an appropriate instrument for health promotion? If so, what are the optimal conditions for success, and in what ways might the use of the spatial planning systems in megacities be exploited?

In setting the context for that consideration, the development of London during the past 100 years will be described; in particular how changes in the city during the last 20 years or so have affected the perception of health conditions. A concern for the health of Londoners was embedded in the duties of the new mayor in 2000 and was subsequently articulated in the Spatial Development Strategy, known as the "London Plan." I will examine the ways in which those London Plan policies have been implemented and use a major redevelopment project—the massive King's Cross regeneration scheme—to examine the role of different actors in the realm of health and health outcomes. In doing so, I will attempt to answer the following questions:

- What distinguishes London as a megacity?
- What particular circumstances in London give rise to a specific intensity and pattern of ill health and inequality?
- What paradigms have been used to define the interface between health and planning?
- To what extent can the health-improving aspirations of the London Plan be said to have been successful?

The Growth of London in Early Modern Times

London has long dominated the English economic and political system, but in the nineteenth century it was transformed into the world's largest city and the center of an empire. Its total population increased from one million residents in 1800 to some seven million by 1911, after more than a century of sustained 20% increases every ten years, as measured by the ten-year censuses. Growth then faltered until the population reached a peak in 1940, whence, through out-migration, the population fell to a low point of 6.8 million in 1980. It should be stressed, however, that the population of London has long been fairly elastic, because its administrative boundaries failed to keep up with the way people moved. By 1940, more people lived just outside the metropolitan area of London than within it. Population distribution was influenced by the railways, which from 1836 enabled a gradual spread of people who relied on the city. As the diaspora was sustained, the London region can be said to have become a megacity, and by 2000, the new mayor was recognizing it as such:

> London is part of a metropolitan region of over 18 million people. This forms a "mega-city region" in which there are a vast number of linkages and networks between all the urban settlements. Within this wider region, London performs the functions characteristic of the central city. It is the main generator and source of jobs as well as of

culture, leisure and higher-level shopping activities. The interactions within the mega-city region are increasing. (Greater London Authority 2004, p. 18)

The pattern of growth was increasingly influenced by the growing transport system. From the first railway in 1836 to the first underground in the 1880s, people rapidly followed the railways in successive waves of building. Simultaneously, London remained a massive reception area for immigrants. The river sustained a growing worldwide trade, and the docks and expanding manufacturing industries settled cheek by jowl with working-class districts in the valleys of the Lee and the Wandle Rivers. The middle and wealthier classes settled on higher land in the suburbs of the north and west and, later, south of the river.

By the mid-nineteenth century, the intensification of working and living activity strained the infrastructure of the city to a breaking point. Water supplies were inadequate and increasingly contaminated as larger and larger volumes of sewage were piped into the Thames River. This vicious circle led to repeated and devastating outbreaks of infectious diseases such as typhoid and cholera. That these processes were linked was immediately apparent to many public figures, but it was not until the mid-nineteenth century that the possibility of intervention on a large enough scale—and the scientific rationale for it—began to be realized. John Snow and others pioneered the practice of epidemiology; germ theory slowly overcame the more antediluvian concepts of miasmatic effusions; and bold engineering began to cut through the corrupt and incompetent system of water and sewerage supply (Johnson 2006). Intensely practical steps were taken—in part altruistic and philanthropic and in part self-interested and defensive—as the ruling and middle classes realized the threat of epidemic.

It can be argued that the governance of London—despite its corrupt, parochial, and occasionally shambolic nature—stumbled its way to managing this dysfunctional aspect of the growing city. Although outbreaks of disease were devastating at the neighborhood level, they were not rampant. Living standards rose erratically—for many far less than for some—but health improved substantially. Average life expectancy in London at the turn of the eighteenth century was 30 years, but by 1911 it had risen to 52 years. Infectious diseases such as cholera and typhoid declined markedly in the second half of the nineteenth century as drastically improved water and sewerage systems were installed.

As the population grew so did employment, and by 1911 London had the greatest concentration of manufacturing in the country. The composition of the economy was balanced, but as transport linkages strengthened in the United Kingdom, the Atlantic region, and worldwide, London's share of trade increased, and by the mid-twentieth century it began to attract and grow its finance and business sector. The distribution of wealth in London at that time is hard to determine. Land and property were a very significant component of wealth, and ownership of property appears to have been relatively diffuse despite the existence of high-value, extensive properties in the center. Overall, the richest 5% in England in the nineteenth century earned 41% of the income.

Rents in London rose faster than did wages in the nineteenth century, although rent levels cycled over time and rent increases were exacerbated by the demolition of areas of slum housing. Rents may have equalled 20% of a working family's income in the 1880s. Rents on cheaper properties rose faster than did higher-value ones, for which the price was depressed by the competition offered by the existence of suburban communities. The gradient of rents outward from the center of the city was steep, but low suburban rents were only accessible by long commuting, which was in turn expensive. Wages may have tripled over this time. London's wage structure does not appear markedly different from other urban areas, but employment may have been more stable than in other major cities of the United Kingdom.

The extent of poverty in the city has been a matter of continuous debate since the early nineteenth century. Booth (1889) estimated that between 30 and 40% of the population lived in poverty, but he estimated that those in real want—that is, with no surplus—made up only 8-12%, in the East End. The reasons for these levels of poverty were seen by some as functions of the local labor market and personal behavior. As the problem became better understood, more national perspectives on the issues of poverty and wages developed and a more sophisticated understanding of causal pathways—family circumstances, illness, large families, and old age—emerged. Poverty was initially an inner London phenomenon but gradually spread eastward to Bethnal Green, Stepney, and Greenwich. Wealth, however, remained concentrated in the West End. Nevertheless, there were safeguards against complete destitution, albeit harsh, and the workhouse and the practice of in-relief—that is, providing work and subsistence within the institution of the workhouses—meant that dire poverty and starvation were not widespread problems in London (Ball and Sunderland 2001).

London was in some respects approaching its zenith as the twentieth century opened. It continued to grow as a manufacturing and financial center and maintained its dominance in the U.K. economy.

Modern London: The Emergence of a Global City

In the 1960s, London was still a city with a manufacturing base and a large working-class population. Total population was on a long downward trend as people moved to the periphery. The city was still characterized by extensive areas of two- and three-story terraced housing, some of which was valuable and some far less so. A large crescent of manufacturing extended to the east and west of the city. Although the docks were still vibrant and busy, much of the riverside was declining economically. The following 30 years saw massive changes—physical, economic, social, and political—as London, perhaps as never before, reinvented itself and became what is now called a world city. This transition was complex, and a more detailed analysis of this transition is outside the scope of this chapter.

The emergence of a network of world cities has been extensively documented. In essence, the analysis suggests that the initiation and growth of neoliberal financial regimes and the "Washington consensus" were crucial enabling factors. Neoliberalism replaced the postwar consensus based on Keynesian and welfare economics and introduced a lessening of restrictions on trade, money flows, and financial systems. The Washington consensus describes the broad agreement between the major Western governments. These changes created the conditions for a network of centers of commerce and of financial businesses that overcame the friction of distance through electronic and other means. Although this is characterized as a global and, to some extent, spatial phenomenon, Massey has rightly pointed out that "the local also creates the global" (Massey 2007, p. 84). In London, therefore, the conditions were created, intentionally and unintentionally, to enable the city to take advantage of the opportunities in the global financial system in a manner different from that of other western European cities such as Paris, where neither financial nor physical constraints were lessened to such a degree.

The ramifications of this transformation were manifold. The physical nature and shape of large parts of inner London changed radically. Despite immigration controls in the European Union (EU) and United Kingdom, the composition of the population continued to diversify. Since 2000, the population decline has dramatically reversed, and 800,000 more people are forecast to be living in London by 2016 than in 2006. The nature of social change is perhaps more contested. Some argue that the rise of a middle class has forced out the working class and changed the composition of London (Hamnett 2003). London has long experienced poverty side by side with extreme wealth, and income inequality increased markedly both in the United Kingdom and London after 1980. There is some support for Sassen's view that the city has become polarized (Sassen 2006):

> This division is made worse by job growth being concentrated in higher paid and in lower paid occupations. In 1980, the top 10 per cent of fulltime male earners in London had weekly earnings just over twice as high as those in the bottom 10 per cent. In 2000, the ratio had grown to nearly four times. (Greater London Authority 2004, p. 35)

Others, however, argue that the almost exponential growth in income at the top end was accompanied by growth in middle incomes and that polarization did not result (Hamnett 2003).

Health of Londoners

London was for most of its long history a focus of disease and ill health, as exemplified by the plague of the 1660s, high rates of infant mortality, periodic epidemics, alcohol abuse, crime, and violence. In the nineteenth century, the rapid growth in population— the addition of more than 4 million people, and growth rates of 20% every ten years—resulted in the intensification of infectious disease as the water and waste systems in essence broke down. The story of the emergence of public health, the discovery of waterborne pathogens, and engineering, housing, and clinical responses has been told in detail (Johnson 2006). London overcame many of its pathogenic characteristics, and the rate of infectious disease declined markedly.

In the then most-deprived borough of Tower Hamlets, life expectancy in 1900 was 55 years, and by 2000 had risen to 70 years. By 2000, the standardized mortality rate varied from 87 per 100,000 Bromley (a suburban borough in the southeast) to 109 per 100,000 the deprived east. Life expectancy was 75 years in Bromley compared to 70 years in Tower Hamlets, although the gap in healthy life expectancy—that is, the number of years of life free from illness— was larger, perhaps 11 years. Leading causes of death were heart disease (23%), cancer (24%), and stroke (9%). The distinctive feature here was the geographical pattern of disease, premature death, and ill health: hospitalization figures as measured by the Department of Health showed high rates in Tower Hamlets, Newham, and Hackney and the fringes of Lewisham, Lambeth, Southwark, and Haringey. This pattern will be familiar from the description of deprivation outlined previously and essentially correlates with the social determinants of health.

General practitioners (GPs) provided (and still do) the front-line first contacts for the National Health Service (NHS). London had a similar rate of provision of GPs as did the rest of the country, but they were in very poor-quality premises and far more of them were working in single-physician practices. The cost of health provision in London was much higher than elsewhere, due in part to higher unit costs—for example, salaries—and in part the preponderance of acute beds in London and the fact that London's teaching hospitals served a much wider catchment area. The Turnberg report, published in 1998, described health services in London as woeful and made numerous recommendations for improvement, including an increase in the number of GPs (Department of Health 1998). This disparity between needs and the level of services and the true costs to the NHS of deprivation in London have been at the heart of the resources argument ever since, with some contending that the allocation of resources fails to match the true needs that arise from the deprived nature of the population in parts of London (Davies and Kendall 1999). In presenting the Turnberg report (one of 20 in the twentieth century) the government stated,

> The report recognises that in many parts of London, particularly in the most deprived areas, primary care, mental health, intermediate care and community services are simply not up to the standard to which everyone in our country is entitled. It proposes a range of measures to bring things up to scratch. We will be providing an additional investment of at least £140 million in these services for London over the lifetime of this Parliament. An extra £30 million will be targeted on these services in the coming financial year. (House of Lords 1998)

Surveys of health on the cusp of the twenty-first century found that the health of Londoners was in many ways not dissimilar to that of individuals in the rest of England and the other metropolitan areas. In some respects, London benefitted from the "southern effect"—that is, the fact that on the whole, the health of the population in the south of England is significantly better than that of the north; as an example, Londoners' health was better for those older than 65 years. It was the health status of those younger than 65 years, and the concentration of ill health and premature death in the deprived areas of London that, if anything, made it distinctive from its regional context. Nevertheless, analysts and commentators repeatedly stressed that London was unique and by implication worthy of more resources (Davies and Kendall 1999). But it would seem that this uniqueness resided in its pure size, which was inarguable, and increasingly its ethnic diversity. From being overwhelmingly White even in the 1960s, London had become the most diverse city in the United Kingdom, and some boroughs were approaching ethnic majority populations.

There is no doubt that some Londoners experienced significant deprivation. When in the 1990s deprivation first came to be measured systematically, 13 of the London boroughs were judged to be among the most deprived 20 boroughs in the country. The concentration of deprivation is clearly visible in any spatial analysis of key social and economic indicators and has been persistent, centering as it does on the boroughs in an eastern arc—Hackney, Tower Hamlets, and Newham. Many boroughs in London demonstrate a gradient in deprivation and its components—income, education, health, and unemployment. London is a city of cities, that is, a complex web of centers and hinterlands coalescing into a metropolitan whole, but by no means homogeneous.

The science of complex systems argues that such systems are characterized by emergent qualities—"quantum" changes that occur at certain stages of growth— and that they are significantly more than the sum of their parts (Huxley and Huxley 1947). This has been used to explain various "agglomeration" effects of urbanization. So far as London and health is concerned, however, it is difficult to demonstrate such an emergent character. The health of Londoners on the whole is similar to that of the rest of the country. Size and complexity have not produced unique prevalences, patterns, or types of disease. However, it is self-evident that the sheer size of London and the density of economic activity and diversity of its people do pose major challenges to the delivery of health services. The uniqueness therefore may lie in the ability of the system of governance and of service provision to respond.

Transformation of Governance: The Greater London Authority and the Mayor

The governance of London has always required a compromise between the parochial and the metropolitan, distorted by the influence of the royal court on the one hand and the City of London on the other. London is often described as a collection of villages, and local distinctiveness has been one of its defining characteristics, although it is now markedly weaker than previously. Nevertheless, the creation of the London County Council at the end of the nineteenth century at least created the capacity for strategic city management. In the 1980s, this city government, by then reconstructed as the Greater London Council, came into conflict with the national government, and for 15 years, London had to survive without strategic governance, until 2000.

The Greater London Authority Act (GLA Act) of 1999 reinstated London-wide government in a radically different form. An elected mayor—the first in the United Kingdom—was given responsibility (but with almost no power) for strategic overview and an elected assembly was charged with overseeing the activities of the mayor. The new Labour Government commissioned a review of health services in London in the face of a previous policy of reducing acute beds and a specific threat to one of the capital's most historic hospitals. In putting the report forward, the government said,

> The report recognises the need for new arrangements to ensure a London-wide strategy for health and proposes as a medium-term aim a single NHS regional office for London. Without London-wide strategies and action, the necessary improvements in mental health services and the proper integration of services for children and other people will be hard to achieve, if not impossible. (House of Lords 1998).

The year 2000 also marked the inauguration of an NHS Plan, which was to lead to the creation of primary care trusts (PCTs) and reorganization into strategic health authorities (SHAs). London's existing pattern of district health authorities became 31 PCTs, broadly on the same boundaries as the London boroughs, and five SHAs were subsequently created in 2002. Alongside these are 43 NHS Trusts providing hospital (acute) and mental health services. This at least had the virtue of establishing common boundaries between the primary care organizations, PCTs, and 31 London boroughs. The potential of this organizational alignment has, however, still not been fully realized.

The regional, strategic overview of London's health infrastructure and policy and the link to government was to be provided by the NHS regional executive for London. This arrangement was to a large extent overtaken by the creation of the five SHAs, which had responsibility for performance improvement and strategic issues.

In 2007, the five SHAs were disbanded and a single SHA, now known as NHS London, was created. NHS London is essentially a performance management organization with a strong financial bias, and it has adopted a very limited strategic planning role. Latterly, the PCTs in London have begun to create both a confederated structure and a central support unit. A major review of health services, the so-called Darzi review, later known as Healthcare for London, was initiated in 2007. A special-purpose committee was created to steer this project, which has since been absorbed by the PCTs.

This brief overview should be sufficient to demonstrate the extent of change in the "management" arm of the NHS in London (reflecting similar changes in England). However, it is clear that this process is far from complete, as far as the NHS in London or indeed the country is concerned, such is the degree of political interest in it. The responsibility for interface with the public for directing them through the health care system and for procuring or commissioning services lies with the PCTs. Although they provide some services directly, the majority of community health services are provided by GPs who are self-employed and not part of the PCT. Secondary and tertiary services are provided by the NHS acute and mental health trusts. Meanwhile, public health is the responsibility of the PCTs. Regional capacity for public health and health protection exists in the shape of the regional director of public health and a regional public health group that is part of the regional arm of government in London; this mirrors arrangements in the remaining nine regions of England.

The Role of the Mayor in Health

> The GLA will have regard to the effect its powers will have on the health of persons in Gtr London. . . . If it exercises those powers it shall do so in ways that it considers are best calculated to promote improvements in the health of Londoners (clauses 4 and 5). (Department of Health 1998)

The mayor was required to produce eight strategies, including a spatial plan, but health was not one of them, such was the desire to maintain the separation between the NHS and local government. In fact, the GLA was specifically prevented from providing any health services. In 2008, the mayor's powers were extended to include greater power to intervene in dealing with planning applications, and in the process the mayor was required to produce a further strategy, the Health Inequalities Strategy. The draft version of this policy statement, the first mayoral policy statement on health, was published in October 2009.

Considerable concern was expressed in the run-up to the passing of the GLA Act in 1999 regarding the way in which health was to be approached. The King's Fund, a major health think tank and charity, was foremost in making the case for a specific duty to address health and for the mayor's office to have a health unit (Davies and Kendall 1999). In the event, as explained above, the GLA was denied specific health powers, but it was given an obligation to take account of the health implications of what it proposed.

How was effect given to this rather uncomfortable and fragile connection? Those pressuring for a more robust response initiated a health strategy for London which was published in 2000 (National Health Service London Executive 2000). Although this was never formally adopted by the GLA, it did serve to focus attention on the scope that existed for pan-London health policies. The mayor then went on to set up the London Health Commission, which drew its 40 members from across the health sector and which carried out a series of health impact assessments (HIAs) of the eight mayoral strategies, thus fulfilling the GLA's legal duty.

Health and Spatial Planning: The London Plan and the Mayor's Spatial Development Strategy

How did this administration and system of governance define and respond to the broad issue of the health of the population through one of its principal instruments—the Spatial Development Strategy or "London Plan"? The London Plan was the first "spatial" plan in the United Kingdom and as such the forerunner of the new national system that emerged in 2004. Spatial planning as a concept had emerged in Europe with the European Spatial Development Plan. What distinguished the spatial plan from what went before, and what was known in English terms as the *land-use plan*, was its broader scope and strategic approach, less immediately concerned with site-by-site implementation and rules and more with broader vision and policies. To what extent the London Plan actually fulfilled these more abstract criteria is open to question.

The plan was published in 2004. It had three cross-cutting themes: (1) the health of Londoners, (2) equality of opportunity, and (3) its contribution to sustainable development in the United Kingdom. The mayor described it in the following terms:

> This is the strategic plan setting out an integrated social, economic and Environmental framework for the future development of London, looking forward 15–20 years. . . . . . it integrates the physical and geographic dimensions of the Mayor's other strategies, including broad locations for change and providing a framework for land use management and development, which is strongly linked to improvements in infrastructure, especially transport. . . . .the main policy directions remain the same and the same factors are seen as driving change in London—particularly the phenomenal pressures for growth. This rapid expansion, of population and jobs is without parallel in any other UK city, and stems from London's exceptional dynamism, attractiveness and advantages in the new era of economic globalisation. It poses unique opportunities—but also challenges—if the potential benefits are to be maximised and the city's environment, quality of life and historic character are to be preserved and improved. My vision, which guides all my strategies, is to develop London as an exemplary, sustainable world city, based on three interwoven themes:
>
> • strong, diverse long term economic growth
> • social inclusivity to give all Londoners the opportunity to share in London's future success
> • fundamental improvements in London's environment and use of resources. (Greater London Authority 2004, p. xi)

As shown above, the GLA was fully aware of the nature of London's role as a world city:

> London is a world city and acts as one of a very small number of command and control centres in the increasingly interactive network of transactions across the world economy. World cities have very distinctive strategic needs. Although separated by thousands of miles, they are intimately linked as a virtual global entity by the transactions of markets and communications systems. To reflect these links, the Mayor has begun to develop a collaborative relationship with New York and Tokyo. (Greater London Authority 2004, p. 15)

There was no appetite to challenge this trajectory:

London must fulfil its potential as a world city in the national interest as well as that of Londoners. Accommodating the anticipated growth in London would be beneficial both to London and the rest of the UK. This plan seeks to work with the market and to address the potential supplyside constraints in terms of space, transport, environmental quality and education to ensure London is capable of accommodating growth. (Greater London Authority 2004, p. 4)

The mayor was clearly committed to creating the conditions for sustained growth, but recognized that there had been some issues, such as:

- Increased difficulties in traveling around London, with heavy traffic and slow and unreliable journey times
- Upward pressure on business costs, made worse by a shortage of appropriate office space, leading to some of the highest office rents in the world
- Acute housing shortages resulting in rapidly rising house prices, reducing real living standards, disadvantaging people on modest and low incomes, and creating a destabilizing factor in the United Kingdom macroeconomy
- Skills gaps in some sectors, along with social deprivation in many areas and increased economic and social polarization
- Continued social exclusion and discrimination, particularly affecting minority ethnic communities
- Increased pollution, damaged environments, and chronic underinvestment generally and in particular, in the public realm

The Health Dimension in the London Plan

Of the six objectives in the London Plan, two were most relevant to health:

Objective 2: To make London a better city for people to live in. . . .

The key policy directions for achieving this objective are
- Improve the quality of Londoners' lives and the environment through better designed buildings and public spaces . . .
- Achieve targets for new housing, including affordable housing, that will cater to the needs of London's existing and future population and give more people who need it access to homes they can afford

- Address the differing needs of London's diverse population
- Promote public safety, including design measures that improve safety in buildings and the public realm . . .
- Improve, by working with partners, including the community and voluntary sectors, the availability of quality local services particularly education and health

Objective 4: To promote social inclusion and tackle deprivation and discrimination. . . .

The key policy directions for achieving this objective are

- Tackle unemployment by increasing access to high-quality jobs through training, advice, and other support, particularly for those women and young people and minority ethnic groups most in need
- Tackle concentrations of deprivation with the aim of ensuring that no one is seriously disadvantaged by where they live within 10 to 20 years . . .
- Tackle homelessness
- Tackle discrimination, building on the economic and cultural strengths of London's diversity and building a London that is more accessible to disabled people . . .
- Provide a framework for the spatial policies and decisions of learning, health, safety, and other key social and community services
- Ensure that local communities benefit from economic growth and are engaged in the development process (Greater London Authority 2004, pp. 7–9)

These objectives were then intended to be pursued through a large set of more specific policies.

As has been made clear, health was both a statutory focus of the mayor and a cross-cutting theme of the above. The concept of health was holistic and set within the social determinants of health model as the above objectives, as the following extract illustrates:

> . . . Health is far more than the absence of illness; rather it is a state of physical, mental and social wellbeing. A person's health is therefore not only linked to age and gender, but to wider factors such as education, employment, housing, social networks, air and water quality, access to affordable nutritious food, and access to social and public services in addition to health care. The Mayor will, in collaboration with strategic partners, produce additional guidance to boroughs on promoting public health. (Greater London Authority 2004, p. 94)

And the approach was to be based on policy integration:

> The Mayor has concluded that this will best be achieved through the following overall spatial strategy for development: integrating spatial policies with policies for neighbourhood renewal, better health, improved learning and skills, greater safety and better employment and housing opportunities in the Areas for Regeneration. . . . (Greater London Authority 2004, p. 95)

Space does not allow a more detailed description of the policies and their elements. The overarching policy contained the sustainability criteria—a checklist of the performance standards to be applied when developing more detailed policy instruments and in considering planning applications. The impact on the health of the local people was one such criterion.

Of the detailed policies that followed, health figured explicitly in four:

- Seeking to ensure the alignment with health policy (of the NHS) generally
- Identifying locations for health infrastructure
- Requiring boroughs to "have regard to" the health impacts of development
- Identifying health facilities as a priority for financial contributions from development

Health as a consideration or contingent issue or outcome figures in many other policies such as housing, minorities, open space, pollution, and climate change, but there is no space here to give due consideration of the nature of these policies. Overall, though, it is fair to say that the sentiment of the plan reflected a view of health that was holistic and which in essence at least derived from the basic assumptions of the social determinants of health model, thus:

> Health is a critical determinant of the quality of all our lives. A range of factors affect the health of Londoners. . . . Factors such as access to leisure facilities, fresh food or decent living conditions can all lead to healthier, longer lives. Planning decisions have the potential to influence these factors. The starting position was that promoting public health is far more than ensuring access to a high quality health care service. (Greater London Authority 2004, p. A12)

The fundamental or overarching policy of the plan was that containing the "sustainability criteria" (Policy 2A.1) the mayor would use in determining applications and addressing its implementation. These criteria, to a degree, reflected the holistic view expressed above and thus provided scope for a wide interpretation of health. This implicit approach, and an overall sentiment of ambivalence toward health improvement, has been reflected in subsequent use of the plan.

Process and Outcome Evaluation of the London Plan

The London Plan was required to set targets and indicators, as all planning strategies are. In the 2004 plan, no health indicators were set. This was to be remedied in the subsequent review adopted in 2008, but in the event, the measure adopted—the difference in life expectancy between the London average and the Regeneration Areas that the plan identified—proved impossible to measure. As a result, no framework or metric existed up to 2008 that would enable the impact of the plan on the health of Londoners to be measured with any confidence whatsoever. Steps have subsequently been taken to remedy this gap. Following the publication of the draft plan, the London Health Commission carried out a HIA of the policies. The conclusions of a later independent review of that process cast some doubt on the extent to which the process had been objective, in that it essentially reviewed the language of the plan rather than the outcomes (Greater London Authority 2004a).

There is no doubt that this criticism carries some weight and that the subsequent adoption of a wider appraisal system, known as integrated impact assessment, that attempts to combine health, equality, and sustainability has done little to overcome it. The efficacy of HIAs in these circumstances is open to doubt for the following reasons: (1) the engagement with the community is problematic; (2) the health baseline is inadequately defined; (3) the pathways are not fully understood; (4) the iteration of the plan to respond to issues raised is not transparent; and (5) monitoring is inadequate to ensure recommendations are delivered.

Implementation of the London Plan

The analysis so far has shown that there are a number of quite strongly complementary strands in the way in which the health topic emerged in the London Plan as it now stands. The mayor's statutory duty to address the health of Londoners was undoubtedly the key driver, but other forces came into play to broaden and deepen the manner in which health was incorporated, with the result that the objectives policy framework and supporting guidance can be judged to be strongly positive.

Whether this was the optimum framework is, however, open to question, and before we speculate on what such a framework might be, it is important to examine the way in which the strategy was implemented. The London Plan has a myriad of paths of influence, but without doubt one of the key pathways is the consideration by the mayor of strategic planning applications. Briefly, these are proposals for development that are, by stated standards, large, or which for some other reason have strategic implications. The powers of the mayor were until recently only negative; he was able to direct refusal of a planning application. Nevertheless, this introduced an element of uncertainty and gave the mayor significant leverage over an application whether or not he was minded to refuse it. The question for this study is to what extent was this process and influence used to further health objectives and to consistently apply the policies and practice so clearly set out.

Use of Strategic Planning Applications to Further Health in London

The NHS London Healthy Urban Development Unit (HUDU), which was established in 2004 to promote the better integration of health and spatial planning strategies carried out reviews of all of the applications reviewed by the mayor from 2006 to 2008. In 2007, a total of 257 applications were reviewed (NHS London Healthy Urban Development Unit; unpublished data). A view was taken as to whether health issues might reasonably have been expected to have been considered, and the evidence was sought as to the presence or absence of that consideration and its outcome.

Of these applications, 156 (61%) were felt to have potential for impact on health. The review demonstrated that health was, in practice, raised as a strategic consideration in 13 cases (8%) and as a secondary consideration in 67 (42%). One important issue is the use of developers' financial contributions for community infrastructure. Of the 156 applications, 8 (0.5%) had developer contributions.

This review was repeated in 2008—with very similar results but in a slightly different way—and looked at a 16-month period. In total, 400 case reports on housing applications were analyzed; of these proposed developments, 218 were considered to have a potential impact on the wider determinants of health and health care provision and infrastructure based upon the quantum of housing. In total, these applications accounted for over 40,000 potential housing units, representing a very significant quantum of development.

This systematic but necessarily somewhat subjective analysis indicates that in the period up to May 2008, when the revised London Plan was being adopted, the role of health in this strategic review process was very poorly developed, and where it was introduced it was restricted to consideration of access to or capacity of health facilities. This strongly suggests that the health objectives of the London Plan were not being pursued by the mayor's office. Together with the aforementioned lack of indicators for health, this means that the mayor was simply not in a position to judge whether he was fulfilling his statutory obligations in this area. A counterargument could be put that in more actively evaluating and acting on such matters as children's play and sustainable transport in reviewing strategic applications, as seemed to be the case, the mayor was de facto creating conditions for health improvement. However, it can be argued that this was still some way short of a rigorous pursuit of his health obligations, and, given the volume of development, potentially a significant missed opportunity. A further caveat to this analysis is that for reasons of time and resources it did not trace the outcomes of the hundreds of applications that went through the system. Borough councils had the primary role in the process and may in some cases have carried out the health assessments that were missing in GLA interventions. However, indirect evidence (for instance, this borough-level view would be expected to be raised in the mayor's reports) suggests that this was not generally the case.

The mayor produces annual monitoring reports on the implementation of the plan and, taken at face value, these support the above conclusions. Health infrastructure is consistently referred to in the reports but not in any way measured, it has to be said. Health improvement and health inequalities were not addressed until the latest annual monitoring report in 2009, which was the first following the adoption of the health inequalities indicator in the 2008 plan. Unfortunately, those indicators proved incapable of being measured. Notwithstanding the lack of a metric, the report still did not attempt an analysis of, for instance, the scale of health implications of the overall volume of development.

Implications of Spatial Plans for Health

The considerable strength of the London Plan in addressing health has been identified above. The issue of health and inequalities can by any standards be said to be one of its consistent cross-cutting themes. At the same time, the strength of the explicit and specific policies cannot be said to reflect this pervasive concern. This inherent policy weakness was compounded by the long-standing failure to identify metrics for measuring progress, although this has been resolved, to a degree, with the 2008 revision. The subsequent Health Best Practice Guide (Greater London Authority 2007) might have been expected to compensate for this relative weakness (although this was, it has to be said, aimed more at others than the GLA itself). In the event, the enthusiasm for the health objectives of the plan was not reflected in the implementation processes. The above analysis in the aftermath of the plan strongly suggests that implementation and delivery of health policy was a serious lacuna, and on recent more circumstantial evidence remains so. This weakness in implementation or delivery has long been recognized as generic in urban planning (United Nations Human Settlement Programme 2009). It can be said to be exacerbated by the nature of the London Plan, which is in large part advisory and exhortative in tone, leaving boroughs very considerable latitude to stretch or adjust the plan's policy intentions.

The key lesson that emerges from this discussion is that lofty and principled plans are only as strong as the weakest link and, in this case as in many others, the London Plan has failed to exploit—or rather optimize—its influence in achieving its health aspirations. Even if the policy weaknesses were to be remedied, then there is a need for a robust delivery plan that connects effectively with the overall planning and development process and which is consistently and continuously monitored. Such a framework would inform the plan, but equally importantly, it would inform the consistent inquiry as to whether and how health can be improved in the urban situation.

King's Cross: A Case Study of Spatial Planning and Health

The King's Cross area of London is one of the largest brownfield (i.e., land previously occupied by development) redevelopment schemes in Europe and has been clearly identified as being of strategic importance for some years. Planning permission for a mixed-use scheme covering 27 hectares was granted in 2006. This followed a period of more than 30 years during which attempts were made to find new uses for increasingly redundant land (where previous uses had ceased to be viable) adjacent to the historic railway terminals. The successful applicant (Argent) began its proposal in 2003, but progress was only secured when the future of the cross-Channel rail link (which connects London to the mainland European rail network via the Channel Tunnel) was assured.

From the outset, Argent set out to be an exemplary developer, publishing a set of "Principles for a Human City" in 2004. It also publicly committed to extensive and intensive public consultation. Although the principle of redevelopment was probably never in doubt, the policy context was in flux as the application developed and the framework only became clear as Camden Council and the mayor published policies that set the context for the area. Argent was, however, pushing at an open door.

Both the mayor, in pursuing his policy for catalyzing London's global role, and Camden took the view that King's Cross had far more than local significance. Camden wanted to achieve global reach, but with local integration:

> The Council seeks the sustainable development of the King's Cross Opportunity Area which achieves its full potential:
>
> - To support and develop London's role as a world business, commercial and cultural centre;
> - To achieve economic, social and physical integration with surrounding communities;
> - To contribute positively to meeting the full range of housing, social and healthcare needs in Camden and so contribute to meeting London's needs;
> - To create employment and training opportunities both generally and for local people;
> - To maximize opportunities for walking and cycling and the use of existing and proposed public transport facilities, thereby minimising dependence on private car use and traffic generation;
> - To minimize any adverse impact on the environment arising from the development and to secure positive environmental gains;
> - To enhance opportunities for biodiversity; and
> - For community regeneration through innovative processes of community involvement in the planning, design and management of the new development services. (London Borough of Camden 2001, p. 5)

Health as a Consideration in the King's Cross Proposals

Health issues figured in the initial documentation prepared by Argent. These put forward the view that the scheme would be positively beneficial to the local community through the creation of jobs and the renovation of blighted and run-down areas that had for many years been a source of crime, illicit drugs, and prostitution. The notion of a "gateway" to London and from London to the world figured strongly in the descriptions. This, it was said, would attract world-class business and bring visitors and activities to the area. Health was thus a positive outcome of the job opportunities, the leavening of the housing stock, a new sequence of public spaces, and the provision of new social infrastructure, including health. The scheme would knit together what had been a massive rent in the urban fabric of north central London.

Health Impact Assessment in King's Cross

The PCT took an early interest in the scheme and commissioned a HIA from a specialist consultant, but also diverted significant resources to an expert internal team and an external advisory group to steer the process. The HIA process used a variety of rapid appraisal techniques and community consultation and explicitly concentrated on potential effects on the local community. There is some indication that this was not entirely to Argent's liking, as the company argued that the community in King's Cross would essentially be new.

The resulting HIA took on a wide scope based on an interpretation of the social determinants model and ranged over the whole gamut of issues in the planning application, from jobs to commercial uses, education, open space, and health facilities. The HIA identified an affected population of some 66,000 that was ethnically diverse, and a large number of community groups and organizations, as well as statutory bodies, that had an interest.

Both boroughs (the site straddled Islington and Camden) were described as deprived and the King's Cross locality as one of the most deprived in England. Low income, high unemployment, poor educational attainment, crime and disorder, poor transport, and poor access to open space and social and community facilities were described in detail. This analysis of the existing conditions formed the foundation for the recommendations that formed the core of the HIA. These emphasized above all the potential of the development to ameliorate the deprivation so long as the needs of the local people were recognized and genuine access was achieved: physical, social, and economic. The recommendations developed at this stage were taken forward by the PCT when the first planning application was submitted in 2004. It proved not to be possible to sustain this level of resources, however, and the involvement of the PCT subsequently has reflected this. Thus, the expectation in the HIA at that time of an ongoing review of impacts has not been fulfilled.

The application was supported by a wide range of material including, as would be expected, an environmental impact statement. This dealt with health in a perfunctory manner lacking either the depth or scope of the HIA. The overall thrust related to beneficial effects through jobs housing and overall improvement. Negative effects in terms of noise and air pollution were judged to be acceptable and manageable. The environmental impact assessment reflected the generic failure of this class of documents to consider the long-term and widespread effects. Thus, the future population was not considered, because the assessment is of the impact of the proposal on the existing situation. The characteristics of the existing population—the 66,000 people who made up the surrounding community—were not adequately reflected either. The HIA ostensibly provided the vehicle for community involvement, and particular community members were trained to carry out parts of the assessment. But it cannot be said that the HIA in itself constituted community engagement, as the mechanisms and structures were simply not in place.

However, Argent itself, as described, set out with the avowed intention of community consultation, and it embarked on a long series of meetings with the plethora of community groups that had been identified. A critique of this process concluded that Argent's approach reflected the prevailing rhetoric in government and from the Camden Council that regeneration had to be inclusive and engage with local communities (Imrie 2009). However, in practice, the process of engagement proved to be far more complex and problematic than this simple rhetoric implies. Tensions within the "community" and between their views and those of the elected councilors resulted in mixed outcomes. There is considerable evidence that community activists were dissatisfied and disillusioned by the entire process. Consultation does not necessarily lead to a response or a desired outcome, and at its worst it results in tokenism. The independent review of the HIA process carried out as part of the National Institute for Clinical Excellence review of such exercises came to similar conclusions: although the HIA had achieved at least one concrete success—the prohibition of 24-hour construction working—it had failed to deliver on a broader agenda and left community members frustrated. The King's Cross Development Forum, set up to channel these community views, reflects that frustration: its Camden Council support was withdrawn and it struggled to maintain momentum.

King's Cross: The Lessons?

The outcome of the massive King's Cross regeneration scheme will take many years to emerge. Whether lessons will or can be learned is open to question. Work has started on the regeneration and the cross-Channel rail link is already well established, creating the gateway so central to the project's concept. The substantive outcomes for health include a prohibition on 24-hour construction working and two health facilities to be built as part of the scheme. The fact that the NHS will, as a result of negotiations, have to pay a commercial rent for the privilege of running these health facilities tends to undermine the value of this concession.

There are potentially many other community, noncommercial, and health-enhancing aspects to the scheme. These include affordable housing, a training scheme for local residents, a primary school, and some community support. However, as clearly understood by the developer at an early stage, there is no community—this is a brownfield site. The effects and outcomes and, importantly, the externalities, will be worked out over a large area, benefiting some—some of whom are not yet residents—and disadvantaging others in complex ways, both subtle and not so subtle. The costs and benefits will be similarly distributed in complex ways. The current disenchantment of the community does the scheme no credit. The tragedy is that it may not be possible to evaluate the impact of this scheme, to subject the aspirations of its promoters and supporters to systematic evaluation. This inability—or rather unwillingness— to set up a learning framework from such massive concentrations of technical and financial expertise means that we continue to take decisions based ostensibly on social environmental and economic criteria on received wisdom and speculation.

Summary

During the nineteenth and into the second quarter of the twentieth century, London was the world's largest city. It experienced a distinctive pattern of growth:

a historic small core surrounded by small and independent communities was rapidly engulfed by successive waves of new development led by railways and structured by a complex pattern of land values, employment, and rents. London evolved or mutated in the context of a modern society and a burgeoning capitalist economic system that established a global network of trade and commerce, but at the same time the city did much to fashion that context both nationally and internationally.

The Victorian city founded on commerce, finance, trade, and manufacturing struggled as the world developed and competitive cities emerged and overtook London during the twentieth century. Its pioneering role was to an extent its undoing, as the ossification of its spatial pattern of activities and its entrenched class divisions created inertia. That is not to say that change did not take place, but in many ways it was a period of stasis, stagnation, and decline. A new transformation emerged from the confluence of world forces in the late 1960s. The changes in the financial markets and flows, the changing population, migration, and the collapse of London's manufacturing and seaborne trade during the previous 20 years created both the catalyst and opportunity for transformation.

London today is markedly different from the London of 1960—perhaps unrecognizable to one who had the misfortune or fortune to have fallen asleep before the swinging 1960s. Vast swaths of what was manufacturing, riverside wharves and docks, and large chunks of the historic city have been occupied by modernist and postmodernist structures and re-energized with new activities. Successive waves of gentrification have displaced large numbers of the working class as the desperate slums of the 1960s have evolved into fashionable and immensely valuable real estate. New sections of the city have been created, Canary Wharf being the epitome.

The context for this change is complex again. The neoliberal economic system and the Washington consensus, the growing population, and migration stimulated the property market in totally new ways. But yet again, London was in large part responsible for that context nationally and internationally.

The population of London lived and died through this massive wave of growth and change spanning two centuries. During the first wave, disease and deprivation was a key emergent characteristic of what increasingly became a dysfunctional settlement. The political, scientific, and yes, market response in the middle and later part of the century was radical and effective, and by the end of the century water and sewerage were largely fixed; the transport system was able to carry large numbers of a new breed of commuters, the housing market was diversifying and spreading reducing rents, and the toll of infectious disease had declined markedly. Despite these changes, vast numbers of people were left stranded, stuck in poor housing, required to be cheek by jowl with work, and barely managing to achieve subsistence wages. The pattern of deprivation was reinforced by geography and the structure of the housing market so that tenanted slums washed around the wealthier quarters across the city. The burden of chronic and noncommunicable disease became more prevalent and ensured that life expectancy was still little more than 50 years as the nineteenth century ended.

This pattern of ill health, deprivation, and premature mortality persisted (Gregory 2009). London and the southeast continued to be far healthier than the northern industrial towns, but within London the hot spots of deprivation persisted and continue to do so. The economic transformation of the last decades of the twentieth century has hardly affected this basic pattern. There is a remarkable congruence between the spatial patterns of 1900 and those of 2001. The devastating epidemics are long gone but have been replaced with a slow toll of lost years and years spent in illness. The gap in male life expectancy for 2004–2008 between the most and least deprived deciles in Westminster, a borough close to the epicenter of world commerce, was 15.6 years (Association of Public Health Observatories 2009).

The response to the emergent pathology of the nineteenth-century city was the public health and town planning movement. Those conditions have changed beyond recognition. Infectious disease and malnutrition are no longer the burden that they were. But huge problems remain; London is still seen as problematic in public health terms. The absolute burden of disease has been replaced by the relative burden structured around groups and neighborhoods. To a large degree, the pattern of poverty and ill health has been sustained. Thus, the East End contains one of the United Kingdom's largest concentrations of deprivation, and the disparity within many boroughs continues to be unacceptable. As the challenge has been transformed, it is hard to conclude that the intervention paradigm has kept pace.

The social determinants of health model, in its many guises, surely offers one of the most powerful if unsophisticated paradigms to explain the persistence of disparities and inequities. The index of deprivation is based on multivariate strands. The map of deprivation to a large degree mirrors that of ill health, however that is measured. The weight of evidence suggests that it is through tackling the social determinants of health that the health gradient will be addressed. Nowhere has this been more forcefully stated than in the report of the World Health Organization Commission on the Social Determinants of Health (Marmot 2008). There is a strong case for arguing that spatial planning is a key activity in addressing the determinants of health, in particular their spatial dimensions. We have seen that the London Plan did indeed adopt the conceptual framework of the determinants of health model, albeit only implicitly. However, there is evidence that the lofty aims of the first mayor have not been carried through into delivery. Thus, the potential of a spatial planning policy framework has not been realized to the degree that it might. This cannot be judged to be a failure of the planning system alone; it also reflects a failure of engagement by the health sector to exploit the previously identified common agenda.

It is sometimes argued that London is unique. In a fundamental sense, this could not be otherwise. However, when used in relation to health, this argument is hard to sustain, and is never made in anything other than generalizations resting on the size and increasingly the ethnic diversity of the city. While it is difficult to argue that ill health continues to be an emergent condition of the city, the uniqueness of the health predicament, if indeed it can be said to exist, is the inadequacy of the governance response. The defining characteristic of the city may thus be inequality, and if that persists, the unequal patterns of disease and premature death are indeed inevitable.

I have argued that in some key respects the potential of the spatial planning system—the strategic and tactical means by which a city is managed—has not been exploited in a way that might enhance health and reduce inequalities. The leverage of the London Plan has hardly been applied to the issue of health enhancement, and the major transformations in the fabric have and continue to be planned and pursued without an explicit health framework and goals. It must be said that this is not the whole story. Some change in the regeneration of public sector housing and the improvement of environmental conditions has doubtless been positive for most if not all of the residents. However, overall, the task of creating the conditions for a healthy population, through the environment, through economic and educational opportunity, and through access to modern health care remains far from complete.

This chapter identifies the need for a new paradigm for the relationship of health and the built environment. The social determinants of health model clearly points to such a new paradigm, whereby health outcomes are the result of the complex interaction of socioeconomic pressures, personal characteristics, and place. Spatial planning has a strong claim to being one of the most effective mechanisms for addressing spatial outcomes. In the United Kingdom, spatial planning is predicated on sustainable development. Health and equity are axiomatic in sustainable development. The necessary common framework can thus be envisaged. The social determinants can be addressed through the spatial planning system with a view to delivering, enabling, or facilitating sustainable development. Properly constructed, such a set of interventions can deliver healthier and more equitable outcomes, a clear win-win situation.

The postmodern story of spatial planning in London demonstrates a reaching out for such a new paradigm. Health and health inequalities were clearly recognized on the cusp of a new political arrangement. Aims were clearly set. Health was explicitly defined as more than the absence of disease and a result of complex pressures across society. However, the administrative political and professional systems failed to secure the necessary degree of synergy. The spatial policy instruments chosen were not calculated to secure optimum health outcomes and the health sector, in turn, failed to formulate its evidence and actions in a spatially intelligent way. As a result, the status quo prevailed. The unique value of the social determinants model was not exploited. As a result, although health has improved, health inequalities persist and massive amounts of development and its associated activity have passed through the system without effective screening for health outcomes.

The solution to this paradox of clear vision and inadequate delivery is "joining up," or vertical and horizontal integration. In London this encompasses the mayor, the regional arm of government, the local borough councils, and the health sector working in a dynamic matrix with the following characteristics:

- A common political purpose rigorously pursued
- Health as an explicit concern
- A consistent performance management framework
- A common and mutually understandable evidence base
- Effective and consistent engagement
- The coproduction of actionable insights

With such a bold collaborative approach, there are in truth few barriers to London becoming an exemplar of a healthy city.

References

Association of Public Health Observatories. 2009. Health Inequalities Indicator for 2009 WCC Assurance Framework. Westminster PCT Summary Charts, 2004–2008. Available at: http://www.apho.org.uk/resource/view.aspx?RID=75050. Accessed January 26, 2011.

Ball M, Sunderland D. 2001. *Economic History of London: 1800–1914*. London, England: Routledge.

Booth C. 1889. *Life and Labour of the People*. London, England: Macmillan.

Commission on Social Determinants of Health. 2008. *Closing the Gap in a Generation: Health Equity Through Action on the Social Determinants of Health*. Final Report. Geneva, Switzerland: World Health Organization.

Communities and Local Government. 2005. *Planning Policy Statement 1: Creating Sustainable Communities*. London, England: Her Majesty's Stationery Office.

Dahlgren G, Whitehead M. 1991. *Policies and Strategies to Promote Social Equity in Health*. Stockholm, Sweden: Institute for Future Studies.

Davies A, Kendall L. 1999. *Health and the London Mayor*. London, England: London Health Commission.

Department for Environment, Food and Rural Affairs. 2005. The U.K. Government Sustainable Development Strategy. Available at: http://www.defra.gov.uk/sustainable/ government/publications/uk-strategy/documents/SecFut_complete.pdf. Accessed November 16, 2010.

Department of Health. 1998. *Health Services in London: A Strategic Review*. The Turnberg Report. London, England: Her Majesty's Stationery Office.

Diderichsen F, Evans T, Whitehead M. 1991. The social basis of disparities in health. In: Evans T, Whitehead M, Diderichsen F, et al., editors. *Challenging Inequities in Health: From Ethics to Action*. Oxford, England: Oxford University:3–11.

Greater London Authority. 2004. *The London Plan*. London, England: Greater London Authority.

Greater London Authority. 2004a. *Sustainability Appraisal of the London Plan*. London, England: Greater London Authority.

Greater London Authority. 2007. *Health Best Practice Guide*. London, England: Greater London Authority.

Gregory I. 2009. Comparisons between geographies of mortality and deprivation from 1900s and 2001: spatial analysis of census and mortality statistics. *BMJ*. 339:b3454.

Hamnett C. 2003. *Unequal City*. London, England: Routledge.

House of Lords (Baroness Jay of Paddington). 1998. London's health services. Hansard HL Debates. 3 February 1998, vol 585 col 519. Available at: http://hansard.millbanksystems.com/lords/1998/feb/03/londons-health-services. Accessed January 25, 2011.

Huxley J, Huxley TH. 1947. *Evolution and Ethics*. London, England: Pilot.

Imrie R. 2009. "An exemplar for a sustainable world city": progressive urban change and the redevelopment of King's Cross. In: Imrie R, Lees L, Raco M, editors. *Regenerating London: Governance, Sustainability, and Community in a Global City*. London, England: Routledge:93–111.

Johnson S. 2006. *The Ghost Map*. London, England: Allen Lane.

London Borough of Camden. 2001. *Kings Cross: Towards an Integrated City*. London, England: London Borough of Camden.

Massey D. 2007. *World City*. Cambridge, England: Polity.

National Health Service London Executive. 2000. *The London Health Strategy*. London, England: National Health Service.

Sassen S. 2006. *Cities in a World Economy*. 3rd ed. London, England: Sage.

Swinburn B, Egger G. 2002. Preventive strategies against weight gain and obesity. *Obes Rev*. 3:289–301.

U.K. Parliament. 1999. *The Greater London Authority Act*. London, England: Her Majesty's Stationery Office.

United Nations Economic and Social Council. 2009. Noncommunicable diseases, poverty and the development agenda. Discussion paper. Geneva, Switzerland: World Health Organization.

United Nations Human Settlement Programme (UN-HABITAT). 2009. Global Report on Human Settlements 2009: *Planning Sustainable Cities*. Nairobi, Kenya: UN-HABITAT. Available at: http://www.unchs.org/downloads/docs/GRHS2009/GRHS.2009.pdf. Accessed January 20, 2011.

11

Suburban Poverty, Diversity, and Health in Megacities: The Case of Los Angeles

Dennis P. Andrulis, PhD, MPH, and Nadia J. Siddiqui, MPH

THE POPULATIONS OF ALMOST all megacities and their trajectory of historical and projected growth have required expansion beyond what were original city limits—a growth that has led to considerable urban sprawl. Although this adaptation has included incorporating nearby areas into the city, in many locations it has also led to major if not explosive growth in the suburbs that surround them. In megacities such as Los Angeles, Mexico City, São Paulo, Buenos Aires, Manila, Shanghai, and Jakarta, nearly all population growth occurred in suburbs surrounding these cities rather than the urban core (Cox 2009).

Although awareness of this global trend is growing, much less is known about the people who live in suburbs and the impact of suburban sprawl on health. Thus, specific information is scant about the demographic and socioeconomic profile of suburban residents versus their urban counterparts, why individuals choose suburban residence, and the kinds of communities they have created. Similarly, little is known about the health status and needs of these residents and the health consequences of suburban living, as well as the health services programs currently in place and their ability to meet needs.

With ever-greater numbers living in suburbs around the world, competence and effectiveness in preventing and treating illness and disease gains increasing urgency. And yet, many questions and concerns arise around access to and quality of suburban public health and health care services and systems: What is the current capacity of these settings to meet current demand for health care services? To what extent are suburban social, health and health-related services and systems prepared to expand, adjust, and adapt to the needs of populations who live and work in these areas? How health care–deficient are these areas and how might they tap into existing efforts or create new efforts to accommodate community and individual needs?

Evidence of the suburban challenges reflected in these questions is likely to be found in most if not all of the current largest cities, as well as in those that will become megacities in the near future. This chapter focuses on one of these major urban areas struggling to find solutions to its suburbanization: Los Angeles. It identifies the sociodemographic shifts driving this change, highlighting in particular the increases in racial/ethnic diversity and poverty and related effects on housing, education, employment, immigration, and crime rates—concerns that extend to many megacities. It considers the health of suburban residents and their communities specifically as well as in the context of factors likely to affect health and access to care—transportation, the physical environment, and food and nutrition. After discussing the ability of current health and health-related resources to meet need and demand, the chapter recommends specific actions to address growing suburban populations' health care priorities.

The Changing Landscape of Megacity Suburbs

Suburbs are often described as areas with widely dispersed populations and low-density development. In much of the developed world, these are places where homes, retail stores, and workplaces are distinct and rigidly separated; where networks of roads are marked by poor access; and where there is a lack of a defining town center or "downtown" (Geller 2003). In the United States, other defining characteristics include very similar if not homogeneous living areas with widely spread-out subdivisions and strip malls (Wilson 2003; Buzbee 2003).

Many assume that suburban sprawl originated in the United States; however, some of the largest cities in Europe and elsewhere also have witnessed this phenomenon. For example, in the nineteenth century and earlier, the suburbs of London, Paris, and others attracted a growing mix of individuals and industries, including those who could not afford to live within the city and work that was too polluting for urban areas (Breugman 2005). With the proliferation of auto- and transit-oriented environments, the predominance of suburban growth has become increasingly characteristic of megacities (Figure 11.1). In fact, today sub-urbs make up the largest part of many megacities in both the developed and developing worlds (Cox 2009). Although suburbs often evoke images of dream homes and plush lawns, at least in the United States (Press 2007), recent data have shattered this suburban myth, suggesting that poverty is becoming deeply entrenched in suburbs. Between 2000 and 2008, the largest cities in the United States witnessed the greatest growth in poverty, and by 2008, more poor resided in suburbs than cities (Kneebone and Garr 2010).

As megacities elsewhere, such as Jakarta and Rio de Janeiro, have rapidly sub-urbanized, they have harbored large impoverished, squatter communities, known as *kampongs* or *favelas,* respectively, on the outskirts of city limits (Goldblum and Wong 2000; Perlman 2005). These troubled suburban communities are beset with problems once found only in big cities: inadequate housing, homelessness, crime, and hunger (Dreier 2004). At the same time, they have far fewer public

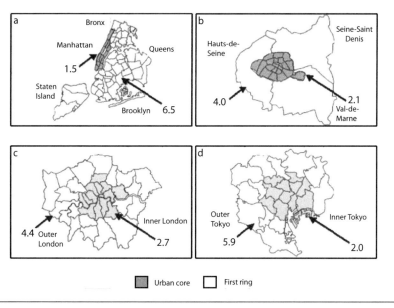

Source: Rodwin and Gusmano 2002.

Figure 11.1 Urban core and first-ring suburban populations (millions) in four megacities: New York City (a), Paris (b), Greater London (c), and Central Tokyo (d).

resources and programs targeting their evolving needs. This has become especially evident in the United States, where suburbs surrounding the largest cities have fewer doctors and health clinics that accept poor, uninsured patients, and social services, subsidized housing, and federal antipoverty programs are scant compared to city centers (Dreier 2004).

Several dynamics likely contribute to the expanding poverty and diversity of suburban communities. These include migrants and immigrants bypassing traditional urban centers and settling in suburban communities that already have concentrations of individuals and families of similar cultural heritage; gentrification in cities that is forcing previously urban residents to find less expensive places to live; lower-skilled employment opportunities; and, in the United States, efforts to improve urban quality of life (e.g., higher-performing schools and lower crime rates; Berube 2007; Andrulis and Siddiqui 2008).

The changing face of suburbs, in particular expanding pockets of poverty, deteriorating infrastructure, dispersed populations, and greater dependence on automobiles raise serious concerns around population health. Research has documented that suburban sprawl affects health in many ways, including greater numbers of traffic fatalities, increased air pollution, fewer opportunities for physical activity, and increasing overweight and obesity among residents (Sturm and Cohen 2004; Reid, Sciber, and Zegeer 2003).

A study of suburban sprawl and physical health in the United States documented the toll on residents (Sturm and Cohen 2004). Using 16 measures of chronic health conditions, the authors asked individuals living in 38 suburban areas, such as those surrounding the city of Los Angeles, to self-report (through interviews) chronic conditions such as diabetes, asthma, and cancer. Their conclusion reaffirmed the health care consequences: "sprawl appears to have a disproportionate impact on the physical health of the elderly and possibly the poor" (Sturm and Cohen 2004 , p494). This results from insufficient resources to lessen the negative factors in their environment, such as fewer parks, greater reliance on transportation, and lack of opportunities to walk to destinations. In addition, suburban sprawl, and in particular automobile commuting, has been linked to mental health problems, including stress and stress-related health concerns such as cardiovascular disease (Frumkin, Frank, and Jackson 2004). Findings from these studies generally seem to support the contention that suburban sprawl is bad for health.

Furthermore, access to health care for those in poverty is a major and grow-ing challenge. In reference to suburban increases in medical care for those with-out insurance, the executive director of the Illinois Public Health Association commented, "As we see poverty grow in these [suburban] areas, we'll see health problems that accompany poverty" (Sundman 1993). The intersection of race, ethnicity, and poverty further compounds care, and concerns have also arisen around tuberculosis and other communicable diseases in these areas.

The Case of Los Angeles

Los Angeles, the ninth largest city in the world, spanning five counties in the state of California—Los Angeles, Orange, San Bernardino, Riverside, and Ventura (Figure 11.2)—was born out of a small mission in the eighteenth century. The city's rapid and sustained growth was fueled by the constant influx of individu-als and industries attracted to the region's vast open space, rich natural resources, and mild climate. The advent of transportation including the railroad and auto-mobiles as well as growing entertainment and manufacturing industries further contributed to this expansion: "The decades leading up to World War II marked the region's rise to prominence and its definitive transformation into a major metropolitan area with significant concentration of economic activity" (Strategic

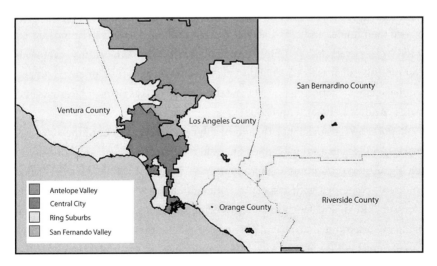

Figure 11.2 Map of Los Angeles and its suburbs.

Economics 2002, p7). By the 1940s, Los Angeles was home to a population of 7 million, 86% of which resided in the city center.

In the years that followed, however, the city experienced continuous deconcentration as newly arriving residents bypassed city centers and city dwellers moved to suburbs and more peripheral regions (Cosby 2004). This shift from concentration to deconcentration happened noticeably earlier than the general American trend (Cosby 2004; Vining Jr. and Strauss 1977). By 2000, of the 16 million people living in the Los Angeles megalopolis, only 58% resided in the urban core and a higher proportion were living in areas surrounding the city than ever before (Strategic Economics 2002).

The sections that follow describe the changing face of suburbs around Los Angeles, highlighting their growth in poverty and diversity, and discussing challenges for the region's health and health care.

Trajectory of Poverty and Diversity

It is generally assumed in many developed and Western countries that suburbs are fairly uniform places settled for the most part by White, middle-class families. The suburbs of Los Angeles were once America's most firmly rooted bastion of middle-income families holding stable jobs and affording top quality education, big homes on large lots, expensive cars, and leisure (Barrett 2009). The San Fernando Valley (in the northern suburban region outside the city) was a prime example of such suburban living, where three of four Valley families owned their homes and nearly 60% of the one million residents were considered middle class (Barrett 2009). But by the start of the twentieth century, suburban communities such as San Fernando Valley had undergone fundamental compositional change, harboring poverty and diversity as well as rising joblessness and crime (Andrulis and Siddiqui 2008).

Reports on the social, health, and health care characteristics of the 100 largest cities and suburbs in the United States found that Los Angeles had one of the ten highest levels of suburban poverty in 2000—almost 15% overall and 19% for children—compared with respective national rates of 9% and 12% for suburbs (Andrulis, Reid, and Duchon 2004). During the 1990s, the number of people living in concentrated poverty nearly quadrupled in the suburbs of Los Angeles County, and by 2000, nearly twice as many poor lived in suburbs compared to the center city (Table 11.1; Matsunaga 2008; McConville and Ong 2003).

Table 11.1   Urban and Suburban Neighborhoods and Total Population, by Poverty Status: Los Angeles, 1970–2000

	Neighborhoods			Total Population		
	Very Poor	Poor	Nonpoor	Very Poor	Poor	Nonpoor
1970						
Urban	29	156	286	80,170	584,696	1,217,379
Suburban	9	98	1,648	5,121	378,830	7,494,680
1980						
Urban	32	239	202	93,196	1,116,886	842,999
Suburban	10	137	1,767	13,521	630,672	8,582,976
1990						
Urban	45	256	168	209,018	1,441,658	767,737
Suburban	18	204	1,857	63,968	1,324,610	10,421,970
2000						
Urban	96	333	147	376,090	1,456,329	653,429
Suburban	61	509	2,131	243,642	2,683,613	10,656,166

Source: McConville and Ong 2003.

Note. Poverty rate is defined as the total number of persons with annual incomes below the U.S. federal poverty level, as a percentage of the total population for whom poverty status is determined. Very poor neighborhoods are defined as having poverty rates of at least 40 percent; poor neighborhoods have poverty rates of at least 20 percent; and nonpoor neighborhoods have rates below 20 percent.

When compared via a Social Deprivation Index—comprised of six indicators including poverty rate, per capita income, percentage speaking a language other than English at home, percentage speaking English not well or at all, unemployment rate, and percentage of population aged 25 years or older without a high school diploma—Los Angeles suburbs ranked among the five worst (Andrulis, Reid, and Duchon 2004). Between 1990 and 2000, they had one of the five lowest rates of increase in high school graduation (4.1%); their unemployment rate was among the bottom ten in 2000, and their violent crime rate was the second highest, behind only Miami (Andrulis, Reid, and Duchon 2004). And by 2008, over 10% of the Los Angeles suburban population lived in poverty, exceeding the national suburban average (9.5%; Kneebone and Garr 2010). Furthermore, during the 2008–2009 recession and housing market collapse, poverty in the Los Angeles area increased 3%, again exceeding the U.S. average of 2% (Kneebone and Garr 2010).

The economic transformation of Los Angeles and other megacity suburbs did not occur overnight. Rather, they are rooted in broad changes characteristic of growing metropolitan societies. Among primary factors are the following:

- *Continued deconcentration of population.* The sheer scale and pace of suburban growth in megalopolises such as Los Angeles—stimulated by opportunities to improve quality of life through affordable housing, better schools, and lower crime rates—has absorbed a broad and diverse economic cross-section of individuals and families (Berube 2007).
- *Suburbanization of employment.* Suburbs of America's largest cities, including Los Angeles, provide more jobs than do their urban counterparts and are increasingly concentrating in lower-wage industries like retail, hospitality, and personal services (Katz and Bradley 2009). These industries have accounted for the bulk of job growth in many fast-growing suburbs in the United States (Gordon and Richardson 1996; Berube 2007).
- *Gentrification of cities.* Observed in large Western cities such as Los Angeles, London, and Paris, the migration of affluent populations from suburbs into city centers is forcing previously urban residents to find less expensive places to live, mainly in older, deteriorating first-ring suburbs.
- *Immigrant settlement in suburbs.* New immigrants to Los Angeles and other large metropolitan areas are bypassing traditional urban centers and settling in suburban communities with concentrations of residents of similar racial, ethnic, and cultural heritage (according to a 2007 U.S. Census Bureau report, 40% of immigrants to large U.S. metropolitan areas are moving directly to the suburbs; Roberts 2007).

Coupled with the growing concentration of poverty is the suburbanization of cultural and linguistic diversity. Evidence suggests that the transformation of the Los Angeles metropolitan region has been ongoing at least since the 1960s, driven by desire to live near friends and family, being with others speaking a common language, employment, and affordable housing (Estrada 1988; McConville and Ong 2003). A report on Los Angeles and 14 other major metropolitan areas found that, by 2000, about half of all African Americans and over 60% of Latinos lived in the suburbs (Orfield et al. 2006). These populations were also more likely to live in "fiscally stressed jurisdictions" with fewer public resources and greater public service needs. In addition, the successive outmigration of Whites, juxtaposed with the continued waves of immigrants to suburbs, has helped create an elderly population that is majority White, a working-age population that is two thirds racial/ethnic minority, and a child population that is predominantly Hispanic and racial/ethnic minority (Frey 2000).

Threats to Health

The unprecedented growth of Los Angeles and its suburbs raises serious concerns for the health of its residents. Problems of poverty such as crowded housing, lack of reliable transportation, limited or dispersed healthy food options, crime, and violence are associated with poor health status and outcomes (Braverman and Egerter 2008). The suburban region of Antelope Valley, 50 miles north of Los Angeles and home to a large and growing low-income, racially and ethnically diverse population, is particularly feeling the brunt. Valley residents have higher rates of chronic conditions, infant mortality, and other poor health indicators than do surrounding areas and in some cases worse than in the city center (Jhawar and Wallace 2005). In addition, poor, racial/ethnic minority women have higher rates of chronic disease and mortality compared with men, and this is true not only in Antelope Valley but also in South Los Angeles and other neighboring suburban communities (Rosenblatt 2007). Furthermore, close to half of these women report little or no physical activity and nearly one in four is obese; the highest levels of obesity were associated with poverty (Rosenblatt 2007). Other findings indicated that nearly one in four adults was diagnosed with hypertension and approximately one in five self-reported their health as fair or poor in these suburban communities of Los Angeles (Jhawar and Wallace 2005). Other data from 1999 to 2003 suggest that Los Angeles and its surrounding suburban counties have some of the highest rates of age-adjusted heart disease mortality in the nation (Braverman and Egerter 2008).

Although suburbs are often associated with open spaces and clean air, this is largely changing in sprawling megalopolises such as Los Angeles, where the heavy reliance on automobiles and closer proximity to expansive highways is resulting in growing air pollution and associated ailments (Frumkin 2002). Air pollution is linked to well-documented health hazards such as higher incidence and severity of respiratory symptoms, including asthma, worse lung function, more emergency room visits, and hospitalizations (Frumkin 2002). A recent study of Los Angeles and its surrounding areas found considerably higher rates of asthma among both children and adults, and this was especially true for Antelope Valley. The rate of asthma among Antelope Valley children was 17.5%, compared with 13.7% in the county and 14.7% in the state (Jhawar and Wallace 2005). Similarly, 14.5% of adults were diagnosed with asthma in the Valley compared with 10.7 and 11.8% in the county and statewide, respectively. Another study of children in the Los Angeles area, including its suburbs, documented the effects of pollution, reaffirming high rates of asthma and significant levels of impaired lung function (Künzli et al. 2003).

As Los Angeles continues to expand and evolve, the health of its residents depends heavily on the availability of and access to social, health, and other public resources. Research suggests that suburban tracts of Los Angeles that experienced significant poverty growth between 1990 and 2000 were proximate to far fewer service providers than central city tracts experiencing such poverty increases (Allard 2004). A recent media report indicated that prenatal medical care for low-income populations is limited in suburbs such as Antelope Valley, resulting in a disproportionate number of problem pregnancies and higher infant mortality (Rivera 2005).

Challenges for Public Health and Health Care in Suburbs of Megacities

The suburban transformation and related health implications identified in previous sections, including the Los Angeles Case Study, pose a set of challenges for public health and health care. These include (1) burden on emergency and trauma care systems, (2) strain on urban and suburban safety net providers, (3) challenges associated with meeting health care needs of diverse populations, and (4) jurisdictional issues in planning for public health and health care.

Burden on Emergency and Trauma Care

Delivery of timely and effective emergency and trauma care represents perhaps one of the more trenchant health care challenges resulting from suburban sprawl in Los Angeles and other megacities. Concentrations of major hospitals in cities, fragmented planning, and failure to adapt to new and expanding populations will likely threaten to leave many and, in particular, poor suburban areas without recourse to services fundamental to effective, timely care. Anecdotal experience from the Los Angeles suburbs of Antelope and Lancaster/Palmdale (Andrulis 2004) has reinforced this deficit especially for poor residents, with individuals stating that "the hospital situation is deplorable—if you get in an accident it would be [very difficult] to get to an effective emergency room" (Andrulis 2004, p5).

As medical directors in the United States have pointed out, housing developments in many suburbs were built before anyone figured out the infrastructure to serve them (Millard 2007). As a result, these areas suffer from poor planning, limited access to major highways because of the lack of an effective grid, and a landscape that looks like "the end of a Scrabble game" (Millard 2007, p71). The consequences for emergency care are significant and, in many cases, life threatening. One study found that the average emergency service response time approached 50% longer for noncity residents (Millard 2007). Houston and other cities approaching megacity capacity have very few Level 1 trauma centers and those they have are located in the urban core. Such arrangements, with little planning, result in ambulances being forced to work in a world of sprawl, facing obstacles in bringing all patients to one city area. In the greater New York City region, some hospitals are further complicating care by moving away from poor areas (Millard 2007). Furthermore, a Joint Commission report found that 21% of patient deaths and permanent injury can be associated with emergency department treatment delays linked to specialist shortages (Joint Commission 2002).

Research in the United States has documented an inverse relationship (not found in cities) between the degree of suburban poverty and the availability and use of essential health care services (Andrulis and Duchon 2007). In 2002, high-poverty suburbs of the nation's largest cities, which represented 44% of the total suburban population, accounted for almost 25% fewer staffed beds, admissions, inpatient days, and outpatient and emergency visits than did the wealthiest suburbs which represented only 26% of the total suburban population. Poor suburbs also had 16 to 33% fewer trauma centers, neonatal intensive care unit beds, and PET scans compared with their affluent counterparts. Indicative of continued concentration of services, affluent suburbs saw a 2,000% increase in PET scans between 1996 and 2002 (Andrulis and Duchon 2007).

Strains on Urban and Suburban Safety Net Providers

The health care safety net is often referred to as providers that deliver health care and other health-related services to poor, underserved, and vulnerable patients (Lewin and Altman 2000). Safety net services in the urban core are generally organized around a large teaching hospital (public or private not-for-profit), supplemented by multiple outpatient primary care providers, such as community health centers, charity clinics, and local health departments. Together, this integrated health care delivery system provides a range of services from primary to secondary and tertiary care.

Few suburbs, however, have an integrated and viable safety net, and many rely on smaller local hospitals or community clinics with a narrow range of services. Others turn to urban providers to fill this void. One study on megacities, including New York City, London, Paris, and Tokyo, found that urban cores had a higher density of physicians than did their outlying suburbs and that city centers accounted for 1.5 to 2.5 times more acute hospital beds per 1000 population than did the suburban fringes (Rodwin and Gusmano 2002). In a recent study of the suburbs of major U.S. cities, findings suggested that "low-income suburban residents had difficulty accessing preventive, primary and specialty care," and patient zip code data revealed an increasing dependence of suburban residents on urban hospitals and services (Felland, Lauer, and Cunningham 2009, p3).

Furthermore, the study showed that physicians, in particular specialty physicians willing to treat poor patients or those with little or no insurance, were difficult to find in suburban areas. A respondent from Harborview Medical Center in Seattle, Washington, noted

> As the safety net hospital for our county, [Harborview Medical Center] has quickly become the safety net hospital for the entire state. We've really had to push back. It wasn't uncommon to get patients from 100 miles away with a nice letter from their physician saying the person lost their insurance and they can't care for the patient anymore. (Felland, Lauer, and Cunningham 2009, p9).

The growing demand for health care among suburban populations, in particular poor and culturally diverse ones, are straining both suburban and urban providers and raising questions for their financial viability. In the United States, the loss of suburban safety net hospitals, where they existed, has exacerbated these circumstances. Between 1996 and 2002, over one quarter of suburban public hospitals were lost (27%), more than any other ownership group, continuing a 47% decline documented between 1980 and 1996 (Andrulis and Duchon 2007).

Challenges Related to Meeting Health Care Needs
of Diverse Populations

As suburbs continue to grow in diversity, expanding access to health care will require addressing barriers related to race, culture, language, and religion, particularly in megacities with significant minority populations such as, London, Paris, Tokyo, and others. Studies have found that even after accounting for socioeconomic factors (such as income or health insurance in the United States), patients who face cultural and linguistic barriers are less likely to have a usual source of medical care and have fewer physician visits and exhibit poorer management of chronic conditions (Mead et al. 2008). Many suburban health care providers lag their urban counterparts in offering culturally and linguistically competent care—care that acknowledges the distinct beliefs and preferences toward medical consultation and intervention among immigrants, rural migrants, and other racial/ethnic minorities as well as their specific health literacy and language needs (Felland, Lauer, and Cunningham 2009).

Beyond an increasing cultural and linguistic diversity, the "graying of the suburbs" is a growing phenomenon in suburbs of major Western metropolitan areas such as Los Angeles. "Aging in place," particularly by early baby boomers born between 1945 and 1955 who settled in suburbs in the latter part of the twentieth century, raises serious concerns regarding the adequate supply of geriatric services; home health care; and transportation to access medical care, rehabilitation, and other services (Frey 2000).

Jurisdictional Issues in Public Health and Health Care Planning

The mismatch in defining and classifying suburban regions raises serious and important questions for building the public health and health care infrastructure, including disease surveillance systems, emergency response capabilities, safety net hospitals, and other health-related programs, in megacity suburbs. For example, the suburban region of Antelope Valley in Los Angeles is considered by the state of California as rural for purposes of health planning, but the U.S. government classifies it as urban, "an action that renders it ineligible for federal health care dollars designated for rural areas" (Rivera 2005). County health officials as well as recent data and reports suggest that it is precisely this rural nature—with a lack of well-connected public transportation and paucity of medical services— but lack of designation and dedicated funding as such, that is feeding poor health outcomes, including high infant mortality and growing prevalence of tobacco use, obesity, asthma, and hypertension (Rivera 2005).

As megacities continue to globalize and expand in economic and political activity, populations in suburbs and other peripheral regions not included explicitly or expansively in public health preparedness planning and funding may be disproportionately more susceptible to being "left behind" in the event of a disease outbreak or disaster. In Los Angeles, New York City, London, and other megacities in which new immigrants are increasingly arriving and settling in outlying areas that are neither urban or rural, this raises concerns regarding adequate public health capacity and resources for essential public health services such as monitoring and containing reemerging communicable diseases (e.g., tuberculosis); providing risk communication and preparedness outreach that is culturally and linguistically appropriate and can be received and understood by new and diverse communities; conducting community health and rapid needs assessment; and other related public health programs.

Future Directions for Public Health and Health Care in Suburbs of Megacities

The challenges to Los Angeles and its suburbs identified here are complex and dynamic, with the consequences of population shifts and major growth in the greater urban areas, as well as doubts about the ability of public health, health care, and broader socioeconomic infrastructure to adapt only beginning to be acknowledged. Adequate planning and response to meet related health and health care needs will not be accomplished by taking incremental steps. Similarly, public health or other single sectors acting alone are likely to fall significantly short of achieving progress. Rather, effective strategies will require active, concerted commitment across a broad spectrum of programs and agencies, levels of government, and these communities.

This section presents initiatives intended to offer megacities in the United States and elsewhere directions and concrete actions for creating high-quality public health and health care programs that meet the challenges of suburban sprawl. Embedded in these recommendations are two fundamental tenets: (1) that achieving related objectives will require collaboration both across sectors and jurisdictions, and (2) that although hospitals and clinics play a central role, ultimately, improving the health of residents will require the engagement of institutions and programs that profoundly influence the well-being of these communities, such as faith-based, social-welfare, cultural, and other community-based organizations.

Creating Regional Systems for Emergency, Trauma, and Other Essential Health Care Services

Responding to suburban health care, trauma, and emergency care needs will require federal and other jurisdictional (e.g., state) leadership in the United States and in other megacities to support and direct local providers and communities in creating regional systems of emergency and trauma care that ensure equitable access in suburban areas, with links to urban providers. To do so will require at least two concerted actions:

- *Linking expertise, staff, and resources of urban emergency departments to suburban, exurban, and rural facilities to enhance regional coordination of emergency care, supportive services, and protocols.* Suburbs with large and growing immigrant and minority populations often lack the infrastructure or specialized services necessary to effectively respond to the needs of these residents generally, but especially in emergency situations. To this end, a regionalized emergency care system could offer the opportunity for suburban hospitals and health care centers to tap into neighboring urban health care facilities with more experience in caring for diverse patients for resources—for example, interpreter services, translated patient information materials, and other culturally competent services—to assure effective communication, timely response (e.g., interhospital transfer), and high-quality care.

  Research has documented that hospitals most frequently located in urban cores that care for higher volumes of patients tend to have more staffing, specialized equipment, treatment protocols, and other resources—and ultimately, better patient outcomes (University of Pennsylvania School of Medicine 2009). Suburban hospitals can draw on urban facilities for expertise and resources to deliver emergency care and relieve the burden of overcrowding by taking in patients with less serious or less acute conditions. Building such "connected" systems of care with shared responsibility, including using suburban facilities as sites for helipads to transport and transfer patients, telemedicine linked to urban facilities, prehospital care, and, most importantly, access to specialists can also work to compensate for the imbalance of sites across urban and suburban landscapes.

- *Promote collaboration on public policy that integrates regional planning for transportation, sprawl, zoning, and other factors that affect the effectiveness of regional emergency care systems.* Regionalization of emergency care and other services will likely benefit from the involvement of emergency physicians and hospitals, along with public health officials and environmental medicine specialists, in planning for community development, particularly on issues pertaining to suburban sprawl and emergency care. For example, research indicates that suburban living contributes to a high prevalence of vehicular trauma. Features of the suburban landscape such as long distances, high speeds, two-lane highways with hazardous curves, suboptimal lighting, and limits to 911 coverage in the United States combine to create hazardous conditions that contribute to collisions and delay out-of-hospital responses. Furthermore, lack of public transportation is cited as a major barrier to accessing emergency and health care services, not only in developed countries such as the United States, but major cities in the developing world as well. The involvement of emergency physicians in public policy on these kinds of issues could help build healthier community infrastructures and complement efforts to develop a coordinated and regionalized emergency care system (Millard 2007).

Supporting a Suburban Public Health and Health Care Safety Net

In megacities such as Los Angeles and other suburban regions, the need to develop, maintain, and sustain a health care safety net through public and other hospitals will remain critical. Evidence from the Institute of Medicine's landmark report, *Unequal Treatment,* and other research has documented that a relatively small number of diverse providers care for many racially and ethnically diverse patients. Moreover, the chronic lack of access for poor populations and the social conditions facing them—including neighborhood issues such as crime, residential segregation, access to healthy food, and other social determinants—may make these patients less attractive to mainstream providers who may be concerned about challenges to adherence to treatment and costs.

In addition, meeting the needs of diverse patients often requires additional services, such as interpreter services and culturally competent care, that are more likely to be found in safety net settings with familiarity in caring for patients from diverse cultural and linguistic backgrounds. Other populations, such as the increasing number of undocumented immigrants, refugees, rural migrants, and other culturally and linguistically isolated populations, may be reluctant to participate in mainstream care. (In the United States, the enactment of health insurance reform is unlikely to be so comprehensive to acknowledge all of these and other population-specific issues.) The presence of a viable safety net can work to assure they are not left out of care.

Building Regional Civic Alliances to Consolidate Resources and Political Power

As isolated entities functioning on their own, smaller jurisdictions and concentrations of residents in suburban megacities attempting to address public health priorities may have insufficient resources and influence to address their public health priorities. However, finding common ground both within and across areas and regions may offer new opportunities to learn from other experiences, share information, collaborate on initiatives, and establish a stronger, more influential position from which to negotiate with governmental agencies engaged in promoting health care and public health programs and policies. In essence, many suburban areas with populations in small towns or dispersed across expanses may benefit significantly by forming collaborations with these communities and, in other cases, bridging to other suburban areas to take advantage of collective resources and build networks. Such regionalization can offer the opportunity to concentrate limited or expensive health care resources locally, while dispersing primary and secondary care more broadly across the region (Amarsingham, Pickens, and Anderson 2005).

In the Los Angeles region, state and private efforts have promoted such alliances to address strategic public health and health-related priorities. For example, the California Department of Public Health has established a community collaborative across the state to address growing concerns around obesity, overweight, and unfit children (California Department of Public Health 2008). Regionally, it has helped to create the Los Angeles Collaborative for Healthy Active Children across the county. Over 100 organizations have joined this effort, including area school districts, health care providers, community-based organizations, department of public health, parks and recreation departments for the city and county, faith-based organizations, chronic disease associations, and food policy advocates. Its work includes development of a "toolbox" to educate residents about nutrition and to encourage ways to curb obesity. It asks participants to work with community organizations to identify barriers to physical activity such as lack of safe walking areas and poorly maintained parks. It is acknowledged as the first countywide initiative to improve physical activity.

Emerging models to address social and economic concerns across suburban areas in jurisdictions other than Los Angeles also offer guidance to megacities in addressing health care needs. For example, suburban areas in and around Gloucester Township in Camden County, New Jersey, which is part of the greater Philadelphia region, have created the First Suburbs Network (Gollway 2008). This initiative brings together towns in the areas that are facing significant challenges in serving new and in many cases increasingly diverse populations, seeking to support and enhance infrastructure, improve quality of life, and improve neighborhoods. Such regional efforts can also address health care as a priority by identifying and developing critical health care infrastructure needs for the region, such as:

> " . . . [establishing] efficient referral and prehospital care, EMS [emergency medical services] patterns . . . [improving] indigent health care reimbursement, [developing] strategies to disperse primary and secondary care . . . and [maintaining] timely access to centralized tertiary services in urban areas" (Amarsingham, Pickens, and Anderson 2005).

Building Capacity Within Suburban Areas

One of the major challenges facing suburban areas of megacities is creating or, in some circumstances, recreating and enhancing the public health-related infrastructure to establish a sustainable, strong set of community services and a community "voice" to address its health priorities. This need may be particularly urgent in areas that have seen major influxes of poorer populations where few health and health-related services are familiar with these individuals, their cultures, and their needs, or where existing agencies and supportive organizations are not prepared for significant increases in these residents.

In California, private eleemosynary sources have stepped up their support to undergird the infrastructure of such communities. A major state foundation, The California Endowment, has launched a Building Healthy Communities Initiative to improve the health of children and youths in low-income areas, with the intention of linking community-based effective programs with state prevention policies. One of their sites for this ten-year initiative is located in the South Los Angeles area, where 40% of households live below poverty and which suffers 17% unemployment as well as widespread substandard housing and poor health care (Los Angeles County Department of Health 2010). This collaboration of community leaders, key political forces, and community-based organizations focuses on reducing racial/ethnic and poverty-related disparities manifest in high rates of lead levels and poor access to care in this area of Los Angeles County. The California Endowment's program will bring South Los Angeles together with other communities, their agencies, and advocacy groups to create opportunities for shared learning with the objectives of improving housing; access to walkable streets, fresh fruits, and vegetables; providing medical homes; and developing strong social networks among participating groups.

Collaborating With Cities to Tap Experience and Resources

Suburban areas with major economic and demographic changes can benefit significantly from developing constructive alliances with their urban counterparts. Municipalities can connect the poor and low-income workers with an array of support including education, child care, and nutrition in ways that reach both suburban and city families (Berube and Kneebone 2006). In many cases, cities have greater experience in addressing the needs of low-income and culturally diverse residents, and in tackling emerging issues affecting health and access such as unemployment and crime. Practically speaking, they most often have health care resources not available in suburban areas, such as teaching hospitals that are critical components to delivery of high-quality care. In addition, cities are more likely to have longer-standing infrastructures to support, advocate, and guide response to need. Local providers, health departments, and health plans, as well as supportive organizations, could draw on these assets to assist in advancing access in suburban areas.

Summary

The urban cores of most megacities are, by their nature, limited in their spatial capacity to expand beyond their borders. Although some incorporation of surrounding areas may provide limited relief to crowded inner cities, population growth and suburban growth for megacities are likely to be inescapable, intimately related trends for the future—a situation reflected in an announcement by President Sarkozy of France of a plan to more closely align the socioeconomic forces of center city Paris with its more isolated suburbs and create a regional "Grand Paris" (Wagner 2010). Unfortunately, as our review has found, awareness of this trend and actions to address the related population and community health needs in general have been limited at best. Because little federal or other major commitment has been evident, our case study city of Los Angeles has had to rely on private foundation incentives and very modest state initiatives for funding of relevant initiatives.

Nonetheless, although our recommendations will require additional resources and political will, they also strongly support reinforcement of existing strengths and political and organizational structures, primarily through collaborations and coordination to identify common priorities of cities and suburbs. Any plans for addressing health, public health, and health care priorities for these areas must recognize the need to work from such a position of mutual benefit. Failure to do so will limit resources and political power, with adverse health consequences that can affect rates of communicable disease, ability to respond to disasters, and other events. These and other negative effects may also extend far beyond the suburbs to affect the well-being of residents in megacity areas generally, in terms of crime, employment, education, safety, and economics for the region. But the benefits of meeting suburban public health and health care challenges will reach far beyond these communities to help create a healthier urban–suburban region for all residents.

References

Allard SW. 2004. *Access to Social Services: The Changing Urban Geography of Poverty and Service Provision.* Washington, DC: Brookings Institution. Available at: http://www.brookings.edu/metro/pubs/20040816_allard.pdf. Accessed September 10, 2010.

Amarsingham R, Pickens S, Anderson RJ. 2005. County hospitals and regional medical care in Texas: an analysis of out-of-county costs. *Tex Med.* June 2004. Available at: http://www.texmed.org/Template.aspx?id=1255. Accessed September 17, 2008.

Andrulis D. 2004. *Pilot Project on Medicaid Managed Care Programs and Racial/Ethnic Enrollees in Suburban Areas.* Princeton, NJ: Center for Health Care Strategies.

Andrulis D, Duchon L. 2007. The changing landscape of hospital capacity in large cities and suburbs: implications for the safety net in metropolitan America. *J Urban Health*. 84:400–414.

Andrulis D, Reid H, Duchon L. 2004. *Quality of Life in the Nations' 100 Largest Cities and Their Suburbs: New and Continuing Challenges for Improving Health and Well-Being*. New York, NY: Downstate Medical Center.

Andrulis D, Siddiqui N. 2008. Health Insurance Coverage Reform: Implications for Improving Access in Suburban America. Presented at: Institute of Medicine; September 23; Washington, DC.

Barrett B. 2009. Middle Class Flight From San Fernando Valley: Will Taxpayers Who Are Leaving "America's Suburb" Behind Doom L.A.? *LA Weekly*. January 29. Available at: http://www.laweekly.com/2009-01-29/news/middle-class-flight-from-san-fernando-valley. Accessed November 23, 2010.

Berube A. 2007. The Geography of U.S. Poverty and Its Implications. Testimony Before the Committee on Ways and Means Subcommittee on Income Security and Family Support. Washington, DC: Brookings Institution. February 13. Available at: http://www.brookings.edu/testimony/2007/0213childrenfamilies_berube.aspx. Accessed September 17, 2008.

Berube A, Kneebone E. 2006. Two Steps Back: City and Suburban Poverty Trends, 1999–2005. Washington, DC: Brookings Institution.

Braverman P, Egerter S. 2008. Overcoming Obstacles to Health: Report From the Robert Wood Johnson Foundation to the Commission to Build a Healthier America. Princeton, NJ: Robert Wood Johnson Foundation.

Breugman R. 2005. *Sprawl: A Compact History*. Chicago, IL: University of Chicago.

Buzbee W. 2003. Urban form, health, and the law's limits. *Am J Public Health*. 93:1395–1398.

California Department of Public Health. 2008. Network for a Healthy California: Champions for Change. Available at: http://www.cdph.ca.gov/programs/CPNS/Pages/default.aspx. Accessed March 25, 2010.

Cosby K. 2004. From mission to megacity: the changing concentration of the Los Angeles city-system [Master's thesis]. Brigham Young University. Available at: http://contentdm.lib.byu.edu/ETD/image/etd415.pdf. Accessed April 15, 2010.

Cox W. 2009. Suburbs and Cities: The Unexpected Truth. *New Geography*. May 16. Available at: http://www.newgeography.com/content/00805-suburbs-and-cities-the-unexpected-truth. Accessed September 9, 2010.

Dreier P. 2004. The Suburbanization of Poverty: The American Dream of Suburbia—Backyard Grilling and Upward Mobility—Rings Hollow in Today's Economy. *The Nation*. September 9. Available at: http://www.alternet.org/story/19828. Accessed April 15, 2010.

Estrada LF. 1988. Hispanic Suburbanization in Los Angeles: Social Arrival and Barrio Formation. Volume IV. 1988–1989: Conference on Comparative Ethnicity: The Conference Papers, June 1988. Los Angeles: University of California–Los Angeles, Institute for Social Science Research. Available at: http://www.escholarship.org/uc/item/6s3927f4. Accessed September 4, 2010.

Felland L, Lauer JR, Cunningham PJ. 2009. *Suburban Poverty and the Health Care Safety Net*. Research Brief No. 13. Princeton, NJ: Center for Studying Health System Change.

Frey WH. 2000. The New Urban Demographics: Race, Space, and Boomer Aging. Washington, DC: Brookings Institution. Available at: http://www.brookings.edu/articles/2000/summer_demographics.aspx. Accessed September 10, 2010.

Frumkin H. 2002. Urban sprawl and public health. *Public Health Rep*. 117:201–217.

Frumkin H, Frank L, Jackson R. 2004. *Urban Sprawl and Public Health: Designing, Planning, and Building for Healthy Communities*. Washington, DC: Island.

Geller A. 2003. Smart growth: a prescription for livable cities. *Am J Public Health*. 93:1410–1415.

Goldblum C, Wong T. 2000. Growth, crisis and spatial change: a study of haphazard urbanization in Jakarta, Indonesia. *Land Use Policy*. 17:29–37.

Gollway T. 2008. Aging Suburbs Start to Address Citylike Challenges. *New York Times*. March 23. Available at: http://www.nytimes.com/2008/03/23/nyregion/nyregionspecial2/23suburbsnj.html. Accessed August 6, 2010.

Gordon P, Richardson HW. 1996. Employment decentralization in US metropolitan areas: is Los Angeles an outlier or the norm? *Environ Plan*. 28:1727–1743.

Jhawar M, Wallace S. 2005. Chronic Conditions of Californians: Findings From the 2003 California Health Interview Survey. Available at: http://www.healthpolicy.ucla.edu/pubs/files/chron_cond05_report.pdf. Accessed September 4, 2010.

The Joint Commission. 2002. Delays in Treatment. Sentinel Event Alert. Oakbrook Terrace, IL: The Joint Commission. June 17. Available at: http://www. jointcommission.org/SentinelEvents/SentinelEventAlert/sea_26.htm. Accessed September 4, 2010.

Katz B, Bradley J. 2009. The Suburban Challenge: Cities, Competitiveness, U.S. Economy, U.S. Poverty, Innovation. Washington, DC: Brookings Institution. January 26. Available at: http://www.brookings.edu/opinions/2009/0126_suburbs_katz.aspx. Accessed April 15, 2010.

Kneebone E, Garr E. 2010. The Suburbanization of Poverty: Trends in Metropolitan America, 2000 to 2008. Metropolitan Opportunity Series, No. 4. Washington, DC: Brookings Institution. January 20. Available at: http://www.brookings.edu/ papers/2010/0120_poverty_kneebone.aspx. Accessed September 10, 2010.

Künzli N, McConnell R, Bates D, et al. 2003. Breathless in Los Angeles: the exhausting search for clean air. *Am J Public Health*. 93:1494–1499.

Lewin ME, Altman S, editors. 2000. *America's Health Care Safety Net: Intact but Endangered*. Washington, DC: National Academies.

Los Angeles County Department of Health. 2010. Los Angeles Collaborative for Healthy Active Children home page. Available at: http://publichealth.lacounty.gov/nut/lacollab/ lacollab.htm. Accessed March 25, 2010.

Matsunaga M. 2008. Concentrated Poverty in Los Angeles. Los Angeles, CA: Economic Roundtable. Available at: http://www.economicrt.org/summaries/Cons_Pov.html. Accessed September 10, 2010.

McConville S, Ong P. 2003. The Trajectory of Poor Neighborhoods in Southern California, 1970–2000. Living Cities Census Series. Washington, DC: Brookings Institution, Center on Urban and Metropolitan Policy.

Mead H, Cartwright-Smith L, Jones K, et al. 2008. *Racial and Ethnic Disparities in U.S. Health Care: A Chartbook*. New York, NY: Commonwealth Fund.

Millard WB. 2007. Suburban sprawl: where does emergency medicine fit on the map? *Ann Emerg Med*. 49:71–74.

Orfield M, Luce T, Mazullo J, et al. 2006. Minority Suburbanization, Stable Integration, and Economic Opportunity in Fifteen Metropolitan Areas. Minneapolis, MN: Institute on Race and Poverty. Available at: http://www.irpumn.org/uls/resources/projects/ Minority_Suburbanization_full_report_032406.pdf. Accessed April 15, 2010.

Perlman JE. 2005. Chronic poor in Rio de Janeiro: what has changed in 30 years? In: Keiner M, Schmid WA, Koll-Schretzenmayr M, editors. *Managing Urban Futures: Sustainability and Urban Growth in Developing Countries*. Hampshire, England: Ashgate.

Press E. 2007. Suburbia: America's Unseen Poverty. *The Nation*. April 11. Available at: http://www.alternet.org/story/50211. Accessed April 13, 2010.

Reid E, Sciber R, Zegeer C. 2003.Urban sprawl as a risk factor in motor vehicle occupant and pedestrian fatalities. *Am J Public Health*. 93:1541–1545.

Rivera C. 2005. A Long Road to Prenatal Medical Care: Antelope Valley Infants Are at Risk From Lack of Readily Available Services. L.A. County Is Worried. *Los Angeles Times*. June 6.

Roberts S. 2007. In Shift, 40% of Immigrants Move Directly to Suburbs. *New York Times*. October 17. Available at: http://www.nytimes.com/2007/10/17/us/17census.html. Accessed September 17, 2008.

Rodwin VG, Gusmano MK. 2002. The World Cities Project: rationale, organization and design for comparison of megacity health systems. *J Urban Health*. 79:445–463.

Rosenblatt S. 2007. Minority Women in LA County Found to Have Higher Rates of Chronic Disease. *Los Angeles Times*. May 24. Available at: http://articles.latimes.com/2007/may/24/local/me-womenhealth24. Accessed September 4, 2010.

Strategic Economics. 2002. Older Suburbs in the Los Angeles Metropolitan Area: Decline, Revitalization, and Lessons for Other Communities. Berkeley, CA: Strategic Economics. Available at: http://www.lgc.org/freepub/docs/community_design/reports/older_suburbs_in_LA.pdf. Accessed April 10, 2010.

Sturm R, Cohen DA. 2004. Suburban sprawl and physical and mental health. *J Royal Inst Public Health*. 118:488–496.

Sundman H. 1993. Suburban Health Care of the Poor Falls Short of Need. *Chicago Reporter*. October. Available at: http://www.chicagoreporter.com/index.php/c/Cover_Stories/d/Suburban_Health_Care_of_the_Poor_Falls_Short_of_Need. Accessed April 15, 2010.

University of Pennsylvania School of Medicine. 2009. 1 in 4 Americans lacks timely access to optimal care during time-sensitive medical emergencies: Penn study points to need for regionalized emergency care system [press release]. Philadelphia, PA: University of Pennsylvania. March 17.

Vining DR Jr, Strauss A. 1977. A demonstration that the current deconcentration of population in the United States is a clean break with the past. *Environ Plan*. 9:751–758.

Wagner J. 2010. Controversy in Paris Makes Regionalism Newsworthy. Up Front Blog [blog]. Washington, DC: Brookings Institution. February 26. Available at: http://www.brookings.edu/opinions/2010/0226_paris_wagner.aspx. Accessed September 9, 2010.

Wilson R. 2003. Centering suburbia: how one developer's vision sharpened the focus of a community. *Am J Public Health*. 93:1416–1419.

12

Primary Care in Megacities of the Developing World

Omar A. Khan, MD, MHS, FAAFP, and Thomas C. Peterson, MD

MEGACITIES, BROADLY DEFINED AS urban centers of population greater than 10 million people, have emerged as a unique phenomenon in global health (United Nations Human Settlements Programme 2009). As health indicators in general seem to suffer in agglomerations of extremely large populations, so must responses be ramped up in scope, intensity, and coverage (Harpham and Stevens 1991). The preceding chapters in this book have dealt with the social determinants of health in megacities, health systems, emergency preparedness, environmental issues, and other concerns. This chapter addresses the provision of primary care: the health services that function to keep individuals and populations healthy, yet which meet with many challenges in the megacity environment.

Primary Care in Megacities

Primary care in developing countries presents a varied set of challenges. Examples from developed settings such as New York City, Singapore, Tokyo, and London suggest that the high population numbers represent an opportunity as well as an obstacle (MRC McLean Hazel and GlobeScan 2007). A high proportion of the population served may reside within a relatively small and defined geographic area; combined with centralized, "one-stop" services, effective and comprehensive primary care may be delivered as well, or better, than is accomplished in suburban or rural settings. However, this has several caveats as applied to the developing setting.

First, "primary care" as defined in the United States usually means comprehensive care from birth to old age and, in the case of family medicine, includes the subdisciplines of pediatrics, gynecology, and adult medicine, and in many settings will include obstetrics, hospital care, nursing home care, and minor surgery. This definition is by nature quite "medical" in the sense that it assumes someone with technical training in medicine is responsible for delivering it, or at the very least is involved directly in its coordination and delivery. The concept of primary care, however, as applied to many settings (especially developing ones) may well use other nonmedical agencies as the locus of health services. The coordinators may be administrators rather than doctors, and the delivery of care may largely be carried out by community health workers rather than physicians.

Second, there is enormous variability regarding the centralization (or lack thereof) in the developing setting. This is best illustrated by a series of examples from both developed and developing countries. In the United States, primary care is a minimally regulated enterprise in comparison with other developed settings. Those who are older than a certain age (usually 65 years) or below a certain income threshold may be recipients of Medicare and Medicaid public health insurance programs, respectively. For the purposes of this discussion, the exact numbers and inclusion criteria are unimportant; it is worth noting, however, that much of the population does not qualify for these two government-funded programs. In addition, even when they are serving recipients of Medicare or Medicaid, the systems of administration and disbursement may involve government or private entities (or some combination) and may vary from state to state. Furthermore, these two are simply insurance and financial systems that reimburse a physician or other provider of services; they are not inherently systems of quality control or evidence-based medicine (although this is changing). At present, there are no "Medicare clinics" or "Medicaid hospitals"; providers of medical care usually have varied patient panels and bill their patient population according to the type of insurance coverage they possess. There are certain federally qualified health centers which aim to serve the lowest-income members of a community, but again, they also have a varied client base and charge patients according to their insurance coverage.

In the United Kingdom, under the National Health Service, reimbursement of care is much more centralized. Although some individuals may possess private insurance or may pay for specialized services out of their pocket, all citizens receive comprehensive health care. The majority of medical providers (individuals, clinics, hospitals) operate as part of the National Health Service. In this system, primary care is a valued and essential part of the system of prevention, treatment, and referral. Typically, however, and in contrast to the U.S. system, general practitioners (there is no exact equivalent of the U.S. family physician) in the United Kingdom do not provide hospital care.

Megacities in developing countries can represent all points along the spectrum including those just mentioned (Freudenberg, Galea, and Vlahov 2006). If there can be such a thing as a "typical" health system in a megacity in a developing country, it can be illustrated by two such urban centers: Karachi, Pakistan, and Dhaka, Bangladesh. In these two cities, coverage for individuals of lower socioeconomic status (SES) is provided not by an insurance plan but by centers which are themselves operated by the government, usually under the Ministry of Health. These centers may include stand-alone clinics for primary care issues such as childhood vaccination and prenatal care; they also may include government-run medical schools and affiliated hospitals. The government facilities are usually low cost, but may not have rigorous quality oversight or clinical excellence characteristics which would make them desirable to those with the ability to pay. Some specific, donor-supported services (e.g., UNICEF for vaccinations, the Global Fund HIV/AIDS, tuberculosis, and malaria) may also be available free of charge or at minimal cost; these may be operated in concert with the government or by nonprofit nongovernment organizations (NGOs). In certain cases, such as those vaccinations deemed a priority by the multidonor Expanded Programme on Immunization, patients can access those vaccinations at participating private clinics for free as well. Meanwhile, there is a thriving industry of fee-for-service, private clinics, hospitals, labs, imaging facilities, and practitioners in all specialties.

Barriers to Primary Care

Much of primary care beyond the very basics, however, is situated in the most underserved areas. Although the governments do in theory provide a basic package of health services, in reality these are utilized only by those of low SES. Even then, there remain barriers to the poor accessing these services. Full coverage of these issues is provided by Reerink and Sauerborn (1996), Tabibzadeh and

Liisberg (1997), and Tabibzadeh, Rossi-Espagnet, and Maxwell (1989), but in brief, the barriers can include access at its most basic: the poor may not be mobile enough to reach a clinic outside of their immediate area; the clinic hours (e.g., 9:00 AM–5:00 PM) may not be adequate for those working during this time. More subtle barriers to seeking care have been described as well, notably a class or culture barrier. If community dwellers feel they are the subjects of health care rather than participants in it, their engagement of the health system is going to be lower as well. Seeing a nurse or physician from a different part of the town or city, who may speak a different dialect, can be another deterrent.

Even in situations where government-run health services may reach the poorest in culturally appropriate ways, other barriers may exist. One example is the legal status of the poorest in many megacities. By nature, megacities represent employment possibility, and attract legal and illegal immigrants. In a slum where a significant minority may be "undocumented" or illegal immigrants, if a government-run facility requires proof of citizenship such as a national ID card, that will further deter many in need of health care services. Government services, for their part, may be hamstrung by regulations promulgated to use taxpayer funds for the benefit of citizens alone.

The argument to use such funds for citizens only misses the point, however. First, the indirect taxation herein taxes the rich and benefits the poor already; citizen or not, the beneficiaries are inherently not those paying the highest taxes. Making a further delineation between legal resident or not is unnecessary. Second, community health does not subdivide itself on lines of national origin. Poor health care does not stop at a certain slum neighborhood, no more than cholera from a nonresident stops at the legal resident's house. Lack of funding for undocumented workers is a shortsighted strategy which may serve political purposes but no health-related ones.

It has been observed that anyone who can afford to do so will go to a private clinic. This observation is related to the general low demand (and supply) of primary care services in these private clinics (including health maintenance and screening for chronic diseases). The common factor is cost—not that it is expensive, but that it is too cheap and therefore not able to compete with expensive diagnostic tests and workups. In a setting of free enterprise medicine, the practitioners most in evidence in these megacities are not family physicians or general practitioners (whose bread-and-butter services include the aforementioned low-cost avenues of health maintenance and screening for chronic diseases), but cardiologists, dermatologists, and pulmonologists—specialists who generally charge higher fees for their services. The second factor is low desirability of general practice as a career (perhaps as a consequence of the first factor). Given the opportunity to enter a more lucrative specialty, medical trainees seem to shun primary care altogether. Along with the medical community's lack of interest in primary care, the public's confidence in the specialty has dropped commensurately.

As an example, if someone self-screens for high blood pressure, they may seek a cardiology consultation and may subsequently receive a stress test or echocardiogram. Someone with a cough may seek pulmonology consultation and receive a chest X-ray, antibiotics, blood work, and spirometry—perhaps even a computed tomography scan. As such, care tends to be episodic rather than continuous, and the concept of having a family doctor has eroded severely in the megaurban settings illustrated here.

The state of affairs is quite different in rural settings, where incomes are not high enough to support the specialty model just described. However, the primary care assignments of the rural areas tend to be regulated by government; as a consequence there are low salaries and general dissatisfaction by physicians, and the sense that specialty care in urban settings would be a more desirable medical career. This is compounded by a "brain drain" drawing skilled workers out of their country of origin to industrialized countries; this phenomenon has been described extensively in the nursing literature and clearly affects physicians as well.

Aligning Community Resources With Community Health Objectives to Support Primary Care

Given the inevitable barriers to change within large (and smaller) populations— knowledge, habits and routines, power and politics, existing and new resource allocations, and belief systems—it seems reasonable to consider a model that focuses less on individual health as a primary goal, but rather takes advantage of community strengths to move toward community health improvement. Such an approach can be led by a small or large collective in the community and spread from there. Significantly, leadership must come from within the community— from an existing health resource, a faith-based organization, a political movement, an industry, or an educational system. External systems with an "idea" or "standard" are less likely to influence primary care health improvement.

A community health development system is easier to measure and build upon, rather than discrete individual improvements such as a hemoglobin A1C measurement or LDL cholesterol level. It builds upon the collective interest and strengths of a community, rather than superimposed metrics used in another area of the world. A community health metric might be the average community body mass index, or the percentage of children who become literate or finish the equivalent of the eighth grade, or the acreage of safe public areas. For primary care to move forward in megacities, it must incorporate a willing investment of community resources, change readiness, and patience.

Such an approach takes advantage of community goals, aspirations, and networking. For example, it makes less sense to approach sexually transmitted illnesses or average blood pressure if the primary (initial) health goal of a community is to improve nutrition or to reduce maternal and infant death during childbirth. Strictly speaking, community health can be improved in some cases without "a clinic"; it might result from better schools, roads, food handling, septic systems, or harvesting techniques—or it could be as straightforward as using vitamin supplementation or vaccination programs. Patience is vital; one health improvement success will cascade into the next, and the inventory of successes will grow and ultimately translate into improved individual health. Progress is more important than is the rate of improvement; a community is made up of individuals living and understanding their milieu—and in many cases aspiring for better health for their children.

The advantages of this approach include building on the strengths and motivation of others in the community, collective decision-making, family values, and community resources. Resources can broadly include schools, employment, food systems, government, belief systems, external factors, and natural resources. A community health approach allows use of more efficient "change effectors," such as community health workers, an eHealth strategy (Table 12.1), and group education.

The challenge is to start the process. The community needs to recognize itself and self-assess for what it values, and what the existing successes are. For an external party to effectively assist, they must endorse the concept of facilitating health improvement based on what the community wants. In the end, internal resources in a megacity are more important than are external resources—they need to be rallied, and then blended with external resources when appropriate.

Table 12.1 The "eHealth" Approach: A Solution for Coordinated Health Care in Megacities?

Information and communication technology (ICT) has brought huge changes in the way megacities function. ICTs such as the Internet and other telecommunication media have connected megacities in developing countries with the developed world, thus increasing global influence on the growth and productivity of these centers.

The use of ICTs to benefit the public's health (also known as "eHealth") gives megacities new hope and new tools for the future. Adopting eHealth has been recommended by the World Health Organization's 58th World Health Assembly eHealth Resolution (WHA58/28) urging member states to consider drawing up a long-term strategic plan for developing and implementing eHealth services in the various areas of the health sector.

The question arises: What can eHealth actually do for the health of inhabitants of a megacity in the developing world? The key principle of eHealth is to address health needs in an equitable, inclusive, participatory, and informed manner, using ICTs that are accessible (which necessarily includes issues of cost). Key features of this approach include (1) recognizing that each part of a megacity, with its unique set of problems (social, economic, health) may require a special approach to address these needs; (2) possessing up-to-date information on demographic characteristics, existing and future infrastructure, and the health issues to be addressed, in terms of what is known about the problems; (3) providing a networked response to current and future issues through effective coordination between health care providers and institutions and other institutions that could influence health; (4) cost reduction in the provision of health services, which could benefit the population as well as the health system; and (5) ensuring the diffusion of health services and benefits to the people living at the bottom of the socioeconomic pyramid through their involvement in decision-making. These features can be summarized as *responsible, pervasive, evidence-based, knowledge-driven, community-centered, networked, decentralized,* and *empowering the vulnerable.*

A typical megacity in a developing country may, for example, require a mix of the following eHealth solutions:
1. An emergency call center to respond to urgent health needs and to coordinate with other health and social sector institutions. This includes services such as counseling and guiding the attendants to handle situations.
2. eHealth-enabled emergency care services with full coordination between call centers, ambulances, police, emergency/trauma care centers, and other agencies involved in disaster response.
3. Telehealth services to link specific community-based health facilities with specialized care centers to provide consultation in the outpatient rather than inpatient setting, where applicable.
4. Providing community health workers with interactive mobile phones to connect with their supervisors, refer to protocols, discuss among peers, and send behavior change messages to the clients.
5. Geographic information system and remote sensing enabled surveillance, tracking and reporting systems for up-to-date health and demographic indicators as well as for real-time biosurveillance and disease monitoring.
6. Learning resource centers for health care providers and communities to enhance their knowledge in health and other areas related to determinants of health. This includes creating digital libraries for easy reference to peer-reviewed and grey literature.

To maximize the benefits of eHealth, it is suggested the system be designed at three levels:
1. A central coordinating site, responsible for networking with health and other agencies for a coordinated approach.
2. Local/district level units such as telehealth centers, learning resource centers, and training centers.
3. Community health workers, essentially a mobile and not geographically limited level of the system. They could be considered the mHealth (mobile Health) system for health promotion, surveillance, and program monitoring at the community level.

The eHealth approach can thus enhance the diffusion of benefits in the megacity communities most in need of health services, and can enable the convergence of resources and energy into a fully networked megacity.

Source: Courtesy of Shariq Khoja and Hammad Durrani, Aga Khan University, Karachi, Pakistan.

Increasing discussion in the United States about the delivery and financing of health care includes "radical" suggestions such as reframing the metrics of care (as described in the previous section). It also includes "supporting community" as having two meanings: the community being supportive of the health interventions it is part of, and the health interventions in turn supporting the community.

This seemingly new idea has been piloted and run for over 40 years in parts of the developing world. Thanks in large part to the work of Dr. Carl Taylor (deceased 2010) and his colleagues, a number of demonstration projects sprang up worldwide to test and assess the model of community-based primary health care (CBPHC). One of the most notable is the Jamkhed Project (http://www.jamkhed.org). At its simplest, the model starts out by assuming the metric of success is community health—not financial success, not patient visits, not even proxy indicators of well-being. It then proceeds to address the social determinants of health (SDH) and development, which include poverty, education, and social class, among others (Arole, Arole, and Taylor 1994).

Projects such as Jamkhed recognized these factors as intuitively important long before the concept of SDH was popularized and given new life by the work of Sir Michael Marmot (Marmot and Wilkinson 2006). The first tier of this model is essentially community development and empowerment. Although this includes strictly health aspects such as immunizations and other preventive care, it may also include economic empowerment programs. The second tier includes the health liaison function, which serves to link the community with centralized care provision and project monitoring. In many CBPHC projects, this tier may provide selected curative services and serve other acute care needs. The third tier provides tertiary care and referral services, which may involve hospitalization and specialized health needs.

In essence, this model allows even rural areas to be served by community health workers who are typically from that village. The concept of community health worker has been put to good use in many South Asian settings that have seen an overall improvement in health status, notably Thailand, China, the Philippines, Bangladesh, and parts of India and Latin America.

The linkage of health and development and the intertwining of primary care cannot be overemphasized. As SDH work has demonstrated, effective primary care exists not in a vacuum, apart from the lives of those its serves, but as part of their existential milieu. Far from being a "soft" concept, it has its roots grounded in theory and demonstrated in practice. Examples of models created to integrate various aspects of development (in this case, economic empowerment) include the Grameen Bank (founded by Nobel Prize winner Muhammad Yunus) and BRAC (founded by Sir Fazle Abed), both in Bangladesh. They have been extensively studied in recent years and their work is being replicated elsewhere as well (Yunus and Jolis 2001).

A 2009 report by Perry and Freeman reviewed the evidence for the CBPHC model in improving child health and family health as a whole. It was clear that CBPHC can effectively provide the primary care services which even in the United States (perhaps especially so in the United States) are fragmented. By treating the health of the family as part of the health of the community, antenatal services can be delivered to villages by community health workers; nutrition education and counseling can be done in what we in the United States now call "group visits" (which in the developing world are essentially community discussions); deliveries can be done safely by trained midwives or by referral to physicians at the health center; and postdelivery counseling on birth spacing and child nutrition is similarly done at the community level.

It is worth reiterating then, that megacities and developing countries contribute something to our understanding of the delivery of primary care—and may indeed help us understand health reform in the West. They can do so by focusing our attention on the metric of improved health rather than on the proximate measures in use in the West: patient revenue (poorly correlated with health) or disease markers (e.g., glycosylated hemoglobin for diabetes). The focus is on community-oriented end-points, not even simply patient-oriented ones, let alone the disease-oriented ones on which many Western health systems focus.

Community health, on the other hand, is fairly simple to measure; a variety of straightforward morbidity and mortality statistics (e.g., maternal and child health and SDH such as violence, substance abuse, employment, percent near ideal body weight) will tell the story better and more effectively than how many revenue units individual physicians generate.

Opportunities for Primary Care in Megacities

Although the health problems faced by inhabitants of megacities in developing countries are variable, certain general conclusions can be drawn. The epidemiologic transition—in which the burden of infectious disease is supplanted by that of chronic disease—is underway in at least bimodal fashion in megacities (World Health Organization 2008; Center for Health Development 2009). Within these cities, social stratification results in the same types of gaps in equity seen in developed countries. The difference is that the poorest remain susceptible to the types of "tropical" infectious diseases—cholera, typhoid, malaria—from which the rich are largely insulated. That is no surprise, considering these are diseases of development; these are also diseases of hygiene, of sanitation, and of the ability to buy a bed net.

Those of a higher SES, meanwhile, find themselves protected from unsafe drinking water, perhaps, but are increasingly victims of their lifestyle: sedentary, with a diet high in fats and carbohydrates. Having escaped malaria, one might now succumb to diabetes, coronary artery disease, or stroke—all the while, driving instead of walking—in which the diseases of underdevelopment trade off for those of overdevelopment.

Nevertheless, increasing SES does bring with it, in general, life expectancy increases and, in particular, reductions in child mortality. The work of many in CBPHC has shown, however, that even in low SES households better outcomes (equating to that of a much higher SES strata) can be achieved with specific interventions such as improved maternal education. Interestingly, that may also mean this lower SES group could be protected from the infectious disease burden while being insulated from the chronic disease burden of the rich.

Primary care has an array of roles to play in this setting, and indeed, where resources are scarce, those needs are required and met just as they are in, say, the United States. The demand then shifts toward "one-stop" care: a family doctor and comprehensive community clinic where concerns relating to pediatrics, maternity, and gynecology can be addressed under the same roof as episodic acute care and minor surgery (Boelen et al. 2002). It is not uncommon for such clinics, located in underserved parts of megacities, to do contraception counseling, IUD placement, vasectomies, and minor surgery along with the usual range of general practice.

An example is a clinic called Shushasthya (pronounced shu-SHAS-tho), in an underserved part of Dhaka, Bangladesh (see http://www.projectbangladeshonline.org). Dhaka is firmly established among the world's megacities in approximately the 13th position, with a balance of strengths and opportunities with regard to health care provision (United Nations Human Settlements Programme 2009a). Shushasthya (which means "good health" in Bangla) was started in the 1980s by a group of alumni from a Dhaka high school. The aim was to provide health care where none existed. Over the past 20 years, the lessons of development were heeded to ensure the clinic was made sustainable without donations from the parent NGO, Project Bangladesh. Two family physicians provide the necessary care, and a variety of issues such as those mentioned earlier are addressed.

However, the services of the clinic would likely not be accessed in wealthier parts of the city. It is likely to be even more fragmented than in the United States—many wealthy Bangladeshis do not have a family doctor, preferring instead to seek episodic and system-specific care from specialists without a coordinating and advising force at the center. In this private-pay system, no referrals are needed. In that sense, then, the promise of CBPHC and of comprehensive medical care has the most to offer those willing to accept it—those who, by circumstance, are poorer and those who in the growing middle class choose a more efficient model. These models may include traditional ones, such as face-to-face medical encounters in a clinic, or newer models of distributed care, accessed via recent advances in information technology (see Table 12.1).

The growth, in our view, may well come from that middle: those who are educated and reasonably well-off, careful of their resources, conscious of the need for health care and, except when compelled to, preferring not to pay for a myriad of specialists for their general care. The middle class in some developing countries is growing, which is generally a good sign for the long-term outlook of primary health care and the community's health in general. They essentially face a choice when accessing services: "upgrade" to the mode of the wealthy or "downgrade" to the services accessed by the poor. Here, then, may lie an interesting opportunity for CBPHC: to serve the growing middle class.

Although CBPHC is an egalitarian concept, it must be understood that clinics intended to serve the lowest SES will carry a stigma for those occupying a higher socioeconomic stratum. Targeting that higher SES, primarily by providing primary care services in a middle-class neighborhood, should prove effective. There are signs that this has begun in some settings, and should be encouraged by government and opinion-leaders as a cost-effective, high-quality means of health care access.

Summary

The cost-effectiveness of primary prevention of health problems is well established, and certainly is applicable within megacities. As argued earlier, primary care ultimately benefits community health—thus, primary prevention efforts (ultimately a finite resource) should be directed toward the values of the megacity community. An understandable approach would emphasize primary prevention efforts that can be directly and contemporaneously linked to an improvement in the quality of community life. Prevention focus in the developing world might differ—based on community ideals—from that in more developed settings; for example, vaccination education might be more important than keeping one's serum LDL cholesterol under 130.

With this approach, key opportunities that might be applicable in a megacity include: basic nutrition strategy; individual and public hygiene information and demonstrations; prevention of infection—wounds, infectious disease, and tropical diseases; injury reduction information and standards; reproductive health knowledge and modeling; school education directed toward tangible employment; and providing mental health education that focuses on behavioral self-care strategies and effective and mindful relationships. These are examples of what the entire network of primary care—physicians and extensions of physicians such as community health workers, school systems, belief organizations, policymakers, and employers—might accomplish.

References

Arole M, Arole R, Taylor C. 1994. *Jamkhed: A Comprehensive Rural Health Project.* London, England: Macmillan.

Boelen C, Haq C, Hunt V, et al. 2002. *Improving Health Systems: The Contribution of Family Medicine.* Singapore: World Organization of Family Doctors and World Health Organization.

Center for Health Development. 2009. *Megacities and Urban Health.* Kobe, Japan: World Health Organization.

Freudenberg N, Galea S, Vlahov D, editors. 2006. *Cities and the Health of the Public.* Nashville, TN: Vanderbilt University.

Harpham T, Stephens C. 1991. Urbanization and health in developing countries. *World Health Stat Q.* 44:62–69.

Marmot M, Wilkinson RG. 2006. *Social Determinants of Health.* London, England: Oxford University.

MRC McLean Hazel and GlobeScan. 2007. *Megacity Challenges: A Stakeholder Perspective.* Munich, Germany: Siemens AG.

Perry H, Freeman P. 2009. *How Effective Is Community-Based Primary Health Care in Improving the Health of Children? A Review of the Evidence.* Washington, DC: Community-Based Primary Health Care Working Group, American Public Health Association.

Project Bangladesh. [n.d.] Home page. Available at: http://projectbangladeshonline.org. Accessed August 15, 2010.

Reerink I, Sauerborn R. 1996. Quality of primary health care in developing countries: recent experiences and future directions. *Int J Qual Health Care.* 8:131–139.

Tabibzadeh I, Liisberg E. 1997. Response of health systems to urbanization in developing countries. *World Health Forum.* 18:287–293.

Tabibzadeh I, Rossi-Espagnet A, Maxwell R. 1989. *Spotlight on the Cities: Improving Urban Health in Developing Countries.* Geneva, Switzerland: World Health Organization.

United Nations Human Settlements Programme (UN-HABITAT). 2009. *Planning Sustainable Cities: Global Report on Human Settlements 2009.* Nairobi, Kenya: UN-HABITAT.

United Nations Human Settlements Programme (UN-HABITAT). 2009a. *State of the World's Cities 2008/2009.* 2009. Nairobi, Kenya: UN-HABITAT.

World Health Organization (WHO). 2008. *The World Health Report 2008: Primary Health Care: Now More Than Ever.* Geneva, Switzerland: WHO.

Yunus M, Jolis A. 2001. *Banker to the Poor: The Autobiography of Muhammad Yunus, Founder of Grameen Bank.* New York, NY: Oxford University.

13

Urban Health Challenges of Megacities: The Case of Mexico City

Carlos Castillo-Salgado, MD, JD, DrPH

DURING THE LAST TWO decades, inequalities in several dimensions of social well-being have continued to increase at unprecedented rates, particularly in megacities, according to reports from national and international agencies (United Nations [UN] Development Programme 1991; World Health Organization [WHO] 1993; Pan American Health Organization [PAHO] 2008; Commission on Social Determinants of Health 2008). The widening gap between the affluent and the deprived is one of the most serious social problems facing modern urban societies, and no public policies have yet managed to adequately address it.

As of 2010, Mexico City, Mexico, is considered one of the largest megacities in the world. The complexity of this megacity is reflected in all areas of human development, from employment opportunities to public health policies, systems, programs, and services. This chapter describes the challenge of establishing more equitable public and health policies and providing health programs and medical health services to the 22 million residents of Mexico City. Achievement of equitable public health interventions will require a new vision of urban human development coupled with renovated equity-focused frameworks and new tools to better address growing unmet urban health needs.

Selected urban health problems in Mexico City provide an opportunity for a case study yielding key lessons learned about delivering public health and health care programs in light of the unique situation of this megacity. These lessons may help other megacities better deal with their own urban health challenges by avoiding predictable mistakes and promoting effective health policies and interventions for important segments of their populations. To this end, I provide a description of the health system organization of Mexico City, illustrating the complex nature of delivering health care through different independent public health service institutions with different standards, policies, and administrations. I then discuss some of the most important urban health policies implemented in Mexico City, especially those directed to the underserved population. Finally, I outline key global urban health initiatives that emphasize the importance of new health information systems, new urban health metrics, and health indicators for the monitoring of local and neighborhood health inequalities and the quality of life in megacities.

Urbanization in the Americas and Mexico City

Many estimates indicate that by 2030, more than 80% of the global population will be living in cities. The population of the Americas is highly urbanized, particularly in the more-developed countries; already, more than 80% of the people living in the Americas—82.6% in 2009 versus 41.0% in 1950—live in urban conglomerates. Some 160 million people live in the 20 largest cities, 55 million of them in the largest metropolitan areas of Mexico City, São Paulo, Brazil, and New York, NY; approximately half of the largest cities in the Americas are in Latin America. However, the current process of urbanization is occurring more rapidly in the less-industrialized countries. The difference in growth rate between urban and rural populations is highest in Brazil at 3.4%, followed by the Andes region at 2.3%, and the Latin Caribbean at 2.2%, indicating a faster urbanization process in these than in other American subregions (PAHO 2008).

For centuries, Mexico City has been recognized as a unique, very large metropolis. Tenochtitlan, as Mexico City was known in 1519 when the Spanish conquistadores arrived, was already considered among the largest cities in the world along with Paris and Constantinople. The population estimates for Tenochtitlan during this era range from 200,000 to 300,000 people. However, it is estimated that the valley of Mexico City and its surroundings was home for an additional 1 million people (Yahoo Encyclopedia 2010). In 1585, 50 years after the Spanish crown declared it the capital of the Viceroyalty of New Spain, it was officially designated it as "the city of Mexico." Over the centuries, this city has been and remains the nucleus of political and economic power in Mexico.

Mexico City is the eighth richest city of the world (Hawksworth, Hoehn, and Tiwari 2009) and the 25th largest economy in the world—ahead of Taiwan and other economically important countries—but it also has one of the most inequitable distributions of wealth and health. In addition, the transition from rural to urban life by thousands of individuals and families in Mexico City has created several new challenges for public health, including the manner of dealing with social determinants of health. Also, building and rebuilding healthier environments and healthier conditions for older and more diverse populations demands new working frameworks and a socioepidemiological approach to assessing urban health problems.

Rapid Urbanization and the Need for a Better Model of Urban Health

Urbanization, as a rapid expansion of urban conglomerates at both the national and global levels, is one of the most striking sociodemographic phenomena of recent decades. As a result of this demographic transformation, the traditional analytical model of public health based on rural dynamics became obsolete. In place of it, a new analytical model is needed to better incorporate the dynamics of the urban health process (Castillo-Salgado 2008). Under a new, equity-oriented model, we should be better able to understand the social and environmental factors that contribute to disease, disability, and health inequalities and the way that the health needs of populations are addressed. The complex dynamics and interactions between different population groups, health determinants, and the institutional response to public health in urban settings require a multisectoral integration of actions and institutional responses (Castillo-Salgado and Gibbons 2010).

In general terms, the mission of those working in urban health is to recognize better ways and innovate policies and practices to improve the health status and conditions of all population groups within urban conglomerates, but with special consideration to underserved communities. Addressing the health needs of urban populations requires a more-comprehensive agenda than the one offered by the conventional provision of health care services for the entire population. It requires the recognition of the unequal distributions of the social determinants of health, which have an impact on the levels of social and epidemiological vulnerability of large segments of the population. Finally, addressing the health needs of urban populations demands new methods of collecting data that account for differences in living conditions, as much of the information currently available is useless for formulating effective, equitable health policies and interventions at the local level.

Mexico City and Its Metropolitan Area

Currently, Mexico City and its metropolitan area form the third largest metropolitan area in the world (UN Population Division 2009), with an estimated population exceeding 21.2 million people (Consejo Nacional de Población 2009); together they are the largest metropolitan area in the Americas (Table 13.1). With a land area of 573 square miles (1485 square kilometers), Mexico City is also one of the most densely populated cities in Mexico.

Mexico City and its metropolitan area include 16 different geopolitical entities called *delegaciones* (boroughs), as well as 36 counties of the surrounding state of Mexico. Table 13.2 lists population size and trends for the 16 *delegaciones* from 2000 to 2010. The urban infrastructure of this megacity includes approximately 30,000 industrial companies, 300,000 businesses and commercial enterprises, and 4 million motor vehicles circulating every day. This impressive infrastructure

Table 13.1   Ranking of the Ten Largest Urban Conglomerates in the Americas, by Population: 2010

Rank	Metropolitan Area	Population
1	Mexico City, Mexico	22,800,000
2	New York, New York	22,200,000
3	São Paulo, Brazil	20,800,000
4	Los Angeles, California	17,900,000
5	Buenos Aires, Argentina	14,800,000
6	Rio de Janeiro, Brazil	12,500,000
7	Chicago, Illinois	9,850,000
8	Lima, Peru	9,200,000
9	Bogotá, Colombia	8,850,000
10	Washington, DC	8,500,000

Source: Adapted from Brinkhoff 2010.

Table 13.2 Population Trends of 16 *Delegaciones* of the Federal District of Mexico: 2000–2010

Delegación	2000	2001	2002	2003	2004	2005	2006	2007	2008	2009	2010
Azcapotzalco	443,535	441,607	439,574	437,256	434,595	431,927	428,320	424,998	421,700	418,413	415,123
Coyoacán	645,385	644,176	642,868	641,176	638,994	636,650	633,200	630,004	626,835	623,672	620,493
Cuajimalpa de Morelos	153,552	157,546	161,549	165,536	169,525	173,630	177,696	181,897	186,087	190,259	194,405
Gustavo A. Madero	1,246,760	1,242,819	1,237,395	1,230,260	1,221,541	1,211,202	1,200,693	1,189,747	1,178,903	1,168,120	1,157,362
Iztacalco	413,953	412,388	410,261	407,550	404,353	400,907	397,148	393,516	389,938	386,399	382,887
Iztapalapa	1,800,177	1,813,788	1,823,619	1,830,238	1,834,751	1,838,005	1,842,819	1,847,666	1,852,251	1,856,515	1,860,402
Magdalena Contreras	224,402	226,423	228,055	229,330	230,349	231,122	232,153	233,102	234,026	234,916	235,765
Milpa Alta	99,578	103,009	106,183	109,223	112,283	115,739	119,110	122,887	126,691	130,518	134,361
Álvaro Obregón	696,056	700,571	704,733	708,290	711,189	713,103	715,307	716,992	718,602	720,112	721,500
Tláhuac	310,024	318,512	325,651	331,935	337,957	344,528	351,652	359,431	367,127	374,728	382,218
Tlalpan	589,709	595,873	601,038	605,218	608,596	610,642	614,092	616,716	619,250	621,674	623,970
Xochimilco	376,491	383,586	389,622	394,884	399,777	404,698	410,234	416,012	421,733	427,383	432,946
Benito Juárez	361,218	361,374	361,845	362,363	362,758	363,251	362,775	362,530	362,264	361,966	361,624
Cuauhtémoc	517,664	518,474	520,674	523,474	526,218	528,518	529,433	530,035	530,565	531,004	531,338
Miguel Hidalgo	353,156	353,720	354,862	356,169	357,317	358,041	358,182	358,063	357,918	357,733	357,499
Venustiano Carranza	465,380	462,933	460,784	458,570	456,053	453,356	449,535	445,827	442,155	438,504	434,859
Total	8,697,040	8,736,799	8,768,713	8,791,472	8,806,256	8,815,319	8,822,349	8,829,423	8,836,045	8,841,916	8,846,752

Sources: Consejo Estatal de Población 2010; Consejo Nacional de Población 2009; Instituto Nacional de Estadística y Geografía 2011.

generated US$390 billion in 2005, representing a third of the Mexican gross domestic product (GDP; Luna-Sanchez et al. 2006).

Despite the impressive contribution to GDP, we can see in Table 13.3 a measure of the degree of social inequality in Mexico City by comparing the extent of high and very high levels of household poverty among the 16 different *delegaciones,* using information from the 2000 census. Overall, 38.2% of households in Mexico City are defined as poor. Of those, 23.9% (521,304) suffer high levels of poverty and 14.3% (311,119) suffer very high levels of poverty (Secretaria de Salud del Distrito Federal 2009a). However, social inequality between and among *delegaciones* is extreme: there are zero poor households in the Benito Juárez *delegación*, which stands in stark contrast with Milpa Alta, in which 78.1% of households suffer a very high level of poverty. With the exception of the Benito Juárez *delegación*, the rest of the *delegaciones* show unacceptable levels of poverty. This high degree of social inequality is demonstrated by the presence of some of the richest individuals in the world. Addressing the social and health inequality of

Table 13.3   Numbers and Percentages of Households in High and Very High Poverty, by *Delegación*: Mexico City, 2000

Delegación	No. High Poverty Households (%)	No. Very High Poverty Households (%)	Total Households
Azcapotzalco	19,612 (17.3)	4,793 (4.2)	113,057
Coyoacán	36,028 (21.4)	13,589 (8.1)	168,486
Cuajimalpa de Morelos	7,503 (21.7)	8,307 (24.1)	34,540
Gustavo A. Madero	80,795 (26.4)	35,840 (11.7)	305,575
Iztacalco	31,635 (30.7)	10 (0.0)	102,998
Iztapalapa	121,999 (28.9)	116,300 (27.5)	422,495
Magdalena Contreras	16,918 (31.3)	16,775 (31.1)	53,977
Milpa Alta	3,464 (15.7)	17,242 (78.1)	22,079
Álvaro Obregón	61,490 (36.0)	18,180 (10.6)	170,917
Tláhuac	32,393 (45.0)	16,206 (22.5)	71,968
Tlalpan	37,843 (26.2)	34,335 (23.7)	144,587
Xochimilco	24,896 (29.0)	26,680 (31.0)	85,971
Benito Juárez	0 (0.0)	0 (0.0)	115,864
Cuauhtémoc	10,400 (6.9)	2,862 (1.9)	151,036
Miguel Hidalgo	12,703 (13.2)	0 (0.0)	96,496
Venustiano Carranza	23,625 (19.7)	0 (0.0)	120,197
Total	521,304 (23.9)	311,119 (14.3)	2,180,243

Source: Secretaria de Salud del Distrito Federal 2010.

Note. High and very high poverty were measured according to the Censo General de Población y Vivienda 2000.

megacities such as Mexico City requires disaggregation of data to recognize the level and intensity of the health differences among the different groups residing in this unique urban conglomerate.

The population size and density, level of poverty, and health care infrastructure of Mexico City show an enormous variation and heterogeneity. For instance, Iztapalapa, with almost 2 million people, is considered the largest and perhaps most complex urban conglomerate of the city; 81.4% of the residents of Iztapalapa are placed in the categories "very high marginality," "high marginality," and "medium marginality" by official statistics. It is identified as having one of the highest levels of violent crime and drug dealing. Also, it is the location of the "Central de Abastos" (Central Wholesale Market). As shown by the information summarized in Table 13.4, this market is one of the largest in the world, covering 752 acres (304 hectares), selling 30% of all the vegetable and fruit production of the country, 30,000 tons of food and produce, and boasting 52,000 motor vehicles daily and 300,000 daily buyers and visitors (Central de Abastos de la Ciudad de México 2010).

The majority of *tianguis* (open air markets or bazaars) are located in the *delegación* of Iztapalapa, where they make up about one third of all markets. This *delegación* contains 304 *tianguis*. In addition, it hosts *El Salado*, one of the largest markets of stolen goods in Mexico. Müller, in describing the "metropolization of crime" in Mexico City, stated that "in 2006, a report from the local Ministry for Social Development (Secretaría de Desarrollo Social del Distrito Federal) identified 63 territorial units, located in 43 neighborhoods, as the principal generators and victims of crime in Mexico City. Nineteen of these territorial units were identified in Iztapalapa, placing it at the top of this list" (Müller 2009, p. 4).

Table 13.4   Basic Indicators of the Central Wholesale Market, Mexico City

Total area	304 hectares (752 acres)
Population served	20 million people
Commercialization	30% of the national production of vegetables and fruits
Operated volume	30,000 tons of food and basic products
Daily traffic volume	52,000 motor vehicles
Visitors	300,000 daily

Source: Central de Abastos de la Ciudad de México 2010.

Most police and news reporters avoid the several "hot" areas of this important but crime-ridden district. The importance of the *delegación* of Iztapalapa was recognized by a major university located in this district, which decided to involve the academic community in addressing some of the most serious health problems. The Autonomous Metropolitan University (UAM–Iztapalapa) is developing a new Urban Health Observatory to collaborate with the local government and different groups of the civil society and monitor the health conditions of the population of this *delegación,* with the assistance of local community leaders and graduate students, with families living in this urban area for several generations (http://www.observatorioensalud.blogspot.com/2010/05/aviso-1.html).

The enormous concentration of resources in Mexico City and the city's strategic role as the seat of federal government and the epicenter of Mexican political forces have not resulted in more equitable distribution of health care services and public health programs. However, in 1997, the government of the city was, for the first time, elected by a direct vote of its citizens, resulting in a new model of governance; previously, city authorities were appointed by the president of Mexico. This resulted in sweeping changes and the polarization of the issue of addressing Mexico City's social and health needs, because the new local governments were elected from political parties opposed to those controlling the federal government. As a result of this new system, several innovative health programs have been implemented with strong community participation in disadvantaged neighborhoods.

Health System Organization in Mexico City

An important task for urban health is to recognize how different key determinants of population health present and interact with specific population groups, particularly highly disadvantaged groups such as those living below the poverty level and in subsistence conditions. Among those determinants are the provision and accessibility of health services, the organization of the health system, and the response of the health system to address the unmet needs of different population groups.

Accessibility of Health Services

Natural disasters provide an excellent example of one such key determinant of public health accessibility. In 1985, Mexico City was severely affected by a major earthquake that left thousands of victims and destroyed most of its infrastructure, including the majority of the larger hospitals and medical centers. More than US$800 million was required for reconstruction of the destroyed health infrastructure (Valdez-Olmedo and Martínez-Narváez 1985). In addition, over the past several years, there have been a series of floods, volcanic eruptions, and other natural disasters that have affected essential public services for and health conditions in this megacity's population.

Geographic and socioeconomic accessibility to health services are two other key determinant of the public's ability to access care. Given the extensive reach of Mexico City's subway system and its low cost (a ticket to any of the stations cost US$0.15 in 2010), there are no important problems of geographic accessibility to health services. However, offering health services according to health need introduces major inequalities in health accessibility. For the same health need, the most disadvantaged groups do not receive the same level of care as do those in the middle class or the more affluent groups. The great heterogeneity of health conditions among the millions of people in disadvantaged areas of the Mexico City metropolitan area has resulted over the years in important public health arrearages. The issue of eliminating or reducing long-standing health problems such as malnutrition and infant and maternal mortality is now coupled with new challenges as obesity, diabetes, injuries, violence, addictions, and noncommunicable chronic diseases. The provision of health care in Mexico City is further affected by the multiplicity, fragmentation, and inefficiencies of the different public health care providers.

Provision of Health Services

Mexico City has a complex and highly fragmented health system organization and infrastructure. In general, the provision of health services in Mexico City follows a pattern similar to that of most of the country. As a result of the several independent public institutions that constitute the Mexican national health system, many institutions provide health services. Health care in Mexico City is provided according to the employment status and payment capability of residents. The system includes several public institutions characterized as "social security institutions." Every person with formal employment is mandated by law to be affiliated with one of these public social security institutions. Table 13.5 presents a list of the main social security institutions providing health care services in Mexico

City. The Mexican Institute of Social Security is the largest institution, covering 80% of employed workers, followed by the Institute of Social Security and Services for Government Employees, Pemex (Petróleos Mexicanos, the national oil company), and the Secretariat of National Defense (SEDENA). The Ministry of Health and the Government of the Federal District cover the population not employed by the formal economy and those without social security.

Several primary health care models have been proposed and implemented in Mexico City with different results. However, most of the primary health care centers are only open Monday through Friday from 8:00 A.M. to 4:00 P.M., creating a major accessibility problem for those individuals without social security coverage.

The provision of services for medical emergencies is a special problem in Mexico City. A new delivery model for medical emergencies was created under a new government agreement, called *Comprehensive System for Medical Emergencies*. During Pope John Paul II's visit to Mexico City in 2002, coordination of all public health agencies for medical emergencies was implemented with great success. In 2003, following this successful endeavor, an interagency program for medical emergencies was formalized by all health care agencies. Under this system, all medical emergency services can be provided by the closest and

Table 13.5   Providers of Health Care Services and Social Security Institutions of Mexico City

	Mexican Institute of Social Security	Institute of Social Security and Services for the Government Employees	Ministry of Health and the Government of the Federal District	Pemex (Petróleos Mexicanos)	Secretariat of National Defense (SEDENA)
Legal nature	Mixed triple organization (government, employers, and workers)	Public institution with legal status and its own resources	Government of the Federal District	Public company independent of federal governance	Mexican Army/ Armed Forces
Sources of funding	Federal government, workers, and employers	Federal government and federal workers	Government of the Federal District budget	Company budget	Federal funds

most adequate hospital or health center, regardless of the health care coverage of the patient. Considering that accidents and violence are among the main causes of death for adolescents and male adults in Mexico City, this program offers great benefit for those individuals requiring emergency treatment.

An important health care problem for the "open" population (those not covered by social security institutions) of Mexico City is the limitation imposed by the current lists of authorized prescriptions and drugs that medical doctors are able to prescribe for the treatment of most health conditions and diagnoses. It is further complicated by serious problems with delivery, shortages, and limited availability of a restricted number of drugs and other necessary medical supplies.

Mexico City has a large indigenous population with minimal access to appropriate health and medical services. Some recent reports estimated that there are more than 500,000 indigenous people in the Federal District, but if estimates include the metropolitan area of Mexico City, that number is raised to several million (Asamblea de Migrantes Indígenas de la Ciudad de México 2010). The *delegaciones* with significant indigenous populations are Iztapalapa, Gustavo A. Madero, and Cuauhtémoc. A major barrier for these groups is the lack of

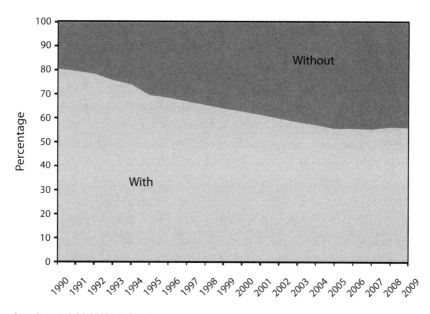

Source: Secretaria de Salud del Distrito Federal 2010.

FIGURE 13.1 Percentage of population with and without social security coverage: Mexico City, 1990–2009.

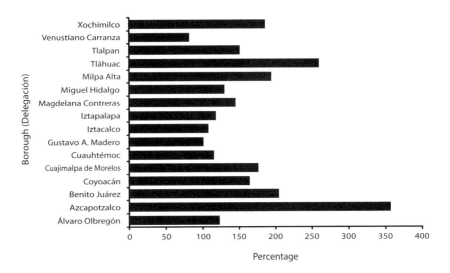

Source: Secretaria de Salud del Distrito Federal 2010.

FIGURE 13.2 Percentage reductions of population with social security coverage, by borough (delegación): Mexico City, 1990–2009.

understanding regarding their rights, in addition to their inability to demand the social and health services to which they are entitled.

Health Protection

A disturbing trend in health protection is emerging in Mexico City as coverage of health services from social security institutions decreases as a result of decreasing employment and subemployment rates. Figure 13.1 presents the trend of population coverage obtained from social security institutions from 1990 to 2009. As shown, the gap in access to health care is widening at a great pace. In 1990, 80% of the population was covered, in contrast to only 69% in 2009. Now, almost 4 million people in Mexico City receive no health protection from any of the social security institutions (Secretaria de Salud del Distrito Federal 2009b). The reduction of population health care protection is more dramatic in Azcapotzalco and Tláhuac *delegaciones*, as illustrated in Figure 13.2. However, all of the *delegaciones* but one have seen increases of 100% or more in the population without health care protection.

An important recent health care initiative linked to Mexican health system reform is the Popular Health Insurance Program (Seguro Popular), which was

Table 13.6   Distribution of Beneficiaries of the Monthly Food Subsidy for Adults Aged Older Than 70 Years: Mexico City, 2006

Rank	*Delegación*	No. Pensioners
9	Álvaro Obregón	27,952
1	Azcapotzalco	24,478
13	Benito Juárez	25,452
2	Coyoacán	33,347
3	Cuadjimalpa de Morelos	4,146
14	Cuauhtémoc	30,908
4	Gustavo A. Madero	64,391
5	Iztacalco	22,342
6	Iztapalapa	57,997
7	Magdalena Contreras	8,836
15	Miguel Hidalgo	18,321
8	Milpa Alta	3,636
10	Tláhuac	8,747
11	Tlalpan	20,953
16	Venustiano Carranza	26,279
12	Xochimilco	13,215
Total		391,000

Source: Consejo de Población del Distrito Federal 2007.

introduced in 2003. The objective of this initiative was to transform the existing health care system and convert it into a public health insurance system. This chapter does not discuss this national health initiative in further detail; Lakin (2010) presents a recent review of the political process and institutional difficulties that Seguro Popular has encountered.

Public Health Policies in Mexico City

As previously stated, several *delegaciones* of Mexico City have a high degree of marginality, with a resulting negative health impact in malnutrition, preventable diseases, drug addictions, and violence. In response to these problems, city authorities, with the participation of various neighborhood and civil society groups, are implementing new, far-reaching health policies and programs. In spite of several major health challenges, Mexico City has been promoting several important policies and initiatives that are globally considered leading examples of health promotion and protection.

A previous city administration created several important health programs directed to assist underserved populations and priority groups. For example, the Food Support and Medical Care Program for the Elderly was formally created in 2007 and is one of the most well-recognized and successful programs for senior citizens. It provides a monthly food subsidy to all residents older than 70 years (Sistema de Información del Desarrollo Social 2007). Table 13.6 shows the number of persons in Mexico City receiving this monthly food pension in October 2006, by *delegación*. In addition, a program providing free medical services and medications for every person older than 70 years was initiated in July 2001, but it was not instituted until May 2006, when the city legislature required its implementation (Asamblea Legislativa del Distrito Federal 2003). By 2009, 430,000 senior citizens were receiving this monthly support, which represented 3.5% of the total budget of the Mexico City government (Terra México 2009).

The 2009 estimated prevalence of smoking among male adults in Mexico City was still very high (59.9% of men 20 to 29 years of age; 46.9% of men 50 to 59 years of age; Menezes et al. 2009). Tobacco cessation policies and regulations have been and continue to be implemented through a network of community health groups and programs to reduce the burden of smoking prevalence. In 2000, the General Health Law and its Federal Regulations, following a 1997 City Ordinance, prohibited smoking in Mexico City's public buildings. Health policies were enacted to promote smoke-free public spaces free from tobacco smoke following the ratification of the WHO Global Framework Convention on Tobacco Control.

Another environmental health policy of great health impact in Mexico City is the mandated monitoring of daily levels of air quality and environmental contamination. City authorities have developed a useful index for monitoring and Web-based reporting of air quality, known as the "IMECA Index" (Air Quality Metropolitan Index). Based on data from the Ambient Air Quality Monitoring System, this index is calculated hourly for five regions around Mexico City from a combination of the local average concentrations of five environmental pollutants: ozone, particulate matter smaller than 10 micrometers (PM_{10}), nitrogen dioxide, sulfur dioxide, and carbon monoxide. Using an open-ended scale in which 100 represents the maximum allowable concentration for each of the five pollutants, it provides a warning system for authorities and the population regarding air-quality-related health risk levels for the population. This advanced monitoring system provides health recommendations for each quality level as well as public measures and alerts (Sistema de Monitoreo Atmosférico 2010a). This environmental monitoring system provides information in "near-time" and it is available to the media and public (at http://www.sma.df.gob.mx/simat2/ingles.php).

An additional environmental policy in Mexico City with great impact on population health is the program *Hoy No Circula* (No Driving Day; Secretaría del Medio Ambiente 2010; Comisión Ambiental Metropolitana 2010a). This program is aimed at decreasing levels of air pollution and traffic congestion in the city by restricting the use of vehicles with specific ending numbers on their license plates during specific days of the week. The official site of IMECA (Secretaria del Medio Ambiente 2010) describes the links between the IMECA Index and the *Hoy No Circula* program. Starting July 1, 2010, the levels of IMECA needed to reach a critical index level and declare an environmental contingency were reduced from 165 (IMECA) in 2008 to 150 in 2011. Specific recommendations are implemented, depending on the contamination level, and one of the key recommendations is for the *Hoy No Circula* program to be extended to two days per week. Also, industrial activities need to be reduced, certain gas power plants shut down, and elementary school hours are modified. The 2009 Report on Air Quality in Mexico City states "From 1989 to 2009, all contaminants showed and maintained a reduction trend, ozone was reduced in 33%, carbon monoxide in 79% and nitrogen dioxide in 13%" (Sistema de Monitoreo Atmosférico 2010b, p. 11). This environmental urban environmental system is a good example of successful urban health policies for any megacity.

Mario Molina, a Nobel Prize laureate, provides a comprehensive review of the air quality in Mexico City, addressing the main forces driving pollutant emissions. This assessment included an analysis of the different factors interacting, such as population, urban and economic growth, the production and consumption of energy, and the sources of erosion and biogenic emissions. It also included a description of the Mexico IMECA Index, the Environmental Contingency Program, and the *Hoy No Circula* program (Molina 2002).

In addition to IMECA and the *Hoy No Circula* program, new traffic routes have been developed in the entire city to speed circulation and have a more rational pattern of transportation routes with coordination of traffic lights. On main city arteries such as Insurgentes, special lanes for public buses and light rail have been implemented to make public transportation more efficient and provide a fast means of transportation across the city. Major investments were recently made for building a new level of the *periferico*, a main highway crossing the city (Gobierno del Estado de México 2010). The first part of this second level was built in less than 2 years and has helped in decreasing traffic congestion.

To address the serious problem of sewage and stormwater runoff, in 1975 the city built a tunnel of 6.5 meters in diameter to serve as the city's "deep sewage system." This is one of the largest deep-water sewage system collectors in the world, consisting of 164 kilometers of tunnel. In 2006, an inspection found major structural problems in the floor of one of the main tunnels and in the shelling and armoring of the system, requiring new re-shelling and protective coverings (BASF 2009). The government completed this major overhaul and avoided a potential major environmental disaster because of the serious storms that the city has experienced recently.

The city authorities, in coordination with the authorities of the state of Mexico, developed a major reforestation plan for the entire metropolitan area of Mexico City. This plan has been identified as the Air Quality Program for the Decade 2000–2010 for the Metropolitan Zone of the Mexico Valley (Comisión Ambiental Metropolitana 2010b; UN Department of Economic and Social Affairs 2004; Soto 2000). This initiative called for the reforestation of the valley of Mexico City and included the planting of nine million new trees in surrounding rural areas during the first year and 14 million trees during the second year. Several community groups have been coordinating the reforestation efforts in the city, and have experienced high levels of volunteer participation from students and members of different communities and neighborhoods.

The unique public response to the 2009 influenza H1N1 pandemic is an example for the rest of the world in how the population of a megacity was able to effectively cooperate with national and local authorities in complying with harsh and demanding public health restrictions. For several weeks during the height of the epidemic, the city was quarantined and all public places, including markets, restaurants, schools, stadiums, movie theaters, offices, and other businesses were closed in an attempt to limit the spread of the virus. Never in the recent history of public health has there been such an impressive collaboration from the population. Bringing the public life of such a large metropolitan area to a halt had never been done before, and while it ultimately cost the city and country many billions of dollars, both the government and population were recognized by the WHO and thousands of public health organizations as global public health heroes.

Role of the Neighborhood Leaders and Communities in Mexico City's Urban Health

The population of Mexico City has been known for its resilience and high participation in community and neighborhood causes and activities. During the 1985 earthquake, thousands of individuals from the community assisted in coordinating traffic, providing food and shelter for the affected population, and volunteering in the recovery efforts. This unprecedented participation of the citizens led to the creation of various nongovernmental organizations interested in greater participation in city governance. In addition, the poor conditions of some Mexico City neighborhoods have stimulated the emergence of folk leaders, such as "Superbarrio" ("Super-Neighborhood"; Kline 1997). Superbarrio has been described as

> a flabby caped crusader in cherry red tights who traverses the streets of Mexico City, defending the lower class. A high school dropout with a humble upbringing, Superbarrio has become one of Mexico City's greatest folk heroes. For the past 10 years, he has stood as the champion of the working class, the poor and the homeless. . . . His role is primarily symbolic as the protector of low-income neighborhoods. But on behalf of squatters and labor unions, Superbarrio leads protest rallies, files petitions and challenges court decisions. (Oddee 2007, p. 1).

The role of Superbarrio in mobilizing the most disadvantaged individuals of Mexico City was recognized by Mexico City's neighborhood assembly (Asamblea de Barrios; Cruz and Sandoval 1997; Corbin 2006). La Asamblea de Barrios has been known as

> a grassroots organization concerned with the egalitarian acquisition and distribution of decent housing for the poor. In the late 1980s, working class women and *amas de casa* [housewives] constituted 70% of the organization. La Asamblea de Barrios was the result of the unification of the representatives of 40 neighborhood unions, which emerged to oppose the city's evictions against the marginal population in Mexico City. (Hemispheric Institute 1988, p.1)

Recently, the Asamblea de Barrios organized several important public health campaigns in Mexico City, including an HIV/AIDS prevention campaign for which it received a national award.

The cultural dimension of the population in megacities should not be neglected when dealing with urban health issues. As a result of the decline in employment rates and an increase in crime during recent years, there has been a dramatic increase in the devotion of thousands of young and poor citizens of Mexico City to Saint Judas Thaddeus, the saint of difficult and impossible causes. On the 28th day of every month and on October 28th in particular, thousands of people attend Catholic Church services to pray and request assistance from this saint.

Regional Urban Health Forum in Mexico City

As discussed previously, addressing the complex nature of urban health in megacities requires the mobilization and participation of multiple sectors, including government, civil and community organizations, academic and scientific groups, the private sector, and international agencies. In 2007, as part of the Forum for Public Health in the Americas, PAHO launched the first meeting of the Regional Urban Health Forum in Mexico City, with the objective of strategically positioning urban health in the public policy agenda of cities and megacities of the Americas. The three key urban health issues selected for this forum were developing urban health metrics, governance in urban settings, and the role of social and environmental determinants in urban health (PAHO 2008). During the forum, there was a consensus that urban health requires tackling the "causes of the causes," as social determinants have been defined by the Global Commission on Social Determinants of Health (Marmot 2007). The main theoretical framework of this forum incorporated the socioepidemiological approach with health equity focus, as recommended by the WHO's Global Commission on Social Determinants of Health.

Governance in urban health was defined as

the decision-making process, resource use, and the formulation of policies that impact the health of urban populations. It involves determination of the necessary actions to forge effective intersectoral partnerships that will combat the current fragmentation and lack of coordination, decision-making and program implementation. (PAHO 2008, p. 26)

An important challenge of governance in megacities such as Mexico City is how to maximize the inclusion of civil society in the formulation and implementation of the governmental public health agenda linked to human development and quality of life, particularly for the city's most vulnerable populations.

During the forum, special attention was given to the discussion of the importance of developing new urban health metrics, in particular those related to health inequalities, promotion of healthy conditions, and performance and accountability of public health programs with equity focus. A major discussion of some of these urban health metrics is presented elsewhere (Castillo-Salgado 2008; Castillo-Salgado and Loyola 2002; Centre for Health Development 2010).

Population health assessments in Mexico City may be sorted into two groups based on time dimension. The first group of assessments deals with health-related events requiring an immediate response. Examples of such events in Mexico City are the 2009 H1N1 influenza pandemic, the 1985 earthquake, and the 2009 floods. These situations required a very rapid accumulation of epidemiological information regarding the affected vulnerable population groups, and the political will to respond to these situations with specific interventions. In these instances, short-term political decisions and immediate interventions needed to be made. The responses to these situations were the result of different competing pressures and negotiations between the main stakeholders of Mexico City. Local and federal governments, private groups and corporations, civil society groups, and other organized groups such as neighborhood associations, workers unions, political parties, and religious groups actively participated depending on the situation. Currently, the new wave of drug-related kidnappings and violence has created a panic mode in several segments of the city's population. Confronting this current social crisis is a major challenge faced by government and population.

The second grouping of population health assessments according to time dimension is the recognition and monitoring of epidemiological and secular data for critical and high-priority health trends. A present example of such a trend is the intensification of the obesity epidemic and the resulting dramatic increase of diabetes mellitus, hypertension, and other related chronic diseases. Currently, in most *delegaciones* of Mexico City the leading cause of death is diabetes mellitus. In a relatively short time, the increase in obesity and diabetes mellitus rates has had a dramatic negative impact on life expectancies and the financial viability of the Mexican health care system.

In 2008, the Global Commission on Social Determinants of Health produced its "Closing the Gap in a Generation" report (Commission on Social Determinants of Health 2008) with recommendations in different knowledge areas, including a comprehensive working framework for urban health, which aims to reduce health inequalities through action on social determinants of health. As part of the work of the Knowledge Network on Urban Settings (Centre for Health Development 2008), the development of the Urban Health Equity

Assessment and Response Tool (Urban HEART; Centre for Health Development 2010) was proposed as a basic measuring instrument of health inequalities. This tool includes a cluster of indicators organized in four policy domains: (1) physical environment and infrastructure, (2) social and human development, (3) economics, and (4) governance and politics. It also includes a list of health outcomes such as life expectancy, infant mortality rate, under-five mortality, maternal mortality ratio, and specific disease morbidity and mortality rates.

Proposed Global City Indicators for Quality of Life/ Health Inequalities and the City Health Profiles Initiative

Developing and using new urban health metrics has become a necessity of the new public health movement. This movement combines the need of measuring local health inequalities with the promotion of healthy conditions for different population groups and spaces in megacities.

The subject of urban health as part of sustainable human development and environmental health has become an important strategic mission for national and international development agencies and civil society organizations. Agenda 21 from the United Nation's Earth Summit of 1992 included a chapter on protecting and promoting human health conditions that recognized the importance of addressing the unmet needs of urban health for achieving sustainable human development (UN Division of Sustainable Development 1993). The role of healthy environments in cities was the center of this important global agenda.

An important urban health agenda was adopted in 2000 under the United Nation's Millennium Development Goals declaration. The United Nations System gave the United Nations Human Settlements Programme (UN-HABITAT; UN 2000) the mission to monitor and gradually attain the Cities Without Slums Target, which is described as "By 2020, to have achieved a significant improvement in the lives of at least 100 million slum dwellers" (UN-HABITAT 2010, p. 8). The UN-HABITAT indicators agenda includes 20 key indicators, eight checklists, and 16 indicators measuring performance and trends. The 20 key indicators are grouped in five domains: shelter, social development and eradication of poverty, environmental management, economic development, and governance (UN-HABITAT 2004).

Another important urban health initiative is the Big Cities Health Inventory of the U.S. National Association of County and City Health Officials (Benbow 2007).

This health inventory is an important compendium of health status indicators produced for the 54 largest metropolitan areas of the United States. Considering the highly diverse urban groups of these metropolitan areas, the indicators are important metrics for understanding the root causes of their health disparities.

Recently, the World Bank and several global institutions have been promoting the use of selected city indicators to recognize the quality of life of the population and the city performance by different levels of government, academia, and civil society. The Global City Indicators Program was designed to help cities monitor quality of life and performance of the city over time (Daniels 2010). These city indicators have been tested in nine pilot cities: Toronto, Montreal, and Vancouver, Canada; São Paulo, Belo Horizonte, and Porto Alegre, Brazil; Bogotá and Cali, Colombia; and Seattle–King County, Washington; currently, there are dozens of cities worldwide implementing the Global City Indicators Program.

Another global urban initiative is the recommendation of preparing health profiles of cities by the WHO. The city health profile has been defined by WHO as "a public health report that brings together key pieces of information on health and its determinants in the city and interprets and analyzes the information. The main function of the profile is to stimulate action that will improve health" (WHO 1998, p. 3). For any megacity such as Mexico City, putting together the required information on health and its determinants is a foremost challenge considering the various spatial, political, economic, cultural, and microenvironmental conditions affecting different areas and population groups living in this complex urban conglomerate. Most health problems in Mexico City are linked to air pollution, inadequate sanitation and solid waste disposal services, substandard housing, insufficient and contaminated drinking water, overcrowding, industrial waste and increased motor vehicle traffic congestion, and the growing stress associated with poverty, unemployment, and violence. The established linkages of health and quality of life of urban populations with these overrepresented factors are demanding more intersectoral strategies and social engineering solutions to tackle urban health issues.

Summary

Urban health has been conceptualized as a branch of public health that studies demographic, social, economic, cultural, and environmental determinants and their effects on health and the quality of life of population groups in cities. Special attention is placed on how urban social relations interact with health promotion and health risk factors in population subgroups.

Urban health and health of megacities are critical knowledge areas of great importance for advancing the new public health of the twenty-first century. Socioepidemiological studies linking different disciplines and multilevel analytical methods are needed to recognize the dynamics of "how" and "why" different neighborhoods in urban conglomerates show different patterns of health outcomes and of quality of life despite being in close spatial proximity. The inner city, the borders, and peripheries of megacities show great heterogeneity in the way factors impacting health. However, the way that conventional statistics measure the health conditions of these diverse groups makes it difficult to recognize the extent and severity of the health gaps that exist in urban areas.

The urban pattern of uncoordinated growth, particularly in megacities, has limited society's ability to adequately meet the human needs of its populations, resulting in growing levels of poverty, poor housing, lack of accessibility to health services, and inadequate diets of large segments of its populations. This pattern of growth is linked with unhealthy effects of pollution and the increase of excessive and avoidable morbidity and mortality.

The ecological and social pressures of rapid urbanization in many megacities have created a major shift in the psychosocial and material pathways and consumption patterns of different populations. Globalization brought high levels of wealth to megacities, but at the same time social exclusion and health inequalities in large segments of the population. Health inequalities have emerged and increased at unprecedented levels during the last two decades. Most megacities are poorly equipped to assess how protective or health risk factors interact in different population groups to affect urban morbidity, disability, and mortality patterns. Improvements in urban health therefore will depend on coordinated action by all levels of government, civil society groups, public health and health care providers, the private sector, and academic and research institutions.

The development of new urban health metrics—the identification of appropriate indicators for analyzing urban health in the context of social inequalities and assessment of the performance of public health programs with a health equity focus—reflects the need for public health assessments that are able to recognize and address specifically the intraurban health gaps. The focus on equity in urban health has prompted steering efforts toward reducing health differences between specific urban areas and the populations that inhabit them. In studying health equity in all megacities one must recognize and address the growing inequalities in health conditions of disadvantaged population groups, and also provide incentives and opportunities for healthy conditions and healthy environments for all population groups.

Considering Mexico City's example, it is important to note that there is more than one way to address the how and why the urban context affects health. A first lesson is that health in megacities may benefit from incorporating a more explicit problem-solving approach for specific disadvantaged populations, while at the same time intensifying the promotion of healthy environments for all. Second, a clearer theoretical framework is needed to guide the recognition of the key social and environmental determinants of urban health. The socioepidemiological framework in particular has emerged as a solid conceptual guideline for the analyses of urban health.

One of the most urgent steps in the effort toward improving urban health is the development of new information systems and urban health metrics. These new assessments require adding more disaggregated local information to better understand the extension and severity of specific health problems in geographic areas and population groups. Current health information systems tend to collect information with large levels of aggregation, which is of limited assistance in identifying the real distribution and severity of key public health problems in urban subpopulations. Multilevel analyses are also needed to recognize the different levels in which the health determinants and risk factors operate in different population groups, from the individual, family, and neighborhood levels to the environmental, cultural, and social levels. Just as multilevel analyses are needed, the responses and interventions to specific urban health problems must include the different source levels: political, social, and environmental, collectively and individually. Intersectoral actions cannot be postponed. Any social, political, or economic sector that neglects to participate in the solutions of the urban health problems creates a new barrier that moves the development of humankind backward.

New dynamics in the urban governance configuration are needed to incorporate different stakeholders in the decision-making process about policies and programs affecting the health of the population in urban centers. Also, new forms of urban governance should provide opportunities for formal and informal agreements requiring greater accountability of governments, grass-roots groups, civil society, the academic and scientific community, and the private sector for promoting healthy environments and improving the quality of life in megacities.

References

Asamblea de Migrantes Indígenas de la Ciudad de México [Indigenous Migrants Assembly in Mexico City]. 2010. Home page. Available at: http://www.indigenasdf.org. mx. Accessed October 11, 2010.

Asamblea Legislativa del Distrito Federal, IV Legislatura [Legislative assembly of the Federal District, IV Legislature]. 2003. Ley que establece el derecho a la pensión alimentaria para los adultos mayores de sesenta y ocho años, residentes en el Distrito Federal [Law recognizing the right of residents of the Federal District of more than 68 years of age to receive a food subsidy]. Mexico City, Mexico: Centro de Documentación Archivo.

BASF. 2009. Drenaje Profundo de la Ciudad de México [Deep Sewage Collector of Mexico City]. Available at: http://www.basf-cc.com.mx/ES/NOTICIAS/Pages/ Drenajeprofundo.aspx. Accessed June 22, 2010.

Benbow N, editor. 2007. Big Cities Health Inventory: the Health of Urban USA. Washington, DC: U.S. National Association of County and City Health Officials. Available at: http://www.who.or.jp/urbanheart/US_Big_Cities_Healt_Inventory_2007. pdf. Accessed January 11, 2011.

Brinkhoff T. 2010. The principle agglomerations of the world. Available at: http://www. citypopulation.de/world/Agglomerations.html. Accessed June 20, 2010.

Castillo-Salgado C. 2008. Development of urban health metrics. In: Pan American Health Organization (PAHO). First Meeting of the Pan American Health Organization's Regional Urban Health Forum. Toward a Conceptual Framework of Urban Health and Agenda for Action in the Americas. November 27–29, 2007; Mexico City, Mexico. Washington, DC: PAHO:59. Available at: http://www.bvsde.ops-oms.org/bvsacd/cd68/ foroeng.pdf.

Castillo-Salgado C, Gibbons MC. 2010. Developing new urban health metrics to reduce the know-do gap in public health. In: Gibbons MC, Bali R, Wickramasinghe N, editors. *Perspectives of Knowledge Management in Urban Health, Healthcare Delivery in the Information Age.* Vol 1. New York, NY: Springer Science:171–186.

Castillo-Salgado C, Loyola E. 2002. Development of the healthy condition index using geographic information systems in health. *Epidemiol Bull.* 23:7–11.

Central de Abastos de la Ciudad de México [Central Wholesale Market of Mexico City]. 2010. Indicadores Básicos [Basic Indicators]. Mexico City, Mexico: Gobierno del Distrito Federal [Government of the Federal District]. Available at: http://www.ficeda. com.mx/indicadoresbasicos.php. Accessed July 20, 2010.

Centre for Health Development, World Health Organization (WHO). 2008. *Our Cities, Our Health, Our Future: Acting on Social Determinants for Health Equity in Urban Settings.* Report of the Knowledge Network on Urban Settings to the WHO Commission on Social Determinants of Health. Geneva, Switzerland: WHO.

Centre for Health Development, World Health Organization (WHO). 2010. Urban Health Equity Assessment and Response Tool (Urban HEART). Geneva, Switzerland: WHO. Available at: http://www.who.or.jp/urbanheart/index.html. Accessed July 22, 2010.

Comisión Ambiental Metropolitana, Secretaría del Medio Ambiente [Metropolitan Environmental Commission, Secretariat of Environment]. 2010a. Comisión Ambiental Metropolitana (CAM). Mexico City, Mexico: Gobierno del Distrito Federal. Available at: http://www.sma.df.gob.mx/sma/index.php?opcion=26&id=60. Accessed June 22, 2010.

Comisión Ambiental Metropolitana, Secretaría del Medio Ambiente. 2010b. Programa para Mejorar la Calidad del Aire de la Zona Metropolitana del Valle de México, 2002–2010 [Program for Improving the Air Quality of the Metropolitan Area of the Valley of México, 2002–2010]. Mexico City, Mexico: Gobierno del Distrito Federal. Available at: http://www.sma.df.gob.mx/sma/download/archivos/proaire_2002-2010. pdf. Accessed June 20, 2010.

Commission on Social Determinants of Health, World Health Organization (WHO). 2008. *Closing the Gap in a Generation: Health Equity Through Action on the Social Determinants of Health. Final Report of the Commission on Social Determinants of Health.* Geneva, Switzerland: WHO. Available at: http://whqlibdoc.who.int/publica tions/2008/9789241563703_eng.pdf. Accessed June 18, 2010.

Consejo de Población del Distrito Federal [Population Council of the Federal District], Secretaria de Gobierno [Secretariat of Government]. 2007. Día Nacional del Adulto Mayor (Agosto, 28 2007) [National Day of the Senior Citizen (August 28, 2007)]. Mexico City, Mexico: Ciudad de México. Available at: http://www.copo.df.gob.mx/ eventos/especiales/dia_nac_adultomayor.html. Accessed January 06, 2011.

Consejo Estatal de Población [National Population Council], Gobierno del Estado de México. 2010. Panorama Socio-demográfico del Estado de México [Sociodemographic Profile of the State of Mexico]. Available at: http://qacontent.edomex.gob.mx/coespo/indicadoressociodemograficos/index.htm. Accessed March 30, 2011.

Consejo Nacional de Población [National Population Council], Gobierno del Estado de México [Government of the State of Mexico]. 2009. Zona Metropolitana del Valle de México [Metropolitan Area of the Valley of Mexico] [brochure]. Available at: http://www.edomex.gob.mx/poblacion/docs/2009/PDF/ZMVM.pdf. Accessed July 30, 2010.

Corbin E. 2006. Habitar: la eficacia de la justicia a través de una intervención de la Asamblea de Barrios y Superbarrio. [Living: the efficacy of justice by an intervention of the Neighborhoods Assembly and Superbarrio]. *E-Misferica* 3.1. Available at: http://hemisphericinstitute.org/journal/3.1/eng/en31_pg_corbin.html. Accessed January 6, 2011.

Cruz L, Sandoval G. 1997. Urban Management in Mexico City? Habitat International Coalition. Available at: http://www.hic-net.org/document.php?pid=2652. Accessed July 20, 2010.

Daniels J. 2010. Global City Indicators home page. Toronto, Ontario: University of Toronto. Available at: http://www.cityindicators.org. Accessed January 11, 2011.

Gobierno del Estado de México. 2010. Viaducto Bicentenario [Bicentennial Beltway]. Home page. Available at: http://www.viaductobicentenario.gob.mx. Accessed June 22, 2010.

Hawksworth J, Hoehn T, Tiwari A. 2009. III—Which are the largest city economies in the world and how might this change by 2025? Annex B. Full City GDP rankings for 2008 and 2025. *Pricewaterhouse Coopers UK Economic Outlook*. Available at: https://www.ukmediacentre.pwc.com/imagelibrary/downloadMedia.ashx?MediaDetailsID=1562. Accessed January 06, 2011.

Instituto Nacional de Estadística y Geografía [National Institute of Statistics and Geography]. 2011. Información Estadística [Statistical Information]. Available at: http://www.inegi.org.mx/inegi/default.aspx?s=est&c=4337&e=00&i=. Accessed April 21, 2011.

Kline C. 1997. Defender of Justice Superbarrio Roams Mexico City. CNN Interactive: World News: Story Page. Available at: http://www.cnn.com/WORLD/9707/19/mexico.superhero. Accessed June 22, 2010.

Lakin JM. 2010. The end of insurance? Mexico's Seguro Popular, 2001–2007. *J Health Polit Policy Law*. 35:313–352.

Luna-Sánchez G, De la Fuente JC, Terán-Álvarez A, Negrete-Rodríguez OI. 2006. Perfil sobre Salud Urbana de la Ciudad de México [Urban Health Profile of Mexico City]. Working Document. Washington, DC: Pan American Health Organization/World Health Organization.

Marmot M. 2007. Achieving health equity: from root causes to fair outcomes. *Lancet.* 370:1153–1163.

Menezes AM, Lopez MV, Hallal PC, et al. and the PLATINO team. 2009. Prevalence of smoking and incidence of initiation in the Latin American adult population: the PLATINO study. *BMC Public Health.* 9:151. Available at: http://www.biomedcentral. com/1471-2458/9/151. Accessed June 20, 2010.

Molina L, editor. 2002. *Air Quality in the Mexico Megacity: An Integrated Assessment.* Alliance for Global Sustainability Book Series. Vol 2. Amsterdam, Netherlands: Springer.

Müller MM. 2009. (In)security and policing in a marginalized Mexico City neighborhood: perceptions, experiences and practice [draft]. Paper prepared for the interdisciplinary workshop on Crime, Insecurity, Fear in Mexico: Ethnographic and Policy Approaches, Columbia University, New York, NY, November 13–14, 2009. Available at: http://ilas.columbia.edu/images/uploads/workingpapers/Muller_Paper.pdf. Accessed February 17, 2011.

Oddee. 2007. 10 Real-Life Superheroes (Masks, Capes and All!) [blog]. Available at: http:// www.oddee.com/item_87762.aspx. Accessed June 22, 2010.

Pan American Health Organization (PAHO). 2007. Health in the Americas 2007, Population Characteristics and Trends. Washington, DC: PAHO.

Pan American Health Organization (PAHO). 2008. First Meeting of the Pan American Health Organization's Regional Urban Health Forum. Toward a Conceptual Framework of Urban Health and Agenda for Action in the Americas. November 27–29, 2007; Mexico City, Mexico. Washington, DC: PAHO. Available at: http://www. bvsde.ops-oms.org/bvsacd/cd68/foroeng.pdf. Accessed April 21, 2011.

Secretaría de Salud del Distrito Federal [Secretariat of Health of the Federal District]. 2009a. Agenda Estadística 2009 [Statistical Agenda 2009]. Cuadro 1.4. Grado de Marginación por Delegación y Número de Hogares, 2000 [Table 1.4. Level of social deprivation by borough and number of households, 2000]. Mexico City, Mexico: Gobierno del Distrito Federal. Available at: http://www.salud.df.gob.mx/ssdf/media/ Agenda_2009/index.html. Accessed July 30, 2010.

Secretaría de Salud del Distrito Federal. 2009b. Agenda Estadística 2009. Cuadro 1.10. Población total, sin seguridad social y usuaria por delegación, 2009 [Table 1.10. Total population without social security and user by borough, 2009]. Mexico City, Mexico: Gobierno del Distrito Federal. Available at: http://www.salud.df.gob.mx/ssdf. Accessed October 11, 2010.

Secretaría del Medio Ambiente [Secretariat of Environment]. 2010. Hoy No Circula [No Driving Day]. Mexico City, Mexico: Gobierno del Distrito Federal. Available at: http://www.sma.df.gob.mx/sma/index.php?opcion=83. Accessed June 20, 2010.

Sistema de Información del Desarrollo Social [Information System of Social Development]. 2007. Pensión Alimentaria para adultos mayores de 70 años, residentes del Distrito Federal [Food subsidy for adults more than 70 years of age, residents of the Federal District]. Mexico City, Mexico: Gobierno del Distrito Federal. Available at: http://www.sideso.df.gob.mx/index.php?id=82. Accessed June 20, 2010.

Sistema de Monitoreo Atmosférico, Secretaría del Medio Ambiente [Ambient Air Quality Monitoring System, Secretariat of Environment]. 2010a. Air Quality Metropolitan Index (IMECA). Mexico City, Mexico: Gobierno del Distrito Federal. Available at: http://www.sma.df.gob.mx/simat2/ingles.php?opcion=1. Accessed June 20, 2010.

Sistema de Monitoreo Atmosférico, Secretaría del Medio Ambiente. 2010b. Informe 2009. Calidad del Aire en la Ciudad de México [2009 Report. Air Quality in Mexico City]. Mexico City, Mexico: Gobierno del Distrito Federal. Available at: http://www.sma.df.gob.mx/simat2/informe2009. Accessed January 08, 2011.

Soto G. 2000. *Mexico City's 10 Year Plan for Improving Air Quality*. Arlington, VA: Pew Center on Global Climate Change. Available at: http://www.pewclimate.org/docUploads/soto_presentation.pdf. Accessed June 22, 2010.

Terra México. 2009. Aumenta GDF pensión alimentaria para adultos mayores [Government of Federal District increases the food subsidy for senior citizens]. Available at: http://www.terra.com.mx/noticias/articulo/782945/Aumenta+GDF+pension+alimentaria+para+adultos+mayores.htm. Accessed June 20, 2010.

United Nations (UN) Department of Economic and Social Affairs. 2004. Improving Air Quality—Mexico City, Mexico. In: Commission on Sustainable Development, Twelfth Session, April 14–30, 2004. Local Government Action on Water, Sanitation, and Human Settlements: Case Summaries. New York, NY: UN:10–12. Available at: http://www.un.org/esa/sustdev/csd/csd12/Background5.pdf. Accessed June 22, 2010.

United Nations (UN) Development Programme. 1991. *Cities, People and Poverty: Urban Development Cooperation for the 1990s.* New York, NY: UN.

United Nations (UN) Division of Sustainable Development. 1993. Earth Summit Agenda 21: The United Nations Programme of Action From Rio. New York, NY: UN. Available at: http://www.un.org/esa/dsd/agenda21. Accessed July 20, 2010.

United Nations Human Settlements Programme (UN-HABITAT). 2004. Urban Indicator Guidelines: Monitoring the Habitat Agenda and the Millennium Development Goals. Nairobi, Kenya: UN-HABITAT. Available at http://ww2.unhabitat.org/programmes/ guo/documents/urban_indicators_guidelines.pdf. Accessed September 1, 2010.

United Nations Human Settlements Programme (UN-HABITAT). 2010. Cities Without Slums—Sub-Regional Initiative. Nairobi, Kenya: UN-HABITAT. Available at: http:// www.unhabitat.org/content.asp?cid=4568&catid=310&typeid=13&subMenuId=0. Accessed July 20, 2010.

United Nations (UN) Population Division. 2009. World Urbanization Prospects: The 2009 Revision Population Database. New York, NY: UN. Available at: http://esa.un.org/ wup2009/wup/source/country.aspx. Accessed June 20, 2010.

United Nations (UN). 2000. United Nations Millennium Declaration. Resolution adopted by the General Assembly. New York, NY: UN. Available at: http://www.un.org/millen nium/declaration/ares552e.htm. Accessed July 20, 2010.

Valdez-Olmedo C, Martínez-Narváez G. 1985. El Terremoto de México en 1985: Efectos e Implicación en el Sector Salud [The Mexico City Earthquake of 1985: Effects and Implications for the Health Sector). 15 de Diciembre de 1985. Centro de Documentación y Archivo. Mexico City, Mexico: Secretaría de Salud del Distrito Federal. Available at: http://desastres.unanleon.edu.ni/pdf/2003/septiembre/Envio1/ pdf/spa/doc7499/doc7499-contenido.pdf. Accessed January 06, 2011.

World Health Organization (WHO). 1993. *The Urban Health Crisis: Strategies for Health for All in the Face of Rapid Urbanization.* Geneva, Switzerland: WHO.

World Health Organization (WHO). 1998. City Health Profiles: A Review of Progress. Copenhagen, Denmark: WHO Regional Office for Europe. Available at: http://www. euro.who.int/__data/assets/pdf_file/0010/101062/E59736.pdf. Accessed July 20, 2010.

Yahoo Encyclopedia. 2010. Tenochtitlán. Available at: http://education.yahoo.com/refer ence/encyclopedia/entry/Tenochti. Accessed June 18, 2010.

About the Authors

Omar A. Khan, MD, MHS, FAAFP

Dr. Khan has active interests in global health, medical education, and clinical practice (primary care). He received his BA and MA from the University of Pennsylvania, completed his MD and residency at the University of Vermont College of Medicine, and received his MHS in public health from the Johns Hopkins University School of Public Health. He is board-certified in family medicine.

Dr. Khan's experience includes serving as a faculty member at the Johns Hopkins School of Public Health and at the University of Vermont, where he directs the global health electives for family medicine. He is presently on the active staff of the Departments of Family Medicine at the University of Vermont, the Christiana Care Health System, and the Department of Pediatrics at A. I. duPont Hospital for Children. Dr. Khan holds faculty appointments with the Departments of Family Medicine at the University of Pennsylvania and the University of Vermont.

Dr. Khan is on the referee panels for the *American Journal of Public Health*, *British Medical Journal*, *JAMA*, *Lancet*, *AIDS*, *American Family Physician*, and several other journals. Additionally, he is on the editorial boards of several journals including *BMC Public Health*, *BMC International Health & Human Rights*, and the *International Journal of Health Geographics*. He has authored or coauthored 5 books in the area of global health, and has authored over 60 articles and book chapters.

He currently serves as cochair for the International Health Program at the American Public Health Association (APHA) Annual Conference and on the Science Board of APHA. He is president-elect of the state chapter of the American Academy of Family Physicians. He serves on the Board of Trustees and the Board of Directors of Christiana Care Health System, one of the largest health systems in the United States. He also serves on the directorial boards of several other organizations, including Medscape/WebMD, the Delaware Academy of Medicine, and Project Bangladesh. He is cofounder of the non-profit Writers Without Borders, a mentor with the International Association of National Public Health Institutes, and a speaker on the issues of medical education, global health, scientific writing, and mentorship.

In 2009, Dr. Khan was named as a "Top Doc" by *Philadelphia* magazine. He has received the Executive Director's Citation from APHA, the Alumnus of the Year Award and teaching awards from the University of Vermont, the AAFP/Pfizer Teaching Award, and the Leonard F. Tow Humanism in Medicine Award from the Arnold F. Gold Foundation.

Gregory Pappas, MD, PhD

Dr. Pappas currently serves as senior deputy director for HIV/AIDS in the Washington, DC, Department of Health. He has broad experience in U.S. domestic and global public health with a focus on health disparities, health systems, and policy. He served as chairman of the Department of Community Health Sciences at the Aga Khan University, including a community health program which provided clinical and development services in three slums of Karachi. As senior policy advisor to U.S. Surgeon General/Assistant Secretary Dr. David Satcher, Dr. Pappas assisted in planning and convening the National Coalition to Eliminate Racial and Ethnic Health Disparities.

Dr. Pappas has fought the global HIV/AIDS epidemic for decades, including being a principal author of the *PEPFAR Five-Year Plan: A Report to Congress*. As deputy director of Demographic and Health Surveys for ORC Macro, he brought important innovations to global health surveys, including adding HIV testing. Dr. Pappas directed the Office of International and Refugee Health for the Department of Health and Human Services, where he also served as a member of the Executive Board of UNICEF. For almost ten years Dr. Pappas was an analyst at the National Center for Health Statistics working on a wide variety of health issues and data systems. He serves on the faculty of the Johns Hopkins Bloomberg School of Public Health and Howard School of Medicine. Dr. Pappas received his MD and PhD (Anthropology) from Case Western Reserve in Cleveland, Ohio.

Dennis P. Andrulis, PhD, MPH

Dr Andrulis is a senior research scientist at the Texas Health Institute and associate professor at the University of Texas School of Public Health. He leads the development of national, state, and community-based research and policy analysis on vulnerable populations, urban and suburban health, and racial and ethnic disparities and cultural competence in health care. He is a cofounder of a nationally and internationally recognized, biennial conference series, Quality Health Care for Culturally Diverse Populations. He is also lead author of a book published of the American Hospital Association Press entitled *The Social and Health Landscape of Urban and Suburban America*. Dr. Andrulis frequently presents testimonies before the Institute of Medicine on the regionalization of urban and suburban health care. Among his more recent publications are "Integrating Literacy, Culture and Language to Improve Health Care Quality for Diverse Populations" in the *American Journal of Health Behavior*, "Preparing Racially and Ethnically Diverse Communities for Public Health Emergencies" in *Health Affairs*, and "The Changing Landscape of Hospital Capacity in Large Cities and Suburbs: Implications for the Safety Net in Metropolitan America" in the *Journal of Urban Health*. Dr. Andrulis has a PhD in educational psychology from the University of Texas–Austin and an MPH from the University of North Carolina–Chapel Hill.

Neil Blackshaw, BA (Hons), MA

Mr. Blackshaw began his career as a town planner in the north of England. He held a variety of senior roles in local government and was county director for a major environmental charity. He was appointed head of the London Healthy Urban Development Unit (HUDU) in 2005. Under Neil's leadership, HUDU gained a strong reputation for connecting the health and planning agendas in the context of unprecedented growth in London. The unit published a range of guidance and influenced and advised a wide range of bodies in and outside London. Its guidance was awarded the Royal Town Planning Institute's planning award in 2008. Neil has recently advised the World Health Organization. He is currently an independent consultant continuing to work on health and planning. Neil has a planning degree (BA Hons) from Manchester University and a master's in urban design from Newcastle University, together with management qualifications.

Carlos Castillo-Salgado, MD, JD, DrPH

Dr. Carlos Castillo-Salgado is currently a professor of epidemiology in the Department of Epidemiology, Bloomberg School of Public Health, with joint appointments in several schools of public health in Latin America, the United States, and Spain. He has been the director of the Health Situation and Trend Assessment Unit of the Pan American Health Organization and the special advisor for the Regional Forum for Public Health in the Americas. He was the team leader of the "Urban Health Metrics" Task Force of the First Meeting of the Pan American Health Organization Regional Urban Health Forum, launched in Mexico City in November 2007. His areas of expertise include epidemiological methods for planning and evaluation of health services, health impact assessment, global health surveillance, and developing new equity-focused health metrics.

Zafar Fatmi, MBBS, FCPS

Mr. Fatmi is an associate professor and head of the Division of Environmental Health Sciences in the Department of Community Health Sciences of Aga Khan University in Karachi, Pakistan. He directs research and academic activities pertaining to environmental health, including on health effects of ambient air pollution, indoor air pollution and coronary syndrome and immunity, arsenic and its health effects, and risk assessment in the environment. He also serves as director of the fellowship program in community medicine (public health) at Aga Khan University. Additionally, he teaches and supervises the work of MSc students of public health, epidemiology, and health policy. He has many peer-reviewed publications and has been listed as "Productive Scientist of Pakistan" by the Pakistani Ministry of Science and Technology. Dr. Fatmi is a medical graduate and completed his fellowship (FCPS) in Community Medicine at the College of Physicians and Surgeons—Pakistan.

Linda Young Landesman, DrPH, MSW

Dr. Landesman is a national expert on the role of public health in disaster preparedness and response and a leader in health care policy and administration. She has edited and authored six books, including the landmark book, *Public Health Management of Disasters: The Practice Guide*, now in its second edition, and has developed national standards for emergency services response. Dr. Landesman earned her BA and MSW degrees from the University of Michigan and practiced clinical social work for ten years. She received her DrPH in health policy and management from the Columbia University Mailman School of Public Health. Dr. Landesman has been an assistant vice president, Office of Professional Services and Affiliations, at the New York City Health and Hospitals Corporation since 1996. She is also on the faculty of the Public Health Practice Program at the University of Massachusetts–Amherst, where she teaches research methods and public health emergency management online. Dr. Landesman has served as chair of the Executive Board of the American Public Health Association and the Editorial Board of the *American Journal of Public Health*.

Thomas C. Peterson, MD

Dr. Peterson is chair of the Department of Family Medicine at the University of Vermont. He is a graduate of the University of California–Santa Barbara (BA degree in biochemistry and molecular biology), the University of Rochester School of Medicine and Dentistry (MD), and the University of Vermont for residency training in family medicine. Dr. Peterson has previously served as residency director, vice-chair, and interim chair for the Department of Family Medicine. He has served as principal investigator for Health Resources and Services Administration grants for the department, and plays a lead role in regional and national committees on primary care. Dr. Peterson has been honored as one of the "Best Doctors in America," the Vermont Family Physician of the Year, and the Department's Teacher of the Year. He is on the Board of the Vermont Academy of Family Physicians and the Dean's Advisory Council of the University of Vermont.

Dr. Peterson has participated in peer review for several journals, including the *Journal of Family Practice*, *Family Medicine*, and the *Journal of the American Board of Family Medicine*. His professional interests include cultural diversity in medicine, practice system development, electronic health records, underserved health care, immigrant health, and palliative care.

Khondkar Ayaz Rabbani, MSc

Mr. Rabbani completed his BS (Honors) in chemistry from the University of Toronto and then went on to complete his MSc from the University of Illinois–Urbana-Champaign. He is a lecturer in the School of Environmental Science and Management at Independent University, where he teaches undergraduate and postgraduate courses in chemistry, environmental pollution, environmental science, and environmental health. His research interests include urban air pollution, water and wastewater chemistry, trace chemical detection methods, and analytical chemistry.

M. Omar Rahman, MD, DSc, MPH

Dr. Rahman is currently pro-vice-chancellor, professor of demography, and executive director of the Center for Health, Population and Development at Independent University, Bangladesh. Prior to that, he was an associate professor of epidemiology and demography at Harvard University and a research fellow in psychiatry at Harvard Medical School. He remains an adjunct professor of demography at Harvard University and a fellow at Harvard Medical School.

Dr. Rahman completed his AB in biochemical sciences from Harvard University, his MD from Northwestern University Medical School, and his MPH and his DSc in epidemiology and demography from Harvard University. Dr. Rahman trained in psychiatry at Harvard Medical School and is a board-certified psychiatrist.

He is the author of multiple peer-reviewed articles, has edited two books and written several chapters. He has been the principal investigator on a number of projects funded by the U.S. National Institutes of Health, United Nations Population Fund, the Global Health Forum, and others. His research interests are migration and urbanization, social networks and their impact on health, gender differences in aging and development, health policy in the developing world, and mental health issues in the developing world.

Irshad Shaikh, MD, PhD, MPH

Dr. Shaikh is a faculty member with the department of international health, and an associate at the Center for Refugee and Disaster Response, at Johns Hopkins Bloomberg School of Public Health. He was Commissioner of Health for the City of Chester, Pennsylvania, from 1994 through 2005.

Nadia J. Siddiqui, MPH

Ms. Siddiqui is a senior health policy analyst at the Texas Health Institute. She conducts evaluation and policy research on national, state, and local programs targeting the health and health care of underserved and vulnerable populations.

She serves as project manager for the National Consensus Panel on Emergency Preparedness and Cultural Diversity. Ms. Siddiqui writes and presents frequently on racial/ethnic disparities in health, health care and emergency preparedness, U.S. health care reform, and access to health care in the suburban United States. Among her recent peer-reviewed publications are "Integrating Racially and Ethnically Diverse Communities into Planning for Disasters: The California Experience" in the *Journal of Disaster Medicine and Public Health Preparedness* (forthcoming) and "Preparing Racially and Ethnically Diverse Communities for Public Health Emergencies" in *Health Affairs*. Ms. Siddiqui has a MPH from the University of Arkansas for Medical Sciences and a BA in economics from the University of Texas–Austin.

Rahat Bari Tooheen, MPH, MDM

Mr. Tooheen completed his BSc in population-environment and MPH degree from Independent University, Bangladesh, and went on to complete a second master's degree in disaster management from BRAC University, Bangladesh. He is a lecturer at the Chittagong Campus of Independent University, Bangladesh. He has taught courses at the graduate and undergraduate levels at the university. His fields of interest include population, environment, public health, and disaster management. He is also a certified trainer on scientific writing from the World Health Organization/Population Council/USAID.

Arpana Verma, MBChB, MPH, MFPH

Dr. Verma is senior lecturer and honorary consultant in public health with the Manchester Urban Collaboration on Health at the University of Manchester, England. She qualified as a doctor from the University of Manchester in 1995. Prior to this she worked in respiratory medicine and adult cystic fibrosis. Her research interests include urban health, hepatitis C, blood-borne viruses, vaccination, and infection control. She set up the Manchester Urban Collaboration on Health, which is part of the Clinical Epidemiology and Public Health Department at the University of Manchester. Dr. Verma is the principal investigator and coordinator of a European Union Commission project (EURO-URHIS 2) investigating urban health indicators in Europe and other countries.

David Vlahov, RN, PhD

Dr. Vlahov is the recently appointed Dean of the University of California, San Francisco School of Nursing. He formerly served as senior vice president for research and director of the Center for Urban Epidemiologic Studies at the New York Academy of Medicine. He is also professor of clinical epidemiology at the Mailman School of Public Health at Columbia University, and adjunct professor in epidemiology at the Johns Hopkins Bloomberg School of Public Health.

Dr. Vlahov has conducted several longitudinal cohort studies for which he received the National Institutes of Health MERIT Award. He has also led epidemiologic studies in Harlem and the Bronx to address social determinants of health. Dr. Vlahov initiated the International Society for Urban Health, serving as its first president. He is a visiting professor at the medical school in Belo Horizonte, Brazil, and is working with the World Health Organization's Urban Health Center in Kobe, Japan. Dr. Vlahov is the editor-in-chief of the *Journal of Urban Health*, and an editor for the *American Journal of Epidemiology* and *Epidemiology*. He has edited three books on urban health and has published more than 600 articles. Dr. Vlahov received his baccalaureate and master's in nursing from the University of Maryland and his doctorate in epidemiology at the Johns Hopkins School of Hygiene and Public Health.

Rodrick Wallace, PhD

Dr. Wallace is a research scientist in the Division of Epidemiology at the New York State Psychiatric Institute. He received a BS in mathematics and a PhD in physics from Columbia University. He is the author of numerous books and peer-reviewed articles on the social production of infectious and chronic disease and is a past recipient of an Investigator Award in Health Policy Research from the Robert Wood Johnson Foundation.

Isaac B. Weisfuse, MD, MPH

Dr. Weisfuse is Deputy Commissioner for the Office of Emergency Preparedness and Response. He has extensive emergency management experience. He served as agency incident commander for a number of events such as the World Trade Center Disaster, the 2003 blackout, and the outbreak of pandemic influenza in 2009. He trained in internal medicine, and was an epidemiologic intelligence officer at the Centers for Disease Control.

Mary E. Wilson, MD

Dr. Wilson is associate professor of global health and population at the Harvard School of Public Health. Her academic interests include the ecology of infections and emergence of microbial threats, travel medicine, tuberculosis, and vaccines. She was chief of infectious diseases at Mount Auburn Hospital for more than 20 years. She has served on the Advisory Committee for Immunization Practices of the Centers for Disease Control and Prevention and is a special advisor to the GeoSentinel Surveillance Network, a global network. She has lectured and published widely, serves on several editorial boards, and is an associate editor for *Journal Watch Infectious Diseases*. She is author of *A World Guide to Infections: Diseases, Distribution, Diagnosis* and senior editor, with Richard Levins and Andrew Spielman, of *Disease in Evolution: Global Changes and Emergence of Infectious Diseases*. She teaches a Harvard course in Brazil.

Index